DICTIONARY OF
Biomedical Optics and Biophotonics

DICTIONARY OF
Biomedical Optics and Biophotonics

Valery Tuchin

PRESS

Bellingham, Washington USA

Library of Congress Cataloging-in-Publication Data

Tuchin, V. V. (Valerii Viktorovich)
  Dictionary of biomedical optics and biophotonics / Valery V. Tuchin.
    p. ; cm.
  Includes bibliographical references and index.
  ISBN 978-0-8194-8973-9
  I. SPIE (Society) II. Title.
  [DNLM: 1. Biomedical Technology--methods. 2. Optical
Phenomena. 3. Ocular Physiological
Phenomena. 4. Terminology. W 15]
  LC classification not assigned
  612.8'40284--dc23
                                                                    2011041852
Published by

SPIE
P.O. Box 10
Bellingham, Washington 98227-0010 USA
Phone: +1 360.676.3290
Fax: +1 360.647.1445
Email: Books@spie.org
Web: http://spie.org

Printed in the United States of America.
First printing

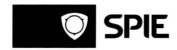

Contents

Preface

This dictionary summarizes the terminology and definitions used in the rapidly developing fields of biomedical optics and biophotonics. It is based on the glossaries of two of my earlier books, *Tissue Optics: Light Scattering Methods and Instruments for Medical Diagnosis* (SPIE Press, 2000) and the second edition of *Tissue Optics: Light Scattering Methods and Instruments for Medical Diagnosis* (SPIE Press, 2007); however, the terms and definitions have been expanded to short articles that serve as brief introductions to biomedical topics. Cross-referenced terms are in bold to facilitate searching.

It is impossible to present definitions of all related terms used in the dictionary, and thus they were selected based on the author's teaching and research experience. As many terms from biomedical optics and biophotonics as possible have been included; both fields are very closely related, however, and the distinction made here is that biophotonics is a broader term that includes biomedical optics as a subset. Researchers, practitioners, and professionals in biomedicine, as well as professionals in other disciplines, such as laser physics and technology, fiber optics, spectroscopy, material science, biology, and medicine will find the book a useful resource. Graduate and undergraduate students studying biomedical physics and engineering, biomedical optics and biophotonics, and medical science would benefit greatly from consulting this reference.

Several Russian and international grants supported this project: 208.2008.2 and 1177.2012.2 of the President of RF "Supporting of Leading Scientific Schools"; 1.4.09, 02.740.11.0770, 02.740.11.0879, and 11.519.11.2035 of the RF Federal Agency of Education; RFBR 11-02-12248-ofi-m and 11-02-00560-a;

224014, PHOTONICS4LIFE of FP7-ICT-2007-2; CRDF RUB1-2932-SR-08; 08-02-92224-RFBR-NNSF (RF–PRC); RFBR-10-02-90039-Bel_a; FiDiPro, TEKES Program (40111/11), Finland; and SCOPES EC, Switzerland/RF/Uzbekistan (2011-14).

I greatly appreciate the cooperation, contributions, and support of all my colleagues from the Optics and Biophotonics Chair and the Research-Educational Institute of Optics and Biophotonics at Saratov State University, the Institute of Precise Mechanics and Control of the Russian Academy of Science, and the Laboratory of Optoelectronics and Measurement Techniques at the University of Oulu, Finland. I have received valuable advice from reviewers, and their input is also appreciated. Last, but not least, I express my gratitude to my family for their support and understanding during my work on this book.

Valery V. Tuchin
Saratov State University

April 2012

Glossary

3-HKG	3-hydroxy-L-kyurenine-0-b-glucoside
$^1O_2$	singlet oxygen
ac	alternating current
ACS	acute coronary syndrome
AFM	atomic-force microscopy
AHA	alpha (a)-hydroxy acid
ALA	aminolevulenic acid
AO	acousto-optic
AOD	acousto-optic deflector
AOM	acousto-optic modulator
AOT	acousto-optic tomography
APD	avalanche photodiode
ATI	above-threshold ionization
ATP	adenosine triphosphate
ATR FTIR	attenuated total reflectance Fourier-transform infrared (spectroscopy)
BBDP	biobreeding diabetes-prone (rat)
BCC	basal cell carcinoma
BEM	boundary-element method
BioMEMS	biomedical microelectromechanical system
BMS	Brillouin–Mandelshtam scattering
BPD	benzoporphyrin derivative
BW	birefringent wedge
CALI	chromophore-assisted light inactivation
CAMs	cell-adhesion molecules
CARS	coherent anti-Stokes Raman scattering
CCD	charge-coupled device
CCT	correlated color temperature

CDI	coherent-detection imaging
CFD	constant-fraction discriminator
CIE	Commission Internationale de l'Eclairage
CIN	cervical intraepithelial neoplasia
CIS	carcinoma in situ
CLASS	confocal-light-absorption and scattering-spectroscopic microscopy
CM	confocal microscopy
CMOS	complementary metal-oxide semiconductor
CNR	contrast-to-noise ratio
CNS	central nervous system
COHb	carboxyhemoglobin
COX	cytochrome c oxidase
CP OCT	cross-polarization (orthogonal-polarized) optical coherence tomography
CPU	central processing unit
CSF	cerebrospinal fluid
CT	computed tomography
CTS	carpal-tunnel syndrome
CW	continuous wave
CW RTT	continuous-wave radiation-transfer theory
D^*	detectivity star
dB	decibel
DBM	double-balanced mixer
DG	delay generator
DIC	differential interference contrast (microscopy)
DIS	double-integrating sphere (technique)
DIW	deionized water
DL	diode laser
DMD	digital micromirror device
DMSO	dimethyl sulfoxide
DNA	deoxyribonucleic acid
DOAS	differential optical-absorption spectroscopy
DOCP	degree of circular polarization
DOF	depth of field
DOLP	degree of linear polarization
DOP	degree of polarization
DOPA	3,4-dihydroxyphenylalanine
DOPE	dioley(o)lphosphatidylethanolamine

DOS	diffuse optical spectroscopy
DOT	diffuse optical tomography
DPS OCT	differential phase-sensitive optical coherence tomography
DPSS	diode-pumped solid-state (laser)
Ds red	Discosomared
DWS	diffusion-wave spectroscopy
ECM	extracellular matrix
EDTA	ethylenediaminetetraacetic acid
EEM	excitation-emission map
EET	electronic energy transfer
EMCCD	electron-multiplying charge-coupled device
EMI	electromagnetic-interference (noise)
EMR	electromagnetic radiation
EMW	electromagnetic wave
ER	endoplasmic reticulum
Er:YAG	erbium:yttrium aluminum garnet (laser)
$f/\#$	f-number
FAD	flavin adenine dinucleotide
FALI	fluorophore-assisted light inactivation
FCS	fluorescence correlation spectroscopy
FD OCT	frequency-domain optical coherence tomography
FD	frequency-domain (spectrometer)
FDA	Food and Drug Administration
fDOT	fluorescence diffuse optical tomography
FDTD	finite-difference time-domain
FFT	fast-Fourier transform (analysis)
FG	function generator
FIR	far-infrared
FLIM	fluorescence-lifetime imaging microscopy
FMN	flavin mononucleotide
FMT	fluorescence molecular tomography
FOV	field of view
FPA	focal plane array
FRAP	fluorescence recovery after photobleaching
FRET	Förster resonance energy transfer
FTIR	Fourier transform infrared (spectroscopy)
FWHM	full width at half maximum
GA	genetic algorithm

Gb/s	gigabits per second
GCF	gingival crevicular fluid
GFP	green fluorescent protein
GHb	glycated hemoglobin
GKPF	Gegenbauer kernel phase function
GRIN	graded index
H_2O	water
H_2O_2	hydrogen peroxide
HAP	hydroxyapatite
HbO_2	oxyhemoglobin
HEM	human epidermal membrane
HgCdTe	mercury cadmium telluride
HGPF	Henyey–Greenstein phase function
Ho:YAG	holmium:yttrium aluminum garnet (laser)
HpD	hematoporphyrin derivative
HPF	high-pass filter
HPV	human papilloma virus
HWHM	half width half maximum
Hz	hertz
IAD	inverse adding-doubling
IC25	Infracyanine®25
ICCD	intensified charge-coupled device
ICG	indocyanine green
ICO	International Commission for Optics
ICV	ileocecal valve
IFN	interferon
IFOV	instaneous field of view
IFS	interfibrillar spacing
IMC	inverse Monte Carlo (method/technique)
IMS	intermolecular spacing
InSb	indium antimonide
IQ	in-phase quadrature (circuit)
IR	infrared
IRFPA	infrared focal plane array
IS	integrating sphere
IVM	intravital microscopy
K_2CrO_4	potassium chromate
KDP	kalium dihydrophosphate
KKM	Kubelka–Munk model

LabVIEW	Laboratory Virtual Instrumentation Engineering Workbench
LAMMA	laser microprobe mass analysis
LASCA	laser speckle contrast analysis
LASEK	laser-assisted epithelial keratomileusis
LASIK	laser-assisted in situ keratomileusis
LC	liquid crystal
LCD	liquid-crystal display
LCW	liquid-core waveguide
LDA	laser Doppler anemometry
LDF	laser Doppler flowmetry
LDI	laser Doppler imaging
LDLS	laser Doppler line scanning
LDM	laser Doppler microscope
LDPI	laser Doppler perfusion imaging
LDPM	laser Doppler perfusion monitoring
LDR	linear dynamic range
LED	light-emitting diode
LIBS	laser-induced-breakdown spectroscopy
LIC	laser-induced coagulation
LIDAR	light detection and ranging
LIF	laser-induced fluorescence
LIHT	laser-induced hyperthermia
LIITT	laser-induced interstitial thermotherapy
$LiNbO_3$	lithium niobate
LIPT	laser-induced pressure transient
LLLT	low-level laser therapy
LMA	laser microspectral analysis
LO	local oscillator
LOC	lab-on-a-chip
LPF	low-pass filter
LSI	laser speckle imaging
LSM	laser scanning microscopy
LSM	light-scattering matrix
LSMM	laser scattering matrix meter
LSPI	laser speckle perfusion imaging
LSS	light-scattering spectroscopy
MAR	modified amino resin
MB	methylene blue
MBG	mean blood glucose

MC	Monte Carlo (method/technique)
MCP	multichannel plate
MCP-PMT	multichannel plate-photomultiplier
MCT	mercury cadmium telluride
MDFI	multidimensional fluorescence imaging
MDTD	minimum detectable temperature difference
MED	minimal erythema dose
MEMS	microelectromechanical system
MFP	mean free path
MI	myocardial infarction
MIN	multiple intestinal neoplasia
MIR	mid-infrared
MONSTIR	multichannel optoelectronic near-infrared system for time-resolved image reconstruction
MOVPE	metal organic vapor phase epitaxy
mrad	milliradian
MRI	magnetic resonance imaging
mRNA	messanger ribonucleic acid
MRT	magnetic resonance tomography
MRTD	minimum resolvable temperature difference
ms	millisecond
msec	millisecond
mTAS	micro total analysis system
MTF	modulation transfer function
MTT	meal tolerance test
NA	numerical aperture
NAD	nicotinamide adenine dinucleotide
NADH	nicotinamide adenine dinucleotide, reduced
NADP	nicotinamide adenine dinucleotide phosphate
NADPH	nicotinamide adenine dinucleotide phosphate, reduced
Nd:YAG	neodymium:yttirum aluminium garnet (laser)
Nd:YAP	neodymium:yttrium aluminium perovskite (laser)
NEMS	nanoelectromechanical system
NET(D)	noise equivalent temperature (distance)
NIR	near-infrared
NIRS	near-infrared spectroscopy
NIST	National Institute of Standards and Technology (US)
nm	nanometer
NO	nitric oxide
NP	nanoparticle

ns	nanosecond
NSOM	near-field scanning optical microscopy
OAT	optoacoustic tomography
OCA	optical clearing agent
OCI	optical coherence interferometry
OCM	optical coherence microscopy
OCP	optical-clearing potential
OCT	optical coherence tomography
OD	optical density
OGTT	oral glucose tolerance test
OLED	organic light-emitting diode
OMA	optical multichannel analyzer
OMAG	optical microangiography
OPC	optical phase conjugation
OPO	optical parametric oscillator
OPS	orthogonal polarization spectroscopy
OPT	optical projection tomography
OR-PAM	optical-resolution photoacoustic microscopy
Osm	osmole
OT	optothermal
OTR	optothermal radiometry
PALM	photo-activated localization microscopy
PAM	photoacoustic microscopy
PAS	periodic acid-Schiff
PBS	phosphate buffered saline
PCA	pyrrolidonecarboxylic acid
PCF	photonic crystal fiber
PCM	phase conjugate mirror
PDD	photodynamic diagnosis
PDF	probability density function
PDT	photodynamic therapy
PEG	polyethylene glycol
PET	positron emission tomography
PEV	pyroelectric vidicon
PG	propylene glycol
PIV	particle image velocimetry
PM	polarization-maintaining
PMF	probability mass function
PMT	photomultiplier tube

POCT	point-of-care testing
POS	polyorganosiloxane
Pp IX	protoporphyrin IX
PPG	polypropylene glycol
PPG	photoplethysmography
PRK	photorefractive keratectomy
PRS	polarized reflectance spectroscopy
PS OCT	polarization-sensitive optical-coherence tomography
PSF	point spread function
PT	photothermal
PTM	photothermal microscopy
PTR	photothermal radiometry
PVDF	polyvinydene fluoride
QD	quantum dot
QELS	quasi-elastic light scattering
r.m.s. (rms)	root mean square
RASH	random access second-harmonic-generation
RBC	red blood cell
RCM	reflection confocal microscopy
rDOI	reflectance diffuse optical imaging
Re	Reynolds number
RET	resonance energy transfer
RF	radio frequency
RFI	radio-frequency interference
RGA	Rayleigh–Gans approximation
RGB	red/green/blue
RI	refractive index
RNA	ribonucleic acid
RNFL	retinal nerve fiber layer
RNS	reactive nitrogen species
ROI	region of interest
ROS	reactive oxygen species
RPS	random phase screen
rRNA	ribosomal ribonucleic acid
RRS	resonance Raman scattering
RTE	radiation-transfer equation
SBMS	stimulated Brillouin–Mandelshtam scattering
SC	stratum corneum
SEM	standard error of the mean

SERS	surface-enhanced Raman scattering
SERS	surface-enhanced Raman spectroscopy
SESAM	semiconductor saturable absorber mirror
SFD-DOI	spatial frequency-domain diffuse optical imaging
SFD-DOS	spatial frequency-domain diffuse optical spectroscopy
SI	structured illumination
SI	Système International d'Unités (International System of Units)
SIM	structured illumination microscopy
SL	sonoluminescence
SLD	superluminescent light diode
SLS	selective laser sintering
SLT	sonoluminescence tomography
SMLB	spatially modulated laser beam
SNOM	scanning near-field optical microscopy
SNR	signal-to-noise ratio
SOA	semiconductor optical amplifier
SOD	superoxide dismutase
SP	selective photothermolysis
SPECT	single photon emission computed tomography
SPIM	selective plane illumination microscopy
SPM	scanning-probe microscopy
SRF	slit response function
SRR	spatially resolved reflectance
SRS	stimulated Raman scattering
ST	Staphylococcus toxin
STED	stimulated emission depletion
STM	scanning-tunneling microscopy
STORM	stochastic optical reconstruction microscopy
TBO	toluidine blue O
TCSPC	time-correlated single-photon counting
TDM	transillumination digital microscopy
TDM	time-division multiplex
TEA	transverse excited atmospheric
TERS	tip-enhanced Raman spectroscopy
TEWL	transepidermal water loss
TGS	thermal gradient spectroscopy
THb	total hemoglobin
THG	third-harmonic generation
THz	terahertz

Ti:Al$_2$O$_3$	titanium sapphire (laser)
Ti:sapphire	titanium sapphire (laser)
TiO$_2$	titanium dioxide
TIR	total internal reflection
TIRF	total internal reflection fluorescence
TiVi	tissue viability imaging
TMFP	transport mean free path
TOAST	time-resolved optical absorption and scattering tomography
TOF	time-of-flight
TOI	tissue optical index
TPF	two-photon fluorescence
TPPSn	sulfonated tetraphenyl porphines
tRNA	transfer ribonucleic acid
TRS	time-resolved spectroscopy
TRT	thermal relaxation time
TSOPC	turbidity suppression by optical phase conjugation
US	ultrasound
UV	ultraviolet
UVA	ultraviolet A
UVB	ultraviolet B
UVC	ultraviolet C
VCSEL	vertical-cavity surface-emitting laser
VOA	variable optical attenuator
VRTE	vector radiative-transfer equation
VRTT	vector radiation-transfer theory
VT-PDT	vascular-targeted photodynamic therapy
WBC	white blood cell
WDM	wavelength-division multiplex
WHO	World Health Organization
WP	Wollaston prism
WST09	TOOKAD®
Yb:YAG	ytterbium:yttrium aluminium garnet (laser)
ZnO	zinc oxide
ZnSe	zinc selenide

0-degree hybrid/splitter: Device that pertains to or notes a current in one of two parallel circuits that have a single-phase current source and equal impedances that produce currents of 0-degree **phase shift**.

3-hydroxy-L-kynurenine-0-β-glucoside (3-HKG): Important age-related **chromophore** of the human eye **lens** that protects the eye mainly from **UVA radiation**.

4Pi-microscope: Confocal **laser** scanning **fluorescence micro-scope** in which **light** is focused ideally from all sides (solid an-gle 4π) in a spot with a diameter smaller than the conventional **laser** focus. It is used to scan an object with this spot point-by-point excitation combined with point-by-point detection. The **4Pi-microscope** has been realized using two opposing high **numerical aperture lenses**. It should be possible to achieve an improved op-tical resolution beyond the conventional limit (~200 nm lateral, ~600 nm axial). In a **4Pi-microscope** of type A, the coherent su-perposition of excitation **light** is used to generate the increased resolution, and the emission **light** is either detected from one side only or in an incoherent superposition from both sides. In a **4Pi-microscope** of type B, only the emission **light** is interfering. When operated in type-C mode, both excitation and emission **light** are allowed to interfere, leading to the highest possible resolution in-crease (~ sevenfold along the optical axis, as compared to wide-field **fluorescence microscopy**). A typical axial resolution of a **4Pi-microscope** is about 100 nm. Typically, **two-photon fluores-cence (TPF) microscopy** is used in a **4Pi-microscope** in com-bination with the emission **pinhole** to lower the sidelobes of the **point spread function (PSF)**.

5-aminolevulinic acid: See **delta (δ)-aminolevulinic acid (ALA)**.

90-degree hybrid/splitter: Device that pertains to or notes a current in one of two parallel circuits that have a single-phase current source but unequal impedances that produce currents of 90-degree **phase shift**.

Abbe refractometer: An instrument for direct determination of the **refractive index** that measures the **total internal reflection**.

abdominal: Related to the abdomen.

abdominal cavity: The human body cavity containing most of the **digestive tract** hollow organs, as well as several solid organs.

abdominal fat: The **adipose tissue** that contains **fat cells** found around the **abdominal organs** such as the **intestines, kidneys**, and **liver**.

abdominal fluid: A number of organs, including the **liver, spleen, pancreas**, and **intestines**, as well as a tiny amount of fluid, are found in the **abdominal cavity**. When the quantity of fluid increases significantly, it is called **ascites**. Inflammation of the **pancreas, liver** disease, and **kidney** failure may cause fluid to accumulate in the abdomen. There may be evidence of a malignancy—for example, marked weight loss in spite of an increasing abdomen. The **white-blood-cell** count in the fluid may be elevated because of an infection. A cytologic examination may reveal the presence of **tumor cells**.

abdominal organs: Hollow **abdominal organs** include the **stomach**, the **small intestine**, and the **colon** with its attached appendix. Solid organs such as the **liver**, its attached **gall bladder**, and the **pancreas** function in close association with the **digestive tract** and communicate with it via ducts. The **spleen, kidneys**, and adrenal **glands** also lie within the abdomen, along with many **blood vessels** including the **aorta** and inferior vena cava. The **urinary bladder, uterus**, fallopian tubes, and ovaries are categorized as either **abdominal organs** or as **pelvic organs**. The abdomen also contains an extensive **membrane** called the **peritoneum**. The **diaphragm** separates the abdomen from the thorax, with the abdomen being posterior to the thorax.

aberration: In optics, this term is applied to certain defects in images formed in optical systems. Descriptions of **aberrations**

are based on geometrical and wave optics. The power series representation allows one to classify different types of **aberrations**. By using the lowest expansion order, the Seidel terms allowing for an analytical description of **aberrations** can be found. The Zernike polynomial approach is also commonly used for **aberration** evaluation and classification. The quality of an optical system can be determined from the form and size of its **point spread function**, or on the basis of its optical transfer function. **Aberration** may be spherical, for example, if the aperture of a concave spherical mirror (**lens**) is large, the rays at the periphery are brought to focus nearer to the mirror than those rays that meet the mirror near the pole, producing a curve (caustic). The primary spherical aberrations are astigmatism, coma, field curvature, and distortion. The dispersion of the optical materials causes the so-called chromatic aberrations that also affect the image quality for nonmonochromatic light. All of the monochromatic aberrations have their chromatic variations, such as colored astigmatism, coma, etc. A white image will therefore have some color. In terms of wave **aberrations**, such definitions as axial color and lateral color were introduced to describe chromatic **aberrations**. Wavefront **aberrations** are precisely measured by means of interferometry.

ablation: Removal of **tissue** or other materials. When **photons** traveling into a **tissue** are absorbed, heat is generated. Depending on the amount of heat deposition, the generated heat can induce several reversible and irreversible effects in **tissue**. Irreversible thermal damage to **tissue** occurs as **tissue** temperature rises past T_{crit} (see **thermal damage**), with **coagulation**, **vaporization**, **vacuolization**, and **pyrolysis** being the basis for photoinduced mechanical and chemical **tissue** destruction. Within a short **light** pulse, these processes develop as explosion or thermal **ablation**. All these phenomena are called **photothermal** mechanisms. During **ablation**, high **pressure** develops in the **tissue** and can result in **shock-wave** formation and mechanical damage to **tissue**, a phenomenon called a "photomechanical mechanism." Due to the increase of the temperature difference between the irradiation and the surrounding **tissue** when using **continuous-wave light**

sources, conduction of heat away from the **light absorption** point and into surrounding **tissue** increases. Coagulation damage to surrounding **tissue** is a disadvantage of **continuous-wave** light-sourced thermal **ablation**. Pulsed **light** delivers sufficient **energy** to ablate **tissue** using a short pulse time, enabling **tissue** removal before any heat is transferred to the surrounding **tissue**. To achieve a precise **tissue ablation**, **lasers** with a very short **penetration depth**, such as an excimer ArF **laser** or **Er:YAG laser**, are used. **CO lasers** and CO_2 **lasers** are also used for precise cellular-depth **ablation**.

ablation by femtosecond NIR lasers: High-**power femtosecond NIR lasers** represent a tool for a precise **tissue ablation** using a nonlinear phenomenon. These **lasers** emit **femtosecond** pulse trains with repetition rates from a few kHz to hundreds of MHz, depending on the **laser** scheme (see **mode-locked laser**). They are used for inducing nonlinear phenomena in **tissues**, which are commonly transparent to **NIR light**. When **laser** pulses are focused in a tiny volume (typical focus spot on the order of a few microns), very high **power** densities are reached ($\sim 10^{13}$ W$\cdot$cm^{-2}), thus inducing nonlinear **multiphoton absorption** that generates free electrons within the focal volume. The free-electron density produced by multiphoton ionization may overcome a threshold value for generating an optical breakdown. In this condition the free electrons absorb **photons** through a process called "**inverse bremsstrahlung absorption**," thus increasing their **energy**. After a certain number of these **absorption** events (depending on the **laser wavelength**), a free electron has acquired sufficient **energy** to produce another free electron by impact ionization (i.e., by collision with a heavy particle). Recurring **inverse bremsstrahlung absorption** and impact ionization give rise to avalanche ionization and **plasma** formation. As a consequence of the very fast **plasma** heating and expansion, **shock waves** and **cavitation**-bubble generation may be observed in **tissues** and **water**. The induced bubbles have a particular dynamic, they grow to a maximum diameter (which can be controlled and limited up to within 5–15 μm) inducing ruptures inside the **tissue**, thus enabling intratissue surgery with a micrometrical precision.

For the production of damage in the target biological structure, there are three major processes (**laser** pulses of 100 fs, 800 nm, focused with a 1.3 NA **objective**): (1) photochemical process due to **multiphoton absorption** (**irradiance** threshold 2.6×10^{11} W $\cdot$ cm^{-2}, electron density per pulse 2.1×10^{13} cm^{-3}), (2) thermoelastic stress (**irradiance** threshold 5.1×10^{12} W $\cdot$ cm^{-2}, electron density per pulse 2.4×10^{20} cm^{-3}), and (3) optical breakdown (**plasma** formation) produced by a combination of multiphoton and cascade ionization processes (**irradiance** threshold 6.5×10^{12} W $\cdot$ cm^{-2}, electron density per pulse 1.0×10^{21} cm^{-3}).

above-threshold ionization (ATI): An extension of multiphoton ionization (see **laser photoionization**), where even more **photons** are absorbed than necessary to ionize the atom or molecule. The excess **energy** gives the released electron higher kinetic **energy** than the usual case of just-above-threshold **photoionization**. The released electron will have an integer number of **photon** energies and more kinetic **energy** than in normal ionization (i.e., lowest possible number of **photons**).

abrasive cream: Cream containing abrasive (hard-mineral) particles. Upon application, it produces **skin peeling** that makes the **skin** surface (***stratum corneum*** layer) smoother and penetrative for medical and cosmetic preparations, such as **liposomes** and nanospheres.

absolute (Kelvin) temperature scale: Thermodynamic temperature scale in which the lower fixed point is **absolute zero** and the interval is identical to that on the Celsius (or **centigrade**) relative scale. The Kelvin unit is equal to 1 °C. 0 K (kelvin) = −273.16 °C. The degree sign and the word *degrees* are not used in describing Kelvin temperatures.

absolute zero: Temperature that is zero on the **absolute (Kelvin) temperature scale**. It is the temperature at which a material is at its lowest **energy** state.

5

absorbance: Ratio of the absorbed **light intensity** to the incident **intensity**. It is a dimensionless quantity. In **spectroscopy**, the **absorbance** A (also called **optical density**) is defined as $A_\lambda = -\log_{10}(I/I_0)$, where I is the **intensity** of **light** at a specified **wavelength** λ that has passed through a sample (transmitted-**light intensity**) and I_0 is the **intensity** of the **light** before it enters the sample or incident-**light intensity**. **Absorbance** measurements are often carried out in analytical chemistry and biochemistry. The **absorbance** of a sample is proportional to its thickness and to the concentration of the absorbing species in the sample, in **contrast** to the **transmittance** I/I_0 of a sample, which varies logarithmically with thickness and concentration.

absorbing medium: Medium that absorbs **light** at certain **wavelengths** or **wavelength** bands. Commonly, an **absorbing medium** consists of **absorption centers** that are particles or molecules that absorb **light**.

absorption: Transformation of **light** (radiant) **energy** to some other form of **energy**, usually heat, as the **light** transverses matter. To characterize **absorption** of a medium, an **absorption coefficient** μ_a is introduced. **Absorption** is just one way in which **light** can interact with the **tissue**. **Absorption** of **UV** and **visible light** in biological materials is due to **electronic excitation** of aromatic or conjugated unsaturated **chromophores**.

absorption band: A range of **wavelengths** in which a medium exhibits stronger **absorption** than it does at adjacent **wavelengths**.

absorption center: A particle or molecule that absorbs **light**.

absorption coefficient: In a nonscattering medium, **absorption coefficient** μ_a is defined as the reciprocal of the distance d over which **light** of **intensity** $I(d = 0) = I_0$ is attenuated (due to **absorption**) to $I(d) = I_0/e \approx 0.37\,I_0$. The units are typically cm^{-1}. Behind this definition is the fundamental process of **photon absorption** that is characterized by a **photon-absorption** cross section.

absorption spectroscopy: Refers to **spectroscopy** techniques that measure the **absorption** of **radiation**, as a function of **wavelength**, due to its interaction with a sample. The sample absorbs **energy** from the radiating field. The strength of the **absorption** varies as a function of **wavelength**, and this variation is the **absorption spectrum**. **Absorption spectroscopy** is performed across the electromagnetic **spectrum** from **x rays** to **terahertz**. It is employed as an analytical biochemistry tool to determine the presence or absence of a particular compound and, in many cases, to quantify the amount of the compound present. **Infrared spectroscopy** and **UV–visible spectroscopy** are particularly common in analytical and biomedical applications.

absorption spectrum: Spectrum formed by **light** that has passed through a medium in which **light** of certain **wavelengths** was absorbed.

absorptive filter: Usually made from glass to which various inorganic or organic compounds have been added. These compounds absorb some **wavelengths** of **light** while transmitting others. The compounds can also be added to plastic (often polycarbonate or acrylic) to produce **gel** filters, which are lighter and cheaper than glass-based filters. **Infrared** (heat-absorbing), **UV**, and neutral-density filters are widely used in **biophotonics**.

absorptivity (*Related term*:absorptance): Proportion (as a fraction of 1) of the **radiant energy** impinging on a material's surface that is absorbed into the material. For a **blackbody**, this is unity (1.0). Technically, **absorptivity** is the internal absorptance per unit pathlength. In thermography, the two terms are often used interchangeably.

acanthocyte: Shrunken **erythrocyte**, also known as spur **cell**, the term is derived from the Greek word "acanthi," meaning "thorn." The **cell** has 5 to 10 irregular, blunt, fingerlike projections that vary in width, length, and surface distribution. Acanthocytes form when **erythrocyte membranes** contain excess **cholesterol**

7

as compared to phospholipid content, which is caused by the increase in **blood cholesterol** content or the presence of abnormal **plasma**-lipoprotein composition.

acceptance angle: Maximum incident angle at which an optical system will transmit **light**.

accuracy of measurement: Maximum that the reading of an instrument will deviate from the acceptable standard reference. It is expressed in percent or as an absolute quantity of the measuring value.

acetic acid: A colorless, pungent, **water**-miscible liquid, CH_3COOH, used in the production of numerous esters that are solvents and flavoring agents.

aceto-whitening effect: Acetic acid is used during **colposcopy** to enhance differences in the **diffuse reflectance** (whitening) of normal and diseased regions of the cervical **epithelium**. Transient whitening of **tissue** after the application of **acetic acid** serves as a simple and inexpensive method for identifying areas that may eventually develop into **cervical cancer**.

achromatic: "Without **color**." Describes a **lens** or optical system that is designed to limit the effects of chromatic **aberration**. **Achromatic lenses** are corrected to bring two **wavelengths** (typically red and blue) into focus in the same plane. The most common type of **achromatic lens** is the **achromatic** doublet, which is composed of two individual **lenses** made from glasses with different amounts of **dispersion**. Usually, one element is a concave **lens** made out of flint glass, having relatively high **dispersion**. The other, a convex element, is made of crown glass, having lower **dispersion**. Typically, **lens** elements are cemented together and shaped so that the chromatic **aberration** of one is counterbalanced by that of the other.

acoustic detector: A transducer that transforms an acoustic signal to an electrical one, such as a **microphone** or **piezoelectric**

transducer. Wideband **piezoelectric transducers**, being low-noise detectors, have proved to be most suitable for **tissue spectroscopy** and tomography.

acoustic wave (*Synonym*: sound wave): Waves produced by a vibrating system where the particles of the medium vibrate in the same direction as the **acoustic wave**. Successive points of high (compressions) and low (rarefactions) **pressures** are formed because of the regular impulses from the vibrating source. **Acoustic waves** may be longitudinally progressive, longitudinally stationary, or transversely stationary. When sound is propagated through a medium (gas, liquid, or solid) it is transmitted by progressive longitudinal waves in that medium. **Acoustic waves** interact with complex and/or moving media with a damping, **refraction**, **diffraction**, **interference**, and/or Doppler shift in **frequency**. Depending on their **frequency**, **acoustic waves** are classified as sound, **ultrasound**, and infrasound. The entire **spectrum** can be divided into three ranges: audio, ultrasonic, and infrasonic. The audio range falls between 20 Hz and 20 kHz, and are those frequencies that can be detected by the human **ear**. The ultrasonic range refers to the very high frequencies, 20 kHz and higher. This range has shorter **wavelengths** that allow for better resolution in imaging technologies. Medical applications such as **ultrasonography** and **elastography** rely on the ultrasonic **frequency** range. The lowest frequencies, lower than 20 Hz, are known as the infrasonic range. **Acoustic detectors** are used to detect **sound waves**.

acousto-optic deflector (AOD): An optical modulator that diffracts a **laser beam** going through a crystal from the incidence angle (order 0) to another angle (order 1). The output angle is proportional to the **laser wavelength** and the frequency of the signal applied to drive the device. It also depends on the structure of the crystal material. By changing the modulation frequency, the angle of a **laser beam** can be scanned in space. Two devices used together allow for XY scanning. High-frequency stability and linearity are required from the driving electronics. Although essentially the same as an **acousto-optic modulator (AOM)**, both the amplitude and frequency are adjusted in an **AOD**, whereas only the amplitude of the **sound wave** is modulated in an **AOM**. Typically, the modulation frequency is in the **radio frequency (RF)** range.

acousto-optic (AO) interaction/effect: Interaction of **ultrasound** and **light beams** within a homogeneous or **inhomogeneous medium**. It occurs through a change in a medium's **optical properties** as a result of compression by the **ultrasound**. See **optical anisotropy** and **photoelasticity**.

acousto-optic modulator (AOM): A device for **intensity modulation** of **light** at certain audio or **radio frequency** using the **acousto-optic interaction/effect**. See **optical anisotropy** and **photoelasticity**.

acousto-optic tomography (AOT): Optical tomography that is based on the acoustic (**ultrasound**) **modulation** of coherent **laser light** traveling in **tissue**. An **acoustic wave** is focused into **tissue**, and **laser light** irradiates the same volume within the **tissue**. Any **light** that is encoded by **ultrasound** contributes to the imaging signal. Axial resolution along the acoustic axis can be achieved with **ultrasound-frequency** sweeping and subsequent application of the **Fourier transformation**, whereas lateral resolution can be obtained by focusing the **acoustic wave**.

acquisition rate: Rate of acquiring experimental data. For example, a particular experimental setup provides data **acquisition rate** of 60 Hz and **acquisition time** of 80 s, (i.e., 4800 measured points), or 100 Hz and 60 s (6000 points). It produces an acceptable level of accuracy for both operation modes, but low data-capture rates of ≤ 40 Hz may underestimate or completely fail to provide an estimate of the measuring value. For optical-imaging systems, such as **optical coherence tomography**, **acquisition rate** is expressed in terms of the number of axial scans per second, which is of a few hundred thousand scans per second for high-speed **swept-laser source/Fourier-domain optical coherence**

tomography systems. Available **analog-to-digital converters** provide high sampling frequencies of 125 MHz to 1 GHz (digital recording systems have typical bands of 2 MHz to 2 GHz and a sustained recording rate of 2.5 to 200 MB/channel). In biology, **acquisition rate** means "rate of susceptibility to," for example, infection or "accumulation of," for example, calcium.

acquisition time: Period of time needed to acquire experimental data, or the amount of time necessary to collect all of the data for a particular sequence. Usually, this does not include the time necessary to reconstruct the image. For example, a standard 10-μm axial resolution optical coherence tomography image with 512 axial scans can be acquired in ~1.3 s, whereas a high-speed, ultrahigh-resolution optical-coherence tomographic image with ~2-μm axial resolution and 2048 axial scans can be acquired in 0.13 s.

acquisition window: Time period within which a living biological subject is stable enough to provide useful diagnostic measurements. For example, the **acquisition window** in the cardiac cycle optimized by the monitoring motion of the **coronary artery** on **magnetic resonance imaging** allows acquisition of good images during diastole with an **acquisition window** of 82 ± 7 ms, and with an **acquisition window** of 51 ± 19 ms during systole.

actinic keratosis: A scaly or crusty bump that forms on the **skin** surface. It is also called solar keratosis, sun spots, or **precancerous** spots.

action spectrum: Rate of a physiological activity plotted against the **wavelength** of **light**. It shows which **wavelength** of **light** is most effectively used in a specific chemical or biological reaction. Producing an **action spectrum** is one method used to identify the **chromophore** mediating a particular physiological reaction.

acute coronary syndrome (ACS): Occurs when an **atherosclerotic plaque** ruptures, leading to thrombus formation within a

11

coronary artery. Patients who develop symptoms consistent with **acute coronary syndrome**, such as **chest pain** and diaphoresis, require timely evaluation to determine the cause. Following recovery from an episode of **acute coronary syndrome**, patients continue to be at heightened risk of **heart attack** and stroke.

acute myocardial infarction (AMI): See **myocardial infarction (MI)**.

acyl group: A functional group derived by the removal of one or more hydroxyl group from an oxoacid. In organic chemistry, the **acyl group** is usually derived from a carboxylic acid of the form R–CO–OH. It therefore has the formula RC(=O)–, with a double bond between the carbon and **oxygen** atoms (i.e., a **carbonyl** group), and a single bond between R and the carbon.

adaptive finite element method: A **finite element method** where discretion of the underlying spatial domain (usually in 2 or 3 space dimensions) and establishing of discrete equations is done using an adaptive mesh refinement scheme for complex structure of the object.

adaptive optics: Generally related to optical systems that improve resolution by compensating for distortions in the optics. Computer-controlled multielement mirrors or liquid-crystal **phase screens** are used as the active compensators. **Adaptive optics** technologies are prospective for applications in **biophotonics**, especially in the sphere of human-vision correction.

adding-doubling method: See **inverse adding-doubling (IAD) method (technique)**.

adenocarcinoma: A **malignant tumor** originating in **glandular epithelium**.

adenoma: A **benign tumor** originating in **glandular epithelium**.

adenomatous: Related to **adenoma** and to some types of **glandular hyperplasia**.

adenosine triphosphate (ATP): A **coenzyme** of fundamental importance found in the **cells** of all organisms. It provides a means of storing **energy** for many cellular activities.

adhesion: Any attraction process between dissimilar molecular species that can potentially bring them in "direct contact." There are several mechanisms of material **adhesion**. These include: *Mechanical adhesion*, when adhesive materials fill the voids or pores of the surfaces and hold surfaces together by interlocking. *Chemical adhesion*, when two materials may form a compound at the join (ionic, covalent, or hydrogen bonding). *Electrostatic adhesion*, when some conducting materials may pass electrons to form a difference in electrical charge at the join. *Diffusive adhesion*, when some materials may merge at the joint by **diffusion** (for mobile and soluble molecules, effective with polymer chains and in **sintering**). *Dispersive adhesion*, when two materials are held together by van der Waals forces. (A drop of liquid on a solid surrounded by air is a typical solid–liquid–gas system, where strong **adhesion** and weak **cohesion** results in a high degree of wetting—a lyophilic condition with low-measured contact angles. In contrast, weak **adhesion** and strong **cohesion** results in lyophobic conditions with high-measured contact angles and poor wetting.)

adiabatic expansion: A curve of **pressure** against volume representing an adiabatic change (curves of equal **entropy**). These lines always slope more steeply than the isothermals that they cross.

adipocyte: A **cell** in which a food reserve is deposited in the form of droplets of **oil**. The quantity of **oil** increases until the **oil** globule formed distends the **cell** and pushes the **nucleus** and **cytoplasm** to one side. A collection of **fat cells** forms **adipose tissue**. **Fat** occupies almost the total volume of a **fatty cell**, as the

cell nucleus is small and is located at the edge. Large **fatty cells** of roundish or many-sided forms are connected among themselves by thin connecting **fibers**. Between **cells** there are spaces where there are small **capillaries** and interstitial liquid. A single **adipocyte** is 95% **fat** by volume. In subjects, **fat-cell** parameters are in the following ranges: **cell** size 15–250 μm, mean **lipid** content in a **cell** 0.3–1.2 μg **lipid/cell**, number of **cells** $(0.2–10) \times 10^{10}$. A great mass of **lipids** in **adipose tissue** are neutral **fats** or triglycerides (90–99%). Other weights consist of diglycerides and monoglycerides (1–3%), phospholipids and glycolipids (0.5–3%), and free-**fat** acids and **cholesterol** (0.5–1.7%). For lean adults, up to 35 billion **adipocytes** are characteristic with each **cell** containing 0.4–0.6 μg of triglycerides. For the seriously obese, the number of **adipocytes** increases fourfold (up to 125 billion), and each **adipocyte** contains twice as much **fat** (0.8–1.2 μg triglycerides). **Adipocytes** possess receptors to cytokines, to **hormones**, factors of growth, and **metabolites**. Functioning of **adipocytes** is driven with biologically active substances (such as catecholamines, which stimulate **lipolysis**).

adipose tissue: A modification of **areolar tissue** in which globules of **oil** are deposited in some of the **cells** (**adipocytes**). The **cells** tend to be grouped together and, in mammals, occur in the **tissues** under the **skin** and around the **abdominal organs** (**kidneys**, **liver**, etc.). This **tissue**-making takes place in a normal range of 15–20% of body weight for men and 20–29% for women and is a metabolically active "organ" supervised by the neuroendocrine system. There are spaces between **fat cells** that contain small **capillaries** and interstitial liquid. Triglycerides of **adipose tissue** are the basic reserve fuel in organisms. The **adipose tissue** of the subject consists of 60–85% of **lipids**, 5–30% **water**, and 2–3% of **proteins**. **Fat** is nonuniformly distributed in the body. When referring to excess weight (see **obesity**), two areas of **fat** should be noted: central and peripheral. The central type of **obesity fat** is positioned mainly in a belly cavity (so-called abdominal **fat**). At peripheral **obesity** it is positioned more under the **skin**.

14

administration: In medicine, the route of **administration** means the path by which a substance is brought into contact with the body.

adventitia: The external covering of an organ or other structure, derived from **connective tissue**, especially the external covering of a **blood vessel**.

African frog: Native to southern Africa. Its Latin name is *Xenopus laevis*.

agarose: Made from agar, a gelatinlike product of certain seaweeds. Used for solidifying certain **cell culture** media, as a substitute for **gelatin**, and as an emulsifier, and such.

agglomeration: Whereby moist, sticky particles collide and adhere to each other due to turbulence, forming agglomerates.

aggregation: A heterogeneous mass of independent but similar units (molecules, **cells**, etc.). The term implies the formation of a whole without an intimate mixing of constituents.

Airy disk: Description of the best-focused spot of **light** that a perfect **lens** with a circular **aperture** can make, limited by the **diffraction** of **light**.

albedo: The probability that a **photon** incident on a small volume element will survive is equal to the ratio of the **scattering** and extinction cross sections and is called the **albedo** for **single scattering**, $\Lambda = \sigma_{sca}/\sigma_{ext} = \mu_s/\mu_t$, where σ_{sca} is the **photon-scattering** cross section, $\sigma_{ext} = (\sigma_{abs} + \sigma_{sca})$ is the **photon-**extinction cross section, σ_{abs} is the **photon-absorption** cross section, μ_s is the **scattering** coefficient, $\mu_t = \mu_a + \mu_s$ is the **attenuation** (extinction) coefficient, and μ_a is the **absorption coefficient**. The **albedo** ranges from zero for a completely **absorbing medium** to unity for a completely **scattering** medium.

albumin: A group of **water**-soluble **proteins** coagulated by heat. They occur in egg white, **blood serum**, milk, and in other animal and plant **tissues**.

albumin blue: A dye used as a quantitative assay to measure **albumin** levels in biological samples including **serum** and urine. The **intensity** of the fluorescent signal is directly proportional to the **albumin** concentration of the sample. **Albumin**-bound dye has a greatly increased excitation, thus the background caused by the emission of any free dye is minimal. **Albumin**-bound dye absorbs **light** at 590 nm and emits **fluorescence** at 620 nm. Long-**wavelength albumin**-blue dyes with **absorption** at 633 nm (AB633) and 670 nm (AB670) are also available and used for selective detection of human-**serum albumin** in **plasma** and **blood**.

alcohol (*Synonym*: spirits): An organic compound that contains one or more hydroxyl groups (–OH). The **alcohols** are hydroxy derivatives of alkanes. They can be classified according to the number of hydroxyl groups: monohydric, C_2H_5OH, **ethanol**; dihydric, $C_2H_4(OH)_2$, **ethylene glycol**; and trihydric, $C_3H_5(OH)_3$, **glycerol**.

Alexa Fluor® **dyes:** Typically used as **cell** and **tissue** labels in **fluorescence microscopy** and **cell** biology. Their excitation and emission spectra cover the **visible spectrum** and extend into the **infrared**. The individual members of the family are numbered roughly according to their excitation maxima (in nm). **Alexa Fluor**® **dyes** are generally more stable, brighter, and less **pH**-sensitive than common dyes (e.g., **fluorescein, rhodamine**) of comparable excitation and emission.

algorithm: A procedure (a finite set of well-defined instructions) for accomplishing some task which, given an initial state, will terminate in a defined end state. The computational complexity and efficient implementation of the **algorithm** are important in computing and depend on suitable data structures.

alpha (α)-globulins: A group of globular **proteins** in **blood plasma** that are highly mobile in alkaline or electrically charged solutions. They inhibit certain **blood** protease and inhibitor activity.

alpha (α)-hydroxy acid (AHA): An acid, such as glycolic, lactic, or fruit acids, that is the mildest of the **skin**-peel formulas and that produces light peels.

α-, β-, and γ-crystallins: The structural **proteins** that are the components of a mammalian **crystalline lens**.

alternating current (ac): An electric current that reverses direction at regular intervals, having a magnitude that varies continuously in a sinusoidal manner.

alveolar bone: A part of upper and lower jaws that holds roots of teeth, which in turn consists of two parts: **alveolar bone** proper (lamina dura)—dense **bone** lining the socket with inserted **periodontal fibers**—and supporting **bone** that is a remaining part of **alveolar bone**. It is composed from highly mineralized (70%), mostly calcium-phosphate (**hydroxyapatite**) crystals, minor amounts of magnesium, sodium, and potassium, osteoblasts and **osteoclasts**, **collagen fibers**, and **proteoglycans**. **Collagen fibers** are made by **osteoblasts**, **mineralization** of **bone** starts in areas within **collagen fibers**. The amount of **alveolar bone** is dependent on the presence of teeth. If teeth are lost and there are no forces on the **bone** from chewing, the **bone** will resorb (see **bone remodeling**). Nutrition is provided by **blood** supply via canals in **bone** or through **bone marrow**.

Alzheimer's disease: A neurodegenerative disease characterized by progressive cognitive deterioration together with declining activities of daily living and neuropsychiatric symptoms or behavioral changes.

ambient temperature: Temperature of the air in the vicinity of the target (target ambient) or the instrument (instrument ambient).

17

ambient-temperature compensation: Correction built into an instrument to provide automatic compensation in the measurement for variations in instrument **ambient temperature**.

ambient-temperature operating range: Range of **ambient temperatures** in which an instrument is designed to operate within published performance specifications.

amide: The organic functional group characterized by a **carbonyl** group (C=O) linked to a nitrogen atom (N). In the **mid-infrared** spectral domain, bands due to the **amide** I, II, III, and A vibrations have been shown to be sensitive to the secondary structure content of **proteins**.

amino acid: Any molecule that contains both amine and carboxyl functional groups. In biochemistry this term refers to alpha (α) **amino acids**. These are molecules where the amino and carboxylate groups are attached to the same carbon, which is called the alpha (α) carbon. The various alpha-**amino acids** differ in which side chain is attached to their alpha carbon. This can vary in size from only a hydrogen atom in glycine, through a methyl group in alanine, to a large heterocyclic group in **tryptophan**. These **amino acids** are components of **proteins**. There are 20 standard **amino acids** used by **cells** in **protein** biosynthesis, and these are specified by the general genetic code. These **amino acids** can be biosynthesized from simpler molecules. The only essential **amino acids** that are obtained from foods are histidine, isoleucine, leucine, lysine, methionine, **phenylalanine**, threonine, **tryptophan**, and valine.

amphiphilic: A term describing a chemical compound possessing both **hydrophilic** and **hydrophobic** properties.

amplifier: An electronic (or optical) circuit that increases the voltage (or **light power**) of a signal fed into it using **power** from an external supply.

amplitude cancellation method (*Related term*: phase cancellation method): Basis for this method is the **interference** of **photon-density waves** [see **interference of photon-density waves (intensity waves)** and **photon-density wave**]. It uses either duplicate sources and a single detector, or duplicate detectors and a single source so that the amplitude characteristics can be nulled and the system becomes a differential.

amplitude-scattering matrix (*Synonyms*: S-matrix, Jones matrix): Consists of four elements (the complex numbers) and provides a linear relationship between the incident and scattered components of an electromagnetic field. Each element depends on **scattering** and azimuthal angles, and optical as well as the geometrical parameters of the **scatterer**. Both field amplitude and phase must be measured to quantify the **amplitude-scattering matrix**.

anabolism: The synthesis of complex organic compounds from simpler organic compounds, such as the synthesis of **proteins** from **amino acids**. The process requires **energy**, mainly supplied in the form of **adenosine triphosphate (ATP)** [see **metabolism**].

anaerobic: In biology, growing without an **oxygen** supply or the lack of **oxygen**. Anaerobic bacterium such as *Propionibacterium acnes* is an aerotolerant anaerobe.

analog-to-digital converter (ADC): A device that converts continuous signals to discrete digital numbers. Typically, an **analog-to-digital converter** is an electronic device that converts an input analog voltage (or current) to a digital number proportional to the magnitude of the voltage or current.

analyzer: A **polarizer** that is placed in front of a detector.

aneurysm: A permanent cardiac or arterial dilation usually caused by weakening of the **vessel** wall.

angiogenesis: A physiological process involving the growth of new **blood vessels** from pre-existing **vessels**. It is a normal and vital process in growth and development, as well as in **wound** healing. However, it is also a fundamental step in the transition of **tumors** from a dormant state to a **malignant** one.

angioplasty: The "reshaping" of **blood vessels** to improve **blood flow**. Different **laser** and fiber-optic technologies are prospectives for **angioplasty**.

angstrom (Å): Unit of length equal to 10^{-10} m.

anhydrous: Having no **water** (for crystal, no **water** for crystallization).

animal model: Refers to a nonhuman animal with a disease or **injury** that is similar to a human condition. These test conditions are often termed *animal models of disease*. The use of **animal models** allows researchers to investigate disease states in ways that would be inaccessible in a human patient, performing procedures on the nonhuman animal that imply a level of harm that would not be considered ethical to inflict on a human.

anionic: Relating to anions, negatively charged ions.

anisotropic crystal: Crystal for which some physical properties (mechanical, optical, magnetic, electrical, etc.) are dependent on direction (not on density or specific **heat capacity**). For example, as **light** propagates through transparent crystals (excluding crystals with a cubic lattice), the **light** undertakes **birefringence** with mutually orthogonal **polarization** of rays propagating in different directions. For crystals with hexagonal, trigonal, and tetragonal structures (e.g., quartz, ruby, and calcite), **birefringence** is maximal along the direction that is perpendicular to the main axis of symmetry and is absent along that axis. Crystals can be uniaxial or biaxial.

anisotropic scattering: A scattering process characterized by a clearly apparent direction of photons that may be due to the presence of large **scatterers**.

anode: A positive electrode towards which the anions (negative ions) move during electrolysis.

anomalous light dispersion: A phenomenon that is closely related to light **absorption** by materials. The **refractive index** of a material changes quickly and anomalously with the **wavelength** ($dn/d\lambda > 0$) within any **absorption band**. See **dispersion, phase-velocity dispersion, fiber material dispersion**, and **Sellmeier equation**.

anomaly: Any indication that deviates from what is expected. Any irregularity, such as a thermal anomaly on an otherwise isothermal surface.

antenna properties of the optical heterodyne system: The narrow **field of view** that provides a high **spatial resolution** for detection and ranging of the medium under study and its image formation.

antibiotic: A drug that kills or prevents the growth of **bacteria**. **Antibiotics** are one class of antimicrobials, a larger group that also includes antiviral, antifungal, and antiparasitic drugs. They are relatively harmless to the host and therefore can be used to treat infections. The term *antibiotic* is also applied to synthetic antimicrobials, such as sulfa drugs. **Antibiotics** are not **enzymes**, but in general are small molecules with a molecular weight of less than 2000 **Da**.

antibody: A **protein** component of the adaptive immune system whose main function is to bind **antigens**, or foreign substances, in the body and to target them for destruction. **Antibodies** can be secreted into the **extracellular** environment or anchored in the **membranes** of specialized B **cells** known as **plasma cells**. An antibody's binding affinity to its target is extraordinarily high.

antigen: Any foreign **protein**, or certain other large molecules, which, when present in a host's **tissues**, stimulates the production of a specific **antibody** by the host. This response leads to rejection of the **antigen** by the host. An **antigen** invades an individual or is injected into an individual. **Antigen** molecules are on the surface of **cells**, **viruses**, **fungi cells**, or **bacteria**. Nonliving substances such as toxins, chemicals, drugs, and foreign particles can be **antigens**. The body's **immune response** recognizes and destroys substances that contain these **antigens**.

anti-reflection coating: A single or multilayered dielectric interferential coating of a lens or other **optical element** surface that reduces light reflection from the surface of the lens or optical element due to reduction of **Fresnel reflection** in a wavelength range defined by refractive index and thickness of the coating layer. To compensate phase shifts of optical fields at reflection on surface—coating and coating—air interfaces of the lens or other optical element, the thickness h of the coating with refractive index n_2 should be $h = \lambda/4n_2$, where λ is the central wavelength of light for which reflection should be minimized. Maximal light transmittance (minimal reflectance) is $(n_2)^2 = n_1 \times n_3$ when amplitudes of reflected fields from two interfaces are approximately equal to each other; here, n_1 and n_3 are refractive indices of the lens material and surrounding media (air), respectively.

anti-Stokes–Raman scattering: A photon interacts with a molecule in a higher vibrational level, thus the energy of the Raman-scattered photons is higher than the energy of the incident photons.

Antrin®: A photodynamic therapy **photosensitizer** that contains motexafin lutetium (pentadentate aromatic metallotexaphyrin). Motexafin lutetium preferentially accumulates in **tumor cells** due to their increased rates of **metabolism**. This drug requires **laser light** of a specific **wavelength** of 742 nm with **fluence** of $75\ \mathrm{J} \cdot \mathrm{cm}^{-2}$ at a **power density** of $75\ \mathrm{mW} \cdot \mathrm{cm}^{-2}$ for activation. It is used to treat **skin** conditions and superficial **cancers**. **Antrin**® has also been tested for use in photoangioplasty (photodynamic-therapy treatment of diseased **arteries**).

antritis: An antral (**antrum**) disorder. Examples include acute **antritis**, which is also known as, or related to, acute **maxillary sinusitis**, and nodular **antritis**, which is defined as antral gastritis with endoscopic findings characterized by a miliary pattern and prominent lymphoid follicles in **biopsy** specimens.

antrum: A general term for a cavity or chamber that may have specific meaning in referencing certain organs or sites in the body. For instance, the **antrum** of the **stomach** (gastric **antrum**) is a portion of the **stomach** located before the outlet. It is lined by **mucosa** (which does not produce acid). The paranasal **sinuses** can be referred to as the frontal **antrum**, ethmoid **antrum**, and maxillary **antrum**.

anxiety: A psychological and physiological state characterized by cognitive, somatic, emotional, and behavioral components. These components combine to create an unpleasant feeling that is typically associated with uneasiness, apprehension, fear, or worry. It is considered a normal reaction to stress. When **anxiety** becomes excessive, it may fall under the classification of an **anxiety** disorder.

aorta: The great **artery** that leaves the left **ventricle**. It conducts the whole of the arterial **blood** supply to all parts of the body except for the **lungs**. In humans, it carries **blood** at the rate of 4 dm^3 per minute.

apatite [*Synonym*: hydroxyapatite (HAP)]: The natural hydroxyapatite crystal, $Ca_5OH(PO_4)_3$. Dental **enamel** consists 87–95% of HAP crystals. **Bone** consists 50–60% of HAP crystals.

aperture: The diameter of a circle of the **optical diaphragm** through which light is allowed to pass. Apertures may be varied and stated as fractions of the **focal length**, e.g., $f/6$ means that the diameter of the **lens** (**aperture**) is $1/6$ of the focal length f. A **pinhole** is an **optical diaphragm** with a small **aperture**.

aphakis subject: A subject with the **crystalline lens** of the eye absent.

apoptosis: The natural, programmed death of a **cell** (for type-I **cell** death, compare **autophagy**) in response to an external signal. The signal induces a chain of biochemical reactions leading to the death of **cells** no longer needed (as in embryonic development).

apparent temperature: The target surface temperature indicated by an **infrared** point sensor, **infrared line scanner**, or **infrared imager** before temperature corrections are made.

aptamer: In general, **aptamers** are oligonucleic acid or peptide molecules that bind to a specific target molecule. **Aptamers** can be used for both basic research and clinical purposes as macromolecular drugs. More specifically, **aptamers** can be classified as **DNA** or **RNA aptamers** and consist of (usually short) strands of oligonucleotides.

aqueous humor: A watery fluid, similar in composition to **cerebrospinal fluid**, that fills the anterior chamber of the **eyeball**, behind the **cornea**. The **iris** and **crystalline lens** lie in it. The **aqueous humor** is continually secreted by the **ciliary body** and absorbed. It helps maintain the shape of the **eyeball** and assists in the **refraction** of **light**.

Ar (argon) laser: A **laser** with a lasing medium composed of ionized argon gas. The emission is mostly in the **UV** and **visible wavelength range** 336.6–363.8 nm, 454.5 nm, 457.9 nm, 488 nm, 514 nm, and 528.7 nm. Ar lasers can be **multimode, single-mode**, and **single-frequency** with a narrow **bandwidth** ($\Delta\lambda \sim 10^{-6}$ nm, when an internal **Fabry–Pérot etalon** is used as a spectral selector). Their **power** ranges from a few milliwatts to tenths of **watts**. These lasers are used in **Raman** and **fluorescence spectroscopy** of biological molecules, as well as to provide photochemical processes in irradiated **tissues**. Ar laser radiation is also widely used for pumping many other types of lasers such as **dye lasers** or **titanium sapphire lasers**.

arachnoid mater: The membrane that covers the **brain** and **spinal cord**. It is interposed between the two other cerebral membranes—the more superficial *dura mater* and the deeper *pia mater*—and is separated from the *pia mater* by the subarachnoid space, where **cerebrospinal fluid** flows.

arc lamp (*Related term*: **flashlamp**): A lamp that uses a luminous and heat emission of plasma bridge formed in a gap between two conductors or terminals when they are separated. **Mercury arc lamps**, **xenon arc lamps**, or **krypton arc lamps** that produce so-called intensive pulse light (IPL) are available and often used in **tissue spectroscopy** and dermatology applications. The output spectrum of an **arc lamp** is a mixed emission spectrum of plasma ions produced from a filling gas. For a high-energy short pulse, the temperature of **arc lamp** plasma can be very high (6000–10000 K), and the dominant emission is provided by heat sources with a spectrum close to blackbody. For CW or long pulse mode, the temperature of arc lamp plasma is relatively low (3000–6000 K), and the emission spectrum has a significant portion of fluorescence **light** in the red and **NIR** spectral range.

areolar tissue: A soft, sometimes spongelike **connective tissue** that consists of an amorphous **polysaccharide**-containing and jellylike ground matrix in which a loose network of **white fibers**, **yellow fibers**, and **reticulin fibers** is embedded. **Fibroblasts** form and maintain the matrix. Areolar **tissue** is found throughout the vertebrate body, binding together organs (by mesenteries) and **muscles** (by **sheaths**), and occurring as **subcutaneous tissue**. Its function is to support or fill in the space between organs or between other **tissues**. The **fibrous** nature of the matrix is modified by variation in the concentration of white, yellow, or

reticulin fibers, which alters the characteristics of toughness, elasticity, and inextensibility to suit the function of the **tissue**. Many modifications of **areolar tissue** occur.

arginine: Abbreviated Arg or R: an α-**amino acid**. The L-form is one of the 20 most-common natural **amino acids**. At the molecular genetic level, within the structure of the messenger ribonucleic acid **mRNA**, CGU, CGC, CGA, CGG, AGA, and AGG are the triplets of nucleotid bases or codons that codify for **arginine** during **protein** synthesis. In mammals, **arginine** is classified as a conditionally essential **amino acid**, depending on the developmental stage and health status of the individual.

arm: In anatomy, an **arm** is one of the upper limbs of a two-legged animal. The term *arm* can also be used for analogous structures, such as one of the paired upper limbs of a four-legged animal. Anatomically, the term refers specifically to the segment between the shoulder and the elbow. The segment between the elbow and **wrist** is the **forearm**.

arteriole: **Arteries** branch repeatedly until their diameter is less than 1/3 mm. They are then called "**arterioles**." **Arteriole** walls are formed from smooth **muscle** under the control of the autonomic **nervous system**. Their function is to control **blood** supply to the **capillaries**.

arteriosclerosis: An arterial disease occurring especially in the elderly. It is characterized by inelasticity and thickening of the **vessel** walls, reducing **blood flow**.

artery: A **blood vessel** conducting **blood** from the **heart** to **tissues** and organs. Lined with **endothelium** (smooth flat **cells**) and surrounded by thick, muscular, elastic walls containing white and yellow **fibrous tissue**. **Arteries** have a complex structure. The medial layer consists mostly of closely packed smooth-**muscle cells** with a mean diameter of 15–20 μm. Additionally, small amounts of **connective tissue**, including **elastin**, collagenous, and reticular **fibers**, as well as a few **fibroblasts**, are located in the **media**. The outer adventitial layer consists of dense **fibrous connective tissue**, and is largely made up of **collagen fibers** 1–12 μm in diameter and thinner **elastin fibers** 2–3 μm in diameter. The cylindrical **collagen** and **elastin fibers** are ordered mainly along one axis, thus causing the **tissue** to be **birefringent**.

artifact: A product of artificial character due to extraneous agency. An error caused by an uncompensated anomaly. In **microscopy**, a structure that is seen in a **tissue** sample under a microscope when it is not present in living **tissue**. It may be caused by improperly used technology in sample preparation or wrong displacement of the sample under the microscope. In thermography, an **emissivity artifact** simulates a change in surface temperature, but not a real change.

A-scan: Axial scan or in-depth scan perpendicular to the sample surface. Typically used in **optical coherence tomography** when a reflectivity in-depth profile is obtained. When moving the mirror in the reference path of the **interferometer**, not only is the depth scanned, but a carrier is also generated.

A-scan-based B-scan: Collecting many **A-scans** for different and adjacent transverse positions. The lines in the generated raster correspond to **A-scans**, in that the lines are oriented along the depth coordinate. The transverse scanner (operating along X or Y, or along the polar angle θ in polar coordinates) advances at a slower pace to build a **B-scan** image. A commercial optical coherence tomography instrument exists that can produce a **B-scan** image of the **retina** in ~1 second.

ascites: Denotes an abnormality where fluid collects in the **abdominal cavity** because of **water** molecules leaking out of capillary **blood vessels** into surrounding **tissues**, caused by decrease of **oncotic pressure** in the bloodstream. This drop in pressure is due to a lack of total **proteins** in the body, most commonly caused by advancing **liver** disease and a corresponding decrease in **protein** production. There are many causes of **ascites**, but the most common is cirrhosis, the chronic scarring of the **liver**. **Ascites** sometimes results from a **malignant tumor** in the peritoneal cavity.

aspirate: Refers to pulmonary aspiration, which is the entry of secretions or foreign material into the **trachea** and **lungs**. It also refers to **lung** infection caused by pulmonary aspiration and needle aspiration **biopsy**, a surgical procedure.

astrocyte: A starlike **cell** of **nervous tissue** macroglia.

astrocytoma: A well-differentiated **glioma**, which consists of **cells** that look like **astrocytes**.

asymmetry parameter (*Synonym*: skewness): Measure of asymmetry in a **probability-distribution function**.

atheroma: Fatty degeneration of the inner walls (**intima**) of the **arteries** in **arteriosclerosis**.

atherosclerotic plaque: An unstable collection of **lipids** (**fatty acids**), white **blood cells** (especially **macrophages**), and sometimes calcium. Accumulates in **arteries** and leads to **occlusion** of the **vessel**.

atomic-force microscopy (AFM) (*Synonym*: scanning-force microscopy): A very high resolution type of scanning-probe **microscopy**, with demonstrated resolution of fractions of a **nanometer**, more than 1000 times better than the optical **diffraction limit**. The precursor to **atomic-force microscopy** was **scanning-tunneling microscopy (STM)**. **Atomic-force microscopy** is one of the foremost tools for imaging, measuring, and manipulating matter at the nanoscale. Information is gathered by "feeling" the surface with a mechanical probe. Piezoelectric elements that facilitate tiny but accurate and precise movements on (electronic) command enable the very precise scanning.

atrium: Refers to the **blood** collection chamber of a **heart**. In humans, there are two atria, one on either side of the **heart**. The **atrium** on the right side holds **blood** that needs **oxygen**. It sends **blood** to the right **ventricle**, which sends **blood** to the **lungs** for **oxygen**. After the **blood** returns, it is sent to the left **atrium**. It is then pumped from the left **atrium** and sent to the left **ventricle** where it is sent out of the **heart** to the rest of the body.

attenuated total reflectance Fourier-transform infrared spectroscopy (ATR FTIR):   Method based on combination of **total internal reflection** technique and Fourier-transform **infrared spectroscopy**.

attenuation: A decrease in **energy** per unit area of a **wave** or beam of **light**. It occurs as the distance from the source increases and is caused by **absorption** or **scattering**, or both, and is characterized by an **attenuation coefficient**.

attenuation coefficient: The reciprocal of the distance over which **light** of **intensity** I is attenuated to $I/e \approx 0.37I$ caused by **light** interaction with both **absorption** and **scattering**. Also referred to as total interaction coefficient, $\mu_t = \mu_a + \mu_s$, where μ_a is the **absorption coefficient** and μ_s is the **scattering** coefficient. The units are typically cm^{-1}.

auscultation: Hearing of sounds of different body structures with diagnostic purposes.

autocorrelation: The **correlation** of an ordered series of observations with the same series in an altered order.

autocorrelation function: The characteristic of the second-order statistics of a random process that shows how fast the random value changes from point to point. For example, the **autocorrelation function** of **intensity** fluctuations caused by **scattering** of a **laser** beam by a rough surface characterizes the size and the distribution of **speckle** sizes in the induced **speckle**

pattern. The **Fourier transform** of the **autocorrelation function** represents the **power spectrum** of a random process.

autoexposure: Camera function that attempts to calculate the optimal exposure time for a camera with user-controllable exposure. This feature is not available on analog cameras. If the camera has a multishot feature, it will attempt to expose each **color** plane separately. When used, the function captures multiple images each time, varying the exposure according to the parameters set on the digital-options property page. It will continue until it gets an image that has the proper dynamic range or until it has exhausted its allowed attempts. On exit, the exposure of the camera will be set to whatever the function calculated.

autofluorescence: Natural **fluorescence** of a **tissue** or a **cell** at excitation of **endogenous** (intrinsic) **fluorophores**.

autophagocytosis: See **autophagy**.

autophagy (*Synonym*: autophagocytosis):   Process where cytoplasmic materials are degraded through the lysosomal machinery. The process is commonly viewed as sequestering organelles and long-lived **proteins** in a double-**membrane vesicle** inside the **cell**, where the contents are subsequently delivered to the lysosome for degradation. **Autophagy** is part of normal **cell** growth and development. For example, a **liver-cell mitochondrion** lasts about 10 days before it is degraded and its contents reused. **Autophagy** also plays a major role in the destruction of **bacteria**, **viruses**, and unnecessary **proteins** that have begun to aggregate within a **cell** and may cause potential problems. When **autophagy** involves the total destruction of the **cell**, it is called autophagic **cell** death (also known as cytoplasmic **cell** death or type-II **cell** death). This is one of the main types of programmed **cell** death (compare **apoptosis**). It is a regulated process of **cell** death in a multicellular organism or in a colony of individual **cells**, such as **yeast**.

avalanche photodiode (APD):   Type of silicon or germanium **photodiode** that uses a phenomenon of the electrical breakdown of a p–n junction that induces collision ionization and avalanche creation of electron–hole pairs. Typically increases the photocurrent up to 10^2–10^3. **Avalanche photodiodes** have a structure similar to regular **photodiodes**, but they are operated with much higher reverse bias. They are usually used in **photon-counting** systems.

average power: A mean value of **light power** received by averaging current values of **power** for some time interval. For a train of pulses of pulsed **light**, the **average power** is calculated as $P_{ave} = E_p \times f_p$, where E_p is the **energy** of a pulse and f_p is the pulse repetition rate.

Avogadro constant: Also called Avogadro's number, it is the number of atoms, molecules, ions, or electrons in one **mole**, which is the number of atoms in exactly 12 grams of carbon-12. $N_A = 6.02214179(30) \times 10^{23}$ mol^{-1}.

axicon lens: A specialized type of **lens** that has a conical surface. It images a point source into a line along the optic axis, or transforms a **laser beam** into a ring. It can be used to turn a **Gaussian light beam** into an approximation of a Bessel beam, with greatly reduced **diffraction**.

axillary: Pertaining to the cavity beneath the junction of the **arm** and the body, better-known as the armpit.

axon (*Synonym*: nerve fiber): A long, slender projection of a **nerve cell**, or neuron that conducts electrical impulses away from the neuron's **cell** body or soma. This is a special cellular filament that arises from the **cell** body at a site called the **axon** hillock and travels for a distance, as far as 1 m in humans or even more in other species. Each **neuron** has no more than one **axon**, which may branch hundreds of times before it terminates.

azure: A methylated thiazine dye, is a metachromatic basic dye ranging from green (to **chromosomes**) and blue (to nucleoli and cytoplasmic **ribosomes**) to red **colors** (to deposits containing **mucopolysaccharides**). There are many methylated homologues used as components of many polychrome stains in combination with **eosin** and methylene blue in **pH**-adjusted solutions. Azure A, also called methylene azur A and asymmetrical dimethylthionine, is a dye used in nuclear and **blood** stain. Azure B, also called methylene azur B, **azure** I, and trimethylthionine chloride, is used in biological stain and a component of polychrome **Giemsa stain** for **blood** protozoa. Azure C, monomethylthionine chloride, is used in staining of mucins and **cartilage**. Azuresin, a complex of **azure** A and carbacrylic **cationic** exchange resin, is used as a diagnostic aid in detection of gastric achlorhydria without intubation. Also of note is Azure II, a mixture of **azure** B and methylene blue in equal amounts.

back-illuminated charge-coupled device: Provides exceptional **quantum efficiency** compared to conventional front-illuminated CCDs, due to their construction. A front-illuminated **charge-coupled device** is thinned to only 15 μm thick and mounted upside down on a rigid substrate. A **back-illuminated charge-coupled device** allows **light** to enter and reach the **pixel** wells without the conventional gate structures blocking the view. **Charge-coupled devices** with backside illumination can boost **quantum efficiency** to over 85%.

background temperature (instrument): The **apparent temperature** of the radiant **energy** impinging on an object that is reflected off the object and enters the temperature-measuring instrument. It originates from the scene behind and surrounding the instrument, as viewed from the target. The reflection of this background appears in the image and affects temperature measurements. Good-quality quantitative thermal sensing and imaging instruments provide a means for correcting measurements for this reflection.

background temperature (target): **Apparent ambient temperature** of the scene behind and surrounding the target, as viewed from the instrument. When the **FOV** of a point-sensing instrument is larger than the target, the target background temperature will affect the instrument reading. It is also called the surrounding temperature or foreground temperature.

backprojection algorithm: Approximate inverse solution to provide efficient tomographic imaging. In **x-ray computed tomography**, the backprojection is reconstructed along the paths of **x-ray** propagation. In optical tomography the backprojection is reconstructed along the paths of **ballistic photons** and/or least-**scattering-photon** propagation. In **optoacoustic tomography**, the backprojection is reconstructed along spherical shells that are centered at the detector and have a radius determined by the acoustic time of flight.

backscattering: The **dispersion** of a fraction of the incident **radiation** in a backward direction.

backscattering coefficient (volume-averaged): The sum of the particle cross sections weighted by their angular-**scattering** functions evaluated at 180 deg.

backscattering Mueller matrix: **Mueller matrix** measured for **light** backscattered by a sample.

bacteria: Unicellular microorganisms that are typically a few **micrometers** long and have many shapes, including spheres, rods, and spirals. **Bacteria** are ubiquitous in every habitat on earth, growing in soil, acidic hot springs, radioactive waste, seawater, and deep in the earth's crust. Some **bacteria** can even survive in the extreme cold and vacuum of outer space. There are typically 40 million bacterial **cells** in a gram of soil and a million bacterial **cells** in a milliliter of fresh **water**. **Gram-positive bacteria** are those that are stained dark blue or violet by **Gram's stain**. This is in contrast to **Gram-negative bacteria**, which cannot retain the **crystal violet** stain, instead taking up the counterstain (**safranin** or **fuchsine**) and appearing red or pink. Gram-positive organisms are able to retain the crystal-violet stain because of the high amount of peptidoglycan in the **cell** wall. Gram-positive **cell** walls typically lack the outer **membrane** found in **Gram-negative bacteria**.

bacterial biofilm: A complex **aggregation** of microorganisms living together in a specific environment marked by the excretion of a protective and adhesive matrix. **Biofilms** are often characterized by surface attachment, structural heterogeneity, genetic diversity, complex community interactions, and an **extracellular matrix** of polymeric substances. **Bacteria** in a **biofilm** can be more resistant to environmental changes, such as introduction of antimicrobial agents, than are **bacteria** in other states.

ballistic imaging: **Optical imaging** methods and techniques that more or less ignore the **diffuse photons** and detect only the **ballistic photons** to create high-resolution (near **diffraction limit**) images through **scattering media**. **Optical coherence tomography** and confocal-scanning **microscopy** are two major techniques based on detection of **ballistic photons**.

ballistic photons (*Synonym*: coherent photons):   A group of unscattered and strictly straightforward-scattered **photons**.

bandgap: Generally refers to the **energy** difference (in electron volts) between the top of the valence band and the bottom of the conduction band, which is found in solid-state materials. It is the amount of **energy** required to free an outer-shell electron from its orbit about the nucleus to become a mobile charge carrier, able to move freely within the solid material. In conductors, the two bands often overlap, so they may not have a **bandgap**. In **semiconductors** and insulators, electrons are confined to a number of bands of **energy**, and are forbidden from other regions. Electrons are able to jump from one band to another. To jump from a valence band to a conduction band, the electron requires a specific minimum amount of **energy** for the transition. The required **energy** differs with different materials. Electrons can **gain** enough **energy** to jump to the conduction band by absorbing either a **phonon** (heat) or a **photon** (**light**).

band-pass filter: Device that passes frequencies (**wavelengths**) within a certain range and rejects (attenuates) frequencies (**wavelengths**) outside that range. The **bandwidth** of the filter is simply the difference between the upper and lower cut-off frequencies (**wavelengths**). In electronics, the shape factor is the ratio of **bandwidths** measured using two different **attenuation** values to determine the cut-off **frequency**. For example, a shape factor of 2:1 at 30/3 **dB** means the **bandwidth** measured between frequencies at 30 **dB attenuation** is twice that measured between frequencies at 3 **dB attenuation**. **Optical filters** are described by the cut-off **wavelength** at 50% of peak. Both types of filters, electronic and optical, also can be created by combining a low-pass **filter** with a high-pass **filter**, or a **long-pass filter** with a **short-pass filter**, respectively. An ideal **band-pass filter** would have a completely flat passband and would completely attenuate all frequencies (**wavelengths**) outside the passband. In practice, no **band-pass filter** is ideal. The filter does not attenuate all frequencies outside the desired **frequency** (**wavelength**) range completely. In particular, there is a region just outside the intended passband where frequencies (**wavelengths**) are attenuated, but not rejected. This is known as the filter roll-off, and in electronics, it is usually expressed in **dB** of **attenuation** per octave or decade of **frequency**. Generally, the design of a filter seeks to make the roll-off as narrow as possible, thus allowing the filter to perform as close as possible to its intended design. Often, this is achieved at the expense of pass-band or stop-band ripple. Some examples: In electronics, an analogue electronic **band-pass filter** is an RLC circuit (a **resistor**–inductor–capacitor circuit). In neuroscience, visual cortical simple **cells** have response properties that resemble a **band-pass filter**. In optics, these are often termed **interference filters**.

bandwidth: Related to electronic or optical instrumentation and characterizes **frequency** or **wavelength** range that is transmitted or amplified by a device. It can be measured on the different levels of the signal, such as **half-width at half-maximum (HWHM)**, **full-width at half-maximum (FWHM)**, or on the level 0.707 (−3 **dB**). In **spectroscopy** it characterizes width of **absorption** or emission bands of molecular or atomic systems in **frequency** or **wavelength** scale, which is defined by transition lifetime (radiative and collisional) and the Doppler-broadening effect of radiating atoms and molecules by gaseous systems.

baroreflex: In cardiovascular physiology, the **baroreflex** or baroreceptor reflex is one of the body's homeostatic mechanisms for maintaining **blood pressure**. It provides a negative feedback loop in which an elevated **blood pressure** reflexively causes **blood pressure** to decrease. Similarly, decreased **blood pressure** depresses the **baroreflex**, causing **blood pressure** to rise.

Barrett's esophagus: Refers to an abnormal change (metaplasia) in the **cells** of the lower end of the **esophagus** thought to be caused by damage from chronic acid exposure, or reflux esophagitis. It is considered to be a premalignant condition and is associated with an increased risk of esophageal **cancer**. The condition is named after Norman Barrett, who described the condition in 1957.

basal cell carcinoma (BCC): The most common **skin cancer**. It can be destructive and disfiguring. Risk is increased for individuals with a high cumulative exposure to UV **light** via sunlight. Statistically, approximately 30% of humans with **Caucasian skin** develop a BCC within their lifetime. In 80% of all cases, BCCs are found on the **head** and **neck**. Treatment involves surgery, **topical**, **x-ray**, **cryosurgery**, **photodynamic therapy**. It is rarely life-threatening but if left untreated, it can be disfiguring, cause bleeding, and produce local destruction (e.g., **eyeball**, **ear**, nose, lip).

basal lamina: A layer of **extracellular matrix**, secreted by the **epithelial cells**, on which **epithelium** sits. It is typically about 40–50 nm thick (with exceptions such as the basal laminae that compose the 100–200-nm-thick glomerular-**basement membrane**) and typically seen with an **electronic microscope**. This includes **proteoglycans**.

36

baseline: Information gathered at the beginning of a clinical study from which variations found in the study are measured. It includes a person's health status before he or she begins a **clinical trial**. **Baseline** measurements are used as a reference point to determine a participant's response to experimental treatment.

basement membrane: Thin sheet of **connective tissue** below the epithelia that usually contains **polysaccharide** and very fine **fibers** of **reticulin** and **collagen**. It regulates the flow of molecules to and from the **epithelium**. **Basal lamina** and reticular lamina together make up the **basement membrane**. Anchoring **fibrils** extend from the **basal lamina** of **epithelial cells** and attach to the reticular lamina by wrapping around the reticular **fiber bundles**. Anchoring **fibrils** are essential to the functional integrity of the dermoepidermal junction. **Basement membranes** are thicker than **basal lamina** and can be seen in **light microscopy**.

beamsplitter: An optical device providing splitting of an optical beam. Outgoing **light beams** diverging from the **beamsplitter** may have different directions of propagation, **wavelengths**, or state of **polarization**. Optical plates, semi-transparent mirrors, **interference filters**, and **prisms** can serve as the **beamsplitters**. See **dichroic (dichromatic) mirror (beamsplitter)**, **epi-fluorescence interference and absorption-filter combinations**, **Glan-Taylor polarization prism**, and **Wollaston prism (WP)**.

beat signal: The signal at the intermediate **frequency** produced by mixing the local- and signal-oscillator beams on a **photodetector**.

bending: See **vibrational modes**.

benign tumor: Nonmalignant **tumor**.

benzoporphyrin derivative (BPD): A **photosensitizer** with an excitation band around 690 nm, it is used in **cancer** diagnostics and photodynamic therapy. Verteporfin® and **Visudyne**® are the commercialized products. At **PDT**, the typical **laser** dose is $100 \, \text{J} \cdot \text{cm}^{-2}$.

Bessel optical beam: An optical beam whose amplitude is described by a Bessel function of the first kind. A true Bessel beam is nondiffractive. This means that as it propagates, it does not diffract and spread out. This is in contrast to the usual behavior of **light**, which spreads out after being focused down to a small spot. As with a plane **wave**, a true Bessel beam cannot be created because it is unbounded and therefore requires an infinite amount of **energy**. Reasonably good approximations can be made, however, and these are important in many optical applications because they exhibit little or no **diffraction** over a limited distance. Bessel beams are also self-healing, meaning that the beam can be partially obstructed at one point, but will re-form at a point farther down the beam axis. These properties together make Bessel beams extremely useful for optical tweezers, as a narrow Bessel beam will maintain its required property of tight focus over a relatively long section of beam, even when partially occluded by the dielectric particles being tweezed. Approximations to Bessel beams are made in practice by focusing a **Gaussian light beam** with an **axicon lens** to generate a Bessel–**Gaussian light beam**.

beta (β) globulins: Group of globular **proteins** in **blood plasma** that are less mobile than **alpha (α) globulins** are in alkaline-charged or electrically charged solutions.

beta-carotene: A provitamin for **retinol (vitamin A)**, it is converted to retinol in the **liver**. It is an antioxidant.

biaxial crystal: Anisotropic crystal characterized by having two optic axes, that is, two axes along which an incoming beam will remain collinear and the **light** of both **polarizations** will propagate at the same speed. Mica is an example.

bile: A secretion of the **liver**. A bitter, slightly alkaline liquid, yellowish-green to golden-brown in **color**, consisting of **bile**

salts, **bile pigments**, and other substances dissolved in **water**. Its function is to assist in the digestion of **fat** and to act as a vehicle for the rejection of toxic or poisonous substances.

bilirubin: Yellow **bile pigment** formed in the breakdown of heme. It has two relatively broad **absorption bands** near 330 and 460 nm.

bimetal nanoparticles: Particularly, **gold nanoparticles** and nanorods that can be used as templates for deposition of a thin silver layer. **Surface-plasmon resonance** of such bimetal particles can conveniently be tuned from **NIR** to VIS through the increase in the silver layer.

bimodal distribution: A distribution having two modes.

binning: A **charge-coupled device** chip is an array of rectangular (generally square) **light**-detecting regions called **pixels**. Sometimes pictures can be taken by combining the information in adjacent **pixels** to create one effective superpixel— this is called **binning** mode. The advantage of **binning** is the subsequent reduction in noise. Noise-reduction occurs because the **signal-to-noise ratio** is proportional to the square of the superpixel and inversely proportional to its square root (because noise is a random process). Thus, the chip acts as if it is more sensitive. A drawback to **binning** is the loss of resolution, because larger **pixel**s detect fewer portions of an object.

biobreeding diabetes-prone (BBDP) rat: A bred strain that spontaneously develops autoimmune type 1 **diabetes**. **BBDP rats** are used as an **animal model** for type 1 **diabetes** because it recapitulates many of the features of human type 1 **diabetes**.

biocompatible: The quality of not having toxic or injurious effects on biological systems.

biofilm: See **bacterial biofilm**.

bioheat equation: Describes the change in **tissue** temperature at a definite point in the **tissue**. It is defined by **tissue** thermal conductivity, metabolic heat-generation rate, and the **heat transfer** caused by **blood perfusion** at this point.

biological cell: Individual unit of protoplasm surrounded by a **plasma membrane** and usually containing a **nucleus**. A **cell** may exhibit all the characteristics of a living organism, or it may be highly specialized for a particular function. **Cells** vary considerably in size and shape, but all have the common features of **metabolism**. Every living organism is composed of **cells**, and every **cell** is formed from existing **cells**, usually by division, but also by fusion of sex **cells**. A **cell** may contain more than one **nucleus**. In prokaiyotic **cells**, the genetic material is not contained in a **nucleus**. Most mammalian **cells** have diameters in the range of 5–75 μm. In the epidermal layer, the **cells** are large (with an average cross-sectional area of about 80 μm^2) and quite uniform in size. **Fat cells**, each containing a single **lipid** droplet that nearly fills the entire **cell** and therefore results in eccentric placement of the **cytoplasm** and **nucleus**, have a wide range of diameters from a few microns to 50–75 μm. There are a wide variety of structures within **cells** that determine **tissue light scattering**. **Cell** nuclei are on the order of 5–10 μm in diameter. Mitochondria, **lysosomes** and peroxisoms have dimensions of 1–2 μm. **Ribosomes** are on the order of 20 nm in diameter. Structures within various organelles can have dimensions up to a few hundred **nanometers**. Usually, the **scatterers** in **cells** are not spherical. Models of prolate ellipsoids with a ratio of the ellipsoid axes between 2 and 10 are more typical.

biological imaging: Related to imaging of various biological species, including **cells**, thin-**tissue** layers, **embryos**, and small animals using imaging modalities based on **microscopy** and tomography. These include scanning-electron **microscopy** (SEM), **atomic-force microscopy (AFM)** and near-field microscopy (NFM), conventional optical microscopes equipped with highly sensitive and high-resolution **charge-coupled device** or com-**plementary metal–oxide semiconductor cameras**, holographic or interferential microscopies, confocal-**reflectance** and **fluorescence** microscopies, **optical coherence tomography**, **optical-projection tomography**, **second-harmonic** and **multiphoton fluorescence scanning microscopies**, and so on. Some of these instruments are destructive and need special preparation of the sample, including dye **labeling**. Others are **noninvasive** and can provide images without **labeling** of target biological components. **Optical coherence tomography**, confocal, second harmonic generation, and multiphoton microscopies belong to **noninvasive** methods. The resolution is also different, as SEM, AFM, NFM, and interferential **microscopy** have a nano scale resolution, and **optical coherence tomography** and **confocal microscopy** have a micro scale resolution.

bioluminescence: A kind of **luminescence** where the production and emission of **light** is provided by a living organism. It is a naturally occurring form of **chemiluminescence** where **energy** is released by a chemical reaction in the form of **light** emission. **Adenosine triphosphate (ATP)** is involved in most instances. **Bioluminescence** occurs in marine vertebrates and invertebrates, as well as in microorganisms and terrestrial animals.

biomedical micro-electromechanical system (BioMEMS): Conceptually, electromechanical is considered as any physical, electrochemical, biochemical, or fluidic phenomenon that provides work at the microscale, including microsensing, microactuation, microassaying, micromoving, and microdelivery. It is a science and technology that aims at more than simply finding biomedical applications for **MEMS** devices and cost-effective solutions to biomedical problems. **BioMEMS** is a platform for the development of nanomedicine (nanoscale medicine) (see **nano-electromechanical system (NEMS)**, **genomics**, and **proteomics**.

biomedical optics: The science and technology of optics applied to life science and health care, such as **cell** and **tissue optics**, **optical spectroscopy**, **light microscopy**, **optical imaging**, **optical tomography**, **optical biopsy**, **nonlinear optics**, and

nonlinear optical imaging. **Biomedical optics** usually considers the interaction of **visible**, **ultraviolet**, and **infrared light** with biological media. The specificity of photobiological processes related to **optical properties** of **cells** and **tissues** is also an area of interest. In biomedical science, all simplified and comprehensive models and theories of optics, such as geometric or ray optics, physical optics based on wave effects (**diffraction**, **interference**, and quantum optics, where **light** is described as a collection of corpuscles, i.e., **photons**) are used successfully. Physiological optics is based on optical science, which is also broadly applied in ophthalmology and optometry.

biophotonics: Photonics as science and technology applied to life science, health care, biotechnology, agriculture, and environmental science. This term is similar to **biomedical optics**, but it is used to describe a broader field of research and applications with a wider **wavelength** range, including **x rays** and **terahertz**. Other devices of interest in **biophotonics** include **heat light sources**, **lasers**, **optical fibers**, **photonic crystal fibers**, **photodetectors**, etc. that have been specially designed or widely used in biology and medicine, as well as different biological and medical instrumentation based on photonic technologies, such as **optical microscopes**, **spectrometers**, **infrared imagers**, and **optical-tomography** systems. The basic physical science for this field is photonics, which deals with the study and generation of photons and their detection, delivery, and manipulation. Therefore, **biophotonics** refers to the emission, **absorption**, **reflection**, modification, and detection of radiation from biomolecules, **cells**, **tissues**, organisms, and biomaterials. Biosensors of different kinds are also important to this field.

biopsy: A medical test involving the removal of **cells** or **tissues** for examination. When only a sample of **tissue** is removed, the procedure is called an incisional **biopsy** or core **biopsy**. When an entire lump or suspicious area is removed, the procedure is called an excisional **biopsy**. When a sample of **tissue** or fluid is removed with a needle, the procedure is called a needle aspiration **biopsy**. **Biopsy** specimens are often taken from part of a **lesion**

when the cause of a disease is uncertain or its extent or exact character is in doubt. Pathologic examination of a **biopsy** can determine whether a **lesion** is benign or **malignant**, and can help differentiate between different types of **cancer**. The margins of a **biopsy** specimen are also carefully examined to see if the disease may have spread beyond the biopsied area. "Clear margins" or "negative margins" mean that no disease was found at the edges of the **biopsy** specimen. "Positive margins" means that disease was found, and additional treatment may be needed.

biospeckle: Speckle formed by coherent **light scattering** from a **cell** or **tissue**.

birefringence: Phenomenon exhibited by certain crystals (or quasi-crystal-**tissue** structures) in which an incident ray of **light** is split into two rays (called an ordinary ray and an extraordinary ray), which are plane (linear) polarized in mutually orthogonal planes.

birefringent: Any material or **tissue** showing **birefringence**.

birefringent wedge (BW): An optical wedge made from **birefringent** material that divides a **light beam** into two orthogonally polarized beams through action of **Snell's law**. With these components, each beam is deviated in the same direction from the original propagation direction. The **polarization** with the larger **refractive index** is deviated by a larger angle.

bit: Denotes the binary value of 1 or 0. An ordered collection of **bits** is a **byte**.

BK7: A borosilicate-crown optical glass that is relatively hard and shows a good scratch resistance. It is commonly used for manufacturing of high-quality optical components. It has high linear-optical transmission in the **visible** range down to 350 nm with **refractive index** of $n_d = 1.51680$ (587.6 nm).

blackbody: An object that absorbs all the **electromagnetic radiation** that falls on the object, regardless of the **radiation wavelength**. Many objects made from condensed materials (for instance, metals, **tissues**) can be considered as blackbodies. All bodies emit **electromagnetic radiation** in the **infrared wavelength** range and with intensities that correspond to their temperature. This is called heat **radiation** or **blackbody radiation** (see **blackbody radiator**, **heat light source**, and **Planck curve**). A **blackbody** is a **Lambertian radiator**, which means that the **radiance** is proportional to the cosine of the viewing angle.

blackbody curve: Plot of spectral radiant exitance ($W \cdot m^{-2} \cdot nm^{-1}$) versus **wavelength** for various temperatures according to **Planck's law**. These curves show the maximum amount of **energy** at any given **wavelength** that can be radiated by an object due solely to its temperature. See also **Planck curve**.

blackbody radiator: A perfect radiator, one that radiates the maximum number of **photons** in a unit time from a unit area in a specified spectral interval into a hemisphere that any body in thermodynamic equilibrium at the same temperature can radiate. It follows that a **blackbody** absorbs all radiant **energy** impinging on it and reflects and transmits none, thus being a surface with **emissivity** of unity (1.0).

bladder: A membranous sac containing or storing fluid.

blister: When the outer (**epidermis**) layer of the **skin** separates from the **fiber** layer (**dermis**), a pool of **lymph** and other bodily fluids collect between these layers while the **skin** regrows from underneath. This is a defense mechanism of the human body. **Blisters** can be caused by chemical or physical **injury**. An allergic reaction is an example of chemical **injury**. A physical **injury** can be caused by heat, frostbite, or friction.

blocking (notch) filter: Filter that blocks the passage of a certain **frequency** (**wavelength**) band. Usually it rejects a narrow-**wavelength** band or part of the **wavelength spectrum** and leaves the rest of the **spectrum** little changed. Filters are used in a variety of applications including **complementary metal-oxide semiconductor (CMOS)** sensor covers for digital imaging, **fluorescence** filters for **microscopy** and cytology, night-vision goggles, and **laser**-line rejection. A variety of coating platforms to provide notch and **blocking filters** ranging from 0.3 nm to 25 μm with **optical density** of more than 6 are available.

blood: A fluid **tissue** contained in a network of **vessels** or **sinuses** in humans and animals. The **vessels** or **sinuses** are lined with **endothelium**. **Blood** is circulated through the network by the muscular action of the **vessels** or the **heart**. **Blood** transports **oxygen**, **metabolites**, and **hormones**. It contains soluble-colloidal **proteins (blood plasma)** and **blood corpuscles**. It assists with temperature control in mammals.

blood cell: One of the various types of **cell** that circulates in **blood plasma**, such as the **red blood cell (RBC)** [**erythrocyte**], **white blood cell (WBC)** [**leukocyte**], and **platelet** [**thrombocyte**]. Normally, **blood** has about 10 times as many **erythrocytes** as **platelets** and about 30 times as many **platelets** as **leukocytes**.

blood corpuscle: See **blood cell**.

blood flow: **Blood** movement along a **blood vessel**.

blood-flow measurement: The clearance of radioactive xenon from **microcirculation** has long been used as a "gold standard" for the measurement of **blood flow**. A tracer of ^{133}Xe is injected intradermally and its elimination from the **microcirculation** of the **skin** provides a measurement of flow in absolute units, (mL/min/100 g of **tissue**). Also, it is often used to image **blood flow** in the **brain**. Other **invasive** methods have been shown to correlate well to this standard method. For instance, in the heat-clearance method, the **skin** is heated to between 2 and 10 degrees above resting levels. When a plateau is reached, the heat is discontinued and the temperature decay is monitored over time. **Skin**-surface-temperature kinetics is measured noninvasively using **infrared cameras** (radiometers), and **blood-flow** rate is calculated based on the phenomenon that for higher **blood flow**, the heat is dissipated at a greater rate. There are a variety of **noninvasive** optical techniques for **blood-flow measurements** based on **dynamic light scattering** and its variants **quasi-elastic light scattering (QELS)** (single-**scattering** techniques) and **diffusion-wave spectroscopy (DWS)** (multiple-**scattering** techniques) [see **Doppler spectroscopy, laser-Doppler imaging (LDI), laser-speckle-contrast analysis (LASCA), Doppler optical coherence tomography, speckle optical coherence tomography, optical microangiography (OMAG)**].

blood microcirculation: The peripheral **blood** circulation, which is provided by the **capillary** network.

blood perfusion: **Blood** pumping (supplying) through an organ or a **tissue**. It is the product of local speed and concentration of **blood cells**.

blood plasma: The clear, waterlike, colorless liquid of **blood**. **Blood plasma** is formed by removing all **blood corpuscles** from **blood**. **Plasma** can be clotted.

blood smear: A well-prepared **blood smear** is necessary for microscopic examination of **blood**. Smears are used to determine **leukocyte** differentials, to evaluate **erythrocyte, platelet**, and **leukocyte** morphology, and, if necessary, to estimate **platelet** and **leukocyte** counts. To give reproducible evaluations, the sufficient reading area, acceptable morphology within the working area, and an even distribution of **leukocytes** should be provided. The wedge technique for preparation of **blood smears** is often used. This method produces a gradual decrease in thickness of the **blood** from thick to thin ends with the smear placed on the slide. The **blood** film occupies the central portion of the slide and has definite margins on all sides that are accessible to examination by **oil**-immersion **microscopy**. The thin end of the film becomes gradually thinner and does not have grainy streaks, troughs, ridges, waves or holes—features that can result in an uneven distribution of **leukocytes**. In typical preparations, the thin section of the smear occupies approximately one-third of the total area and, within that area, **erythrocytes** are distributed in a monolayer. The thickness of the spread is influenced by the angle of spreader slide (the greater the angle, the thicker and shorter the **blood smear**), the size of the drop of **blood**, and the speed of spreading. Glass coverslips are mounted on all **blood smears** to prevent damage to the smear during examination, cleaning, handling, and storage.

blood vessel: A tube through which **blood** flows to or from the **heart**. A general term for a conducting **vessel** for **blood**, it includes **arteries**, **veins**, **arterioles**, **venules**, and **capillaries**.

blood volume: The total **blood** content within the region of a **tissue**. This includes volumes of both oxygenated and deoxygenated **blood**.

bolometer: Type of thermal detector commonly used in uncooled radiometers.

Boltzmann's constant: The ratio of the universal gas constant to the **Avogadro constant**, equal to 1.3803×10^{-16} erg per $°C$.

bone: A **connective tissue** forming the skeleton. It consists of **cells** embedded in a matrix of **bone** salts and **collagen fibers**. The **bone** salts (mostly calcium carbonate and phosphate, **hydroxyapatite** crystals) form about 60% of the mass of the **bone** and give it its tensile strength. **Bone cells** are interconnected by fine protoplasmic processes situated in narrow channels in the **bone**, and are nourished by the bloodstream. This **vascular** nature of **bone** differentiates it from **cartilage**.

bone marrow: The flexible **tissue** found in the hollow interior of **bones**. In adults, marrow in large **bones** produces new **blood cells**.

It constitutes 4% of total body weight, (i.e., approximately 2.6 kg in average adults).

bone remodeling: All living **bones** are in a dynamic process of growth and resorption via a process called "remodeling," which allows the **bone** to adapt to changing mechanical forces and the body's need for calcium balance.

Born approximation: The single-**scattering** approximation when the field affecting the particle does not essentially differ from that of the initial **wave**. This method is used for the computation of cross sections in **scattering** problems. The interactions are treated as perturbations of free-particle systems.

Bouguer–Beer–Lambert law: Exponential law describing **attenuation** of a **collimated** beam by a thin **absorption** layer with **scattering**. A **collimated** (**laser**) beam is attenuated in a thin-**tissue** layer of thickness d in accordance with this law, $I(d) = I_0 \exp(-\mu_t d)$, where $I(d)$ is the **intensity** of transmitted **light** measured using a distant **photodetector** with a small aperture (on-line or **collimated transmittance**) in W $\cdot$ cm^{-2}. I_0 is the incident **light intensity** in W$\cdot$cm^{-2}. $\mu_t = \mu_a + \mu_s$ is the extinction coefficient (interaction or total **attenuation coefficient**).

boundary conditions: A stated restriction, usually in the form of an equation, that limits the possible solutions to a differential equation.

boundary-element method (BEM): A numerical computational method of solving linear partial-differential equations that have been formulated as integral equations (i.e., in boundary-integral form). The method can be applied in many areas of engineering and science including fluid mechanics, acoustics, electromagnetics, fracture mechanics, and **tissue** optics (in electromagnetics, the more traditional term method of moments is often, though not always, synonymous with **BEM**).

Bragg diffraction: Occurs when **electromagnetic radiation** or subatomic-particle waves with **wavelength** λ comparable to atomic spacings d are incident upon a **crystalline** sample, scattered in a **specular** fashion by the atoms in the system, and undergo **constructive interference** in accordance to **Bragg's law**. A **diffraction** pattern is obtained by measuring the **intensity** of scattered waves as a function of **scattering** angle θ. Very strong intensities known as Bragg peaks are obtained in the **diffraction** pattern when scattered waves satisfy the Bragg condition.

Bragg mirror (reflector): A structure that consists of an alternating sequence of layers of two different optical materials. The most frequently used design is that of a quarter-**wave** mirror, where each optical-layer thickness corresponds to one-quarter of the **wavelength** for which the mirror is designed. The latter condition holds for normal incidence. If the mirror is designed for larger angles of incidence, accordingly thicker layers are needed. Each interface between the two materials contributes a **Fresnel reflection**. For the design **wavelength**, the optical pathlength difference between **reflections** from subsequent interfaces is half the **wavelength**. In addition, the **reflection** coefficients for the interfaces have alternating signs. Therefore all reflected components from the interfaces interfere constructively, which results in a strong **reflection**. The reflectivity achieved is determined by the number of layer pairs and by the refractive-index mismatch between the layer materials. The **reflection bandwidth** is determined mainly by the index **contrast**. Dielectric mirrors based on thin-film-coating technology are used in many types of **lasers**. Fiber Bragg gratings are fabricated by irradiating a **fiber** with spatially patterned UV **light** and are often used in **fiber lasers** and other **fiber** devices. **Semiconductor Bragg mirrors** can be produced with lithographic methods and used in **diode lasers**, particularly in surface-emitting and distributed-feedback **diode lasers**. There are other multilayer mirror designs that deviate from the simple quarter-**wave** design. They generally have a lower reflectivity for the same number of layers, but can be optimized, e.g., as **dichroic mirrors** or as chirped mirrors for **dispersion compensation**.

Bragg's law: Describes **specular scattering** (**diffraction**) of **electromagnetic radiation** or subatomic-particle waves from **crystalline** materials. The law is expressed as $2d \sin \theta = n\lambda$, where d is the atomic spacing (interplanar distance between separated lattice planes), θ is the **scattering** angle, and n is an integer determined by the order given. It describes conditions for the **constructive interference** between the scattered (diffracted) fields.

brain: The coordinating center of the **nervous system**. The human **brain** comprises 2% of body weight but requires 20% of total **oxygen** consumption. The **brain** requires this large amount of **oxygen** to generate sufficient **ATP** by oxidative phosphorylation to maintain and restore ionic gradients.

breast (*Synonym*: female breast): The milk-secreting organ of female mammals, which contains a mammary **gland**.

breathing: Transports **oxygen** into the body and carbon dioxide out of the body. Aerobic organisms require **oxygen** to create **energy** via respiration, in the form of **energy**-rich molecules such as **glucose**.

brightness: An attribute of visual perception in which a source appears to emit a given amount of **light**. In other words, **brightness** is the perception elicited by the **luminance** of a visual target. **Brightness** is a subjective attribute/property of an object being observed.

Brillouin–Mandelshtam scattering (BMS): Occurs when **light** in a medium (such as **water** or a crystal) interacts with time-dependent **optical-density** variations and changes its **energy** (**frequency**) and path. The density variations may be due to acoustic modes (such as **phonons**), magnetic modes (such as magnons), or temperature gradients. In optics, when the medium is compressed its **index of refraction** changes and the light's path necessarily **bends**. BMS represents an inelastic-**scattering**

process of **light** with quasi-particles and measures properties such as the elastic behavior on a larger scale. Experimentally, the **frequency** shifts in **BMS** are detected with an **interferometer**.

Brownian motion: The irregular motion of particles in a medium, caused by molecules of the medium bombarding these particles.

Brownian particles: Small particles suspended in a liquid or a gas that undergo irregular motion caused by molecules of the medium bombarding the particles.

B-scan: See **A-scan-based B-scan**.

burn: A type of **injury** to the **skin** caused by heat, cold, electricity, chemicals, or **radiation** (e.g., a sunburn).

burn scar: There are three major types of **burn**-related **scars**: keloid, hypertrophic, and contractures. Keloid **scars** are an overgrowth of **scar tissue**, the **scar** will grow beyond the site of the **injury**. These **scars** are generally red or pink and will become a dark tan over time. Hypertrophic **scars** are red, thick, and raised, however, they differ from **keloid scars** in that they do not develop beyond the site of **injury** or **incision**. A contracture **scar** is a permanent tightening of **skin** that may affect the underlying **muscles** and **tendons**, which may limit mobility and cause possible damage or degeneration of the **nerves**.

burst noise: A noise that consists of sudden steplike transitions between two or more levels (non-**Gaussian statistics**), as high as several hundred millivolts, at random and unpredictable times. Each shift in offset voltage or current lasts for several **milliseconds**, and the intervals between pulses tend to be in the audio range (less than 100 Hz), leading to the term "popcorn noise" for the popping or crackling sounds it produces in audio circuits.

butanediol: 1, 4-**butanediol** ($C_4H_{10}O_2$) is an **alcohol** derivative of the alkane butane, carrying two hydroxyl groups. It is a colorless, viscous liquid. Molecular mass of 90.12 g/mol. Its Melting point is 20 °C, and its boiling point is 230 °C. It is used as an **optical clearing agent** for **tissues**.

butilene glycol: 1, 3-**butilene glycol** is used in **cosmetics**: it gives rigidity and gloss to lipsticks, it retains fragrance on the **skin**, and it provides better smoothness, elasticity, and gloss to **hair**. It also prevents loss of moisture and/or **gain** of moisture. The substance is very safe and nonirritating—it has lower oral toxicity than other glycols/glycerin, and it has the approval of the **Food and Drug Administration (FDA)** and Food Chemical Codex III. Butilene glycol provides more inhibition of microorganisms than other glycols. Its boiling point is 207.5 °C, and it has neutral **pH**.

byte: A unit of digital information, a **byte** is an ordered collection of **bits**. The size of a **byte** is typically hardware dependent, but the modern standard is 8 **bits**, as this is a convenient **power** of 2. Most of the numeric values used by many applications are representable in 8 **bits**: 1 **byte** = 8 **bits**, 1 kilobyte (KB) = 2^{10} **bytes** = 1, 024 **bytes**, 1 megabyte (MB) = 2^{20} **bytes** = 1, 048, 576 **bytes**, 1 gigabyte (GB) = 2^{30} **bytes** = 1, 073, 741, 824 **bytes**, 1 terabyte (TB) = 2^{40} **bytes** = 1, 099, 511, 627, 776 **bytes**, 1 petabyte (PB) = 2^{50} **bytes** = 1, 125, 899, 906, 842, 624 **bytes**. Signal-processing applications tend to operate on larger values and some digital-signal processors have 16 or 40 **bits** as the smallest unit of addressable storage (on such processors a "**byte**" may be defined to contain this number of **bits**).

caecum: See **cecum**.

calcification: The deposition of lime or insoluble salts of calcium and magnesium in a **tissue**.

calcium fluoride: CaF_2, an insoluble ionic compound of calcium and fluorine, occurs naturally as the mineral fluorite (also called fluorspar).

calf: The fleshy area located on the lower part of the back of a human leg.

calibration: Checking and/or adjusting an instrument such that its readings agree with a standard. **Calibration** removes systematic instrument error and quantifies the instrument random error.

calibration accuracy: The **accuracy of measurement** to which a **calibration** is performed. It is usually based on the accuracy and sensitivity of the instruments and references being used in the **calibration**.

calibration check: A routine check of an instrument against a reference to ensure that the instrument has not deviated from **calibration** since its last use.

cancer: A general term applied to a **carcinoma** or a **sarcoma**. The typical symptoms are a **tumor** or swelling, a discharge, a **pain**, an upset in the function of an organ, a general weakness, and a loss of weight.

cancerous: Related to **cancer** conditions.

candela: A measure of a photometric quantity, luminous **intensity**. **Candela** (cd) is a number of **lumens** per steradian (lm/sr).

canine: A dog or any animal of the *Canidae*, or dog family, including wolves, jackals, hyenas, coyotes, and foxes.

capillary: A minute hairlike tube (diameter about 5–20 μm) with a wall consisting of a single layer of flattened **cells** (**endothelium**). The wall is permeable to substances such as **water**, **oxygen**, **glucose**, **amino acids**, carbon dioxide, and to inorganic ions. The **capillaries** form a network in all **tissues**. They are supplied with oxygenated **blood** by **arterioles** and pass deoxygenated **blood** to venules. Their function is the exchange of dissolved substances between **blood** and **tissue** fluid.

capsular: Pertaining to a capsule, a membranous sac or integument.

carbamide: See **urea**.

carbohydrate: Simple molecules that are straight-chain aldehydes or ketones with many hydroxyl groups added, usually one on each carbon atom that is not part of the aldehyde or ketone functional group. **Carbohydrates** are the most abundant biological molecules, and serve numerous functions in living things, such as the storage and transport of **energy** (starch, **glycogen**) and structural components (cellulose in plants, chitin in animals). Additionally, **carbohydrates** and their derivatives play major roles in the functioning of the immune system, fertilization, pathogenesis, **blood** clotting, and development. The basic **carbohydrate** units are called monosaccharides, such as **glucose**, galactose, and fructose. The general chemical formula of an unmodified monosaccharide is $(C \cdot H_2O)n$, where n is any number of 3 or greater.

carbon-dioxide (CO_2) laser: A **carbon-dioxide laser** is an **infrared** carbon-dioxide molecular **laser** in which the lasing medium is CO_2 gas with an IR emission from 9.2 to 11.1 μm, the maximal efficiency at 10.6 μm, and a **power** from a few watts to a few kilowatts. Both **continuous-wave** and pulsed regimes are available. **Lasers** are tunable in the limits of the CO_2 molecule spectral range (from 9.2 to 11.1 μm). Because of a high **absorption** of **tissues** in this **wavelength** range, **CO_2 lasers** are mostly used for **tissue ablation**.

carbon-monoxide (CO) laser: A carbon-monoxide laser is an **infrared** carbon monoxide molecular **laser** in which the lasing medium is CO gas with an IR emission from 5 to 6.5 μm with a **power** up to 100 W in **continuous-wave** mode. These **lasers** are tunable in the limits of CO molecule spectral range (from

5–6.5 μm). Because of a high **absorption** of **tissues** in this **wavelength** range, **CO lasers** are mostly used for **tissue ablation**.

carbon nanoparticle: Particles made of carbon with dimensions on the order of billionths of a meter. They have different physical, chemical, electrical, and optical properties than occur in bulk samples, due in part to the increased surface-area-to-volume ratio at the nanoscale. Carbon black is a form of amorphous carbon that has an extremely high surface-area-to-volume ratio, and as such it is one of the first nanomaterials to find common use. Little is known about interaction of **carbon nanoparticles** with human **cells**.

carbon nanotube (CNT): Typical hollow single-walled **carbon nanotubes** used in biomedical-related studies that are around 170-nm long and 1.7 nm in diameter, and have a monotonically decreased **absorption** with increases in the **wavelength**. To provide high **plasmon absorption** in the **near-infrared** range of 850 nm, they can be covered by a thin gold layer. Such carbon–**gold nanoparticles** exhibit high **water** solubility and biocompatibility, low cytotoxicity (due to the protective layer of inert gold around the carbon), and the average dimensions of the particles are around 92 nm in length and 13 nm in diameter. Functionalized particles are used as labels for optoacoustic detection and **ablation** of nonpigmented **breast-cancer cells** in **sentinel lymph nodes**.

carbonyl: A **carbonyl** group is a functional group composed of a carbon atom double-bonded to an **oxygen** atom: C=O.

carboxyhemoglobin (COHb): A stable complex of carbon monoxide and **hemoglobin** that forms in **red blood cells** when carbon monoxide is inhaled or produced in normal **metabolism**. Large quantities will hinder delivery of **oxygen** to the body. Tobacco smoking raises the **blood** levels of COHb by a factor of several times from its normal concentrations. It is bright, cherry red in **color**.

carcinoma *Synonym*: carcinoma *in situ* (CIS): A **malignant** growth of abnormal **epithelial cells**.

cardiovibration (*Synonym*: heartbeat): The rhythmic vibrations and sound of the **heart** pumping **blood**. It has a double beat caused by the sound of ventricles contracting, followed by a shorter, sharper sound of the semilunar valves closing. The atria do not contribute to the sound of the beat.

caries: Dental **caries** is a multifunctional disease. The presence of **dental plaque biofilm**, which contains **bacteria** that are both acid-producing and survive at low **pH** (*Streptococcus mutans* are believed to be the most important **bacteria** in the initiation and progress of dental **caries**), and the availability of **glucose**, which drives bacterial **metabolism** to produce **lactic acid**, influences its progression. Generally **caries** is initiated in the **enamel**, but it may also begin in **dentin** or **cementum**. When acid challenges occur repeatedly, the eventual **collapse** of enough **enamel** crystals (**demineralization**) will result in **cavitation**. Three major factors determine susceptibility of a **tooth** to **caries**, and the interplay of these factors over time is a key in the process: (1) **tooth** morphologic features that allow plaque retention, i.e., presence of pits and **fissures**, interproximal areas, and structural integrity, i.e., how well the **tooth** is mineralized; (2) presence of cariogenic **bacteria**, e.g., *Streptococcus mutans* and *lactobacilli*; (3) presence of food substrate for **bacteria** such as simple **carbohydrates** (**sucrose** and/or **glucose**). Cariogenic **bacteria** are able to produce acid rapidly, thrive under acidic conditions, adhere well to the **tooth** surface, and synthesize sticky **extracellular** polysaccarides. Acid may change local **pH** from 7 (normal) to below 5 within a few minutes of **bacteria** being exposed to food substrate. It can take up to 1 hour for **pH** to get back to 7. Acid slowly diffuses out of plaque, and in spite of buffering in plaque and **saliva**, acid action is not totally neutralized. Frequent and repeated consumption of simple sugars (e.g., soft drinks) will result in the persistence of acid and **tooth demineralization**. Types of **caries** include (1) pit and **fissure** (chewing surface), (2) smooth surface (e.g., **tooth** proximal/interproximal), (3) root

(root surface, in older adults where **gums** have receded, exposing the **cementum** to oral environment), and (4) secondary/recurrent (adjacent to existing restoration). White-spot **lesion** is the earliest **visible** evidence of **enamel caries**, it looks white, opaque (sometimes brown due to **absorption** of **exogenous** material), and/or colored due to increased **porosity** of **enamel** (from mineral loss). Microscopically, it appears as a cone-shaped **lesion**. Surface **enamel** can appear relatively unaffected with subsurface layers showing more mineral loss. **Enamel** remains hard to clinical exam (no appreciable cavity). Decay can be arrested at this early stage and may be partially repaired if intervention (plaque removal, diet modification, fluoride) is done in time. If the **lesion** progresses, clinically apparent **tissue** breakdown and **cavitation** will be seen. Once **cavitation** occurs, the **lesion** can progress faster as plaque can grow relatively undisturbed in cavity. The lesion can move through **enamel** and spread laterally along the dentinoenamel junction into the softer **dentin**. If the decay is not removed, further progression into **pulp** will result. Subject will perceive **pain** once decay reaches **dentin**, and bacterial toxins can travel down dentinal tubules to **pulp**.

carotid: In human anatomy, the common **carotid artery** is an **artery** that supplies the **head** and **neck**. It divides in the **neck** to form the external and internal **carotid arteries**.

carpal-tunnel syndrome (CTS): An entrapment neuropathy of the median **nerve** at the **wrist**, leading to paresthesia, numbness, and **muscle** weakness in the **hand**. It is one of the most common peripheral-**nerve** disorders. Most cases of **carpal-tunnel syndrome** are idiopathic (without known cause), although genetic factors determine most of the risk. The role of **arm** use and other environmental factors is disputed.

cartilage: A strong, resilient, skeletal **tissue**. The simplest and most common form consists of a matrix of a **polysaccharide**-containing **protein** with embedded **cartilage cells** (chondroblasts). The matrix is without structure and without **blood vessels**.

The type known as hyaline **cartilage** is translucent and clear, and occurs in the cartilaginous rings of the **trachea** and bronchi. Elastic **cartilage** (yellow fibrocartilage) contains **yellow fibers** in the matrix. It occurs in the external **ear** and in the epiglottis. White fibrocartilage contains **white fibers** in the matrix and occurs in the disks of **cartilage** between the vertebrae. All types of **cartilage** contain chondroblasts, which deposit in the matrix and become enclosed in the matrix as chondrocytes.

catabolism: The decomposition of chemical substances within an organism. The substances are usually complex organic substances, and the products are simpler organic substances. The process is usually accompanied by a release of **energy** (see **metabolism**).

cataract: An abnormality of the eye characterized by opacity of the **crystalline lens**.

cataractogenesis: The process of **cataract** formation.

cathode: A negative electrode toward which cations (positive ions) move in electrolysis.

cationic: Relating to cations, positively charged ions.

Caucasian skin: White-colored **skin**.

Cauchy's equation: Related to material **dispersion**, it describes the empirical relationship between the **refractive index** n and **wavelength** of **light** λ for a particular transparent material, including **tissue**. The most general form of **Cauchy's equation** is $n = A + B\lambda^{-2} + C\lambda^{-4}\ldots$. For example, refractive-index measurements for fresh animal **tissues** and human **blood** at room temperature and four **laser wavelengths** 488, 632.8, 1079.5, and 1341.4 nm can be presented in a form of a Cauchy **dispersion** equation with λ in **nanometers** as the values of the Cauchy coefficients. For example, as $A = 1.4753, B = 4390.2, C = 923.85 \times 10^6$ (for porcine adipose **tissue**), and $A = 1.3587, B =$

58

1474.4, $C = 1710.3 \times 10^6$ (for human **whole blood**). The empirical equation for human-**blood plasma** valid in the spectral range from 400–1000 nm is $n_{bp}(\lambda) = 1.3254 + 8.4052 \times 10^3 \lambda^{-2} - 3.9572 \times 10^8 \lambda^{-4} - 2.3617 \times 10^{13} \lambda^{-6}$. In general, **Cauchy's equation** is only valid for regions of normal **dispersion** in the **visible wavelength** region. In the **infrared**, the equation becomes inaccurate, and it cannot represent regions of anomalous **dispersion**. The **Sellmeier equation** accounts for anomalous **light-dispersion** regions, and more accurately models material **refractive index** across the **UV**, **visible**, and **IR spectrum**.

cavernous hemangioma: See **port wine stain**.

cavitation: General term used to describe the behavior of voids or bubbles in a liquid.

cavity-dumped mode-locked laser: Laser that uses a specific technology for producing high-**energy ultrashort laser pulses** by decreasing the pulse-repetition rate (see **mode-locked laser**). The **laser**-output mirror is replaced by an optical selector consisting of a couple of spherical mirrors and an acousto- or electro-optical deflector, which extracts a pulse from the cavity after it has passed over a few dozen cavity lengths. The pulse **energy** is accumulated between two sequential extractions: Pulse-repetition rate can be tuned in the range from dozens of hertz to a few megahertz.

cecum (*Synonym*: caecum): A pouch that connects the **ileum** with the ascending **colon** of the **large intestine**. It is separated from the **ileum** by the ileocecal **valve** (ICV) or Bauhin's **valve** and from the **colon** by the cecocolic junction.

cell: See **biological cell**.

cell culture: The complex process by which **cells** are grown under controlled conditions. Based on the concept of maintaining live **cell** lines separated from their original **tissue** source. In practice the term **cell culture** has come to refer to the culturing of **cells**

derived from multicellular **eukaryotes**, especially animal **cells**. Animal-**cell culture** is a common laboratory technique used since the mid-twentieth century.

cell fixation: Killing, making rigid, and preserving a **cell** for microscopic study.

cell membrane: The thin, limiting covering of a **cell** or **cell** part. It regulates the ingress of substances into a **cell** or its parts and may have some other functions that depend on the cell's specialization.

cell-adhesion molecules (CAMs): Proteins located on the **cell** surface that allow their binding to other **cells** or to the **extracellular matrix** in the process called **cellular adhesion**. These **proteins** are typically transmembrane receptors and are composed of three domains: An intracellular domain that interacts with the **cytoskeleton**, a transmembrane domain, and an **extracellular** domain that interacts either with other **cell-adhesion** molecules of the same kind (homophilic binding), with other **cell-adhesion** molecules, or with the **extracellular matrix** (heterophilic binding).

cellular adhesion: The binding of a **cell** to a surface, **extracellular matrix**, or another **cell** using **cell-adhesion** molecules such as selectins, integrins, and cadherins. **Cell-adhesion molecules** involved in the process are first hydrolyzed by **extracellular enzymes**. **Cell adhesion** is directly related to **protein absorption** [see **cell-adhesion molecules (CAMs)**].

cellular organelle: Part of a **cell** that is a structural and functional unit, e.g., a flagellum is a locomotive organelle, a **mitochondrion** is a respiratory organelle. Organelles in a **cell** correspond to organs in an organism.

cellulitis: Considered a disease of the **subcutaneous-fat** layer and appearing mostly in women, it consists of changes in **fat-cell** accumulation along with disturbed lymphatic drainage, affecting the external appearance of the **skin**. Changes are observed in the fibrotic septae between **fat cells** and in a reduction of the metabolic rate, causing the congested **tissue** to affect the external aspect of **skin**. **Skin** surface will appear bumpy and uneven. **Cellulitis** results from a chronic lymphokinesis malfunction, **blood** circulation in **capillaries** of a fatty layer, and fibrosis (incorrectly generated **connective tissue**). At a **cellulitis**, the expanded **fatty cells** impede **blood** circulation, and a **collagen** mesh tries to prevent **water** deducing. The changes in dermal structure in cellulite-affected areas are quite apparent. There are projections of **subcutaneous fat** into the reticular and papillary **dermis**. An increased value of dermal **glycosaminoglycans** in cellulite-affected areas suggests greater **water** binding in these regions. Activity within the **subcutaneous tissues** plays an obvious role in the generation of cellulite.

Celsius temperature scale (centigrade): Temperature scale based on 0 °C as the freezing point of **water** and 100 °C as the boiling point of **water** at standard atmospheric **pressure**. A relative scale related to the Kelvin scale [0 °C = 273.12 K. 1 C° (ΔT) = 1 K (ΔT)].

cementoblasts: **Cells** that form **tooth**-root **cementum**.

cementum: Thin, pale-yellow, calcified, bonelike layer covering root of **tooth**. It contains 45% **hydroxyapatite**, 55% **protein** (**collagen**), and **water**. It is softer than both **dentin** and **bone**. Functions include coverage of the **dentin** tubules and insertion point of **periodontal ligament fibers**. Has ability to develop **cementoblasts** throughout life of **tooth**, which form **cementum** that lie along root surface in the **periodontal ligament** space. Relative softness of **cementum**, as well as its thinness, renders it vulnerable to easy abrasion once it is exposed to the **oral cavity** (see **gingival** recession).

central nervous system (CNS): In vertebrates (such as humans), it contains the **brain, spinal cord**, and **retina**.

centriole: In biology, a barrel-shaped microtubule structure found in most animal **cells**. The walls of each **centriole** are usually composed of nine triplets of **microtubules**. An associated pair of **centrioles**, spatially arranged at right angles, constitutes the compound structure known to **cell** biologists as the centrosome. **Centrioles** are very important in the **cell**-division process.

cerebellum: A region of the **brain** that plays an important role in the integration of sensory perception and motor output. Many neural pathways link the **cerebellum** with the motor **cortex**, which sends information to the **muscles** causing them to move, and to the spinocerebellar tract, which provides feedback on the position of the body in space. The **cerebellum** integrates these pathways, using the constant feedback on body position to fine-tune motor movements.

cerebral cortex: See **cortex**.

cerebral lobe: See **lobe**.

cerebrospinal fluid (CSF): Clear liquid that fills the cavities of the **brain** and **spinal cord** and the spaces between the arachnoid and *pia mater*. The fluid moves in a slow current down the central canal and up the spinal meninges. It is a solution of **blood** solutes of low **molar mass**, such as **glucose** and sodium chloride, but not of the same concentration as in the **blood**. The fluid contains little or no **protein** and very few **cells**. Its function is to nourish the **nervous tissue** and to act as a buffer against **shock** to the **nervous tissue**. The total quantity of **cerebrospinal fluid** in humans is about 100 cm^3.

cervical cancer: A **malignant tumor** of the **cervix** uteri, e.g., a **cervical intraepithelial neoplasia**. **Cervical intraepithelial neoplasia** I and **cervical intraepithelial neoplasia** II are **precancerous**. **Cervical intraepithelial neoplasia** III stage corresponds to **carcinoma** *in situ* (CIS). The next stage is an **invasive cancer**.

cervical intraepithelial neoplasia (CIN): Cervical intraepithelial neoplasia I and **cervical intraepithelial neoplasia** II are **precancerous**, and correspond to slight and moderate displasia. **Cervical intraepithelial neoplasia** III stage corresponds to marked displasia or **carcinoma *in situ*** (CIS).

cervical smear: Thin specimen of the cytologic material taken from the female cervical channel. It is usually received as a smear on a glass plate and is fixed and stained before being examined.

cervical tissue: Multilayered **tissue** consisting of the upper-**epithelial cell** layer, basal layer (basal **membrane**), and **stromal layer**. Depending on the area of the **cervix**, the **epithelium** may be in one of two forms: squamous or columnar.

cervix: A short tube leading from the vagina to the **uterus**.

C–H group: As the simplest diatomic (linear) structure, the carbon-hydrogen functional molecular group has only one bond, which provides a stretching **vibrational mode**.

chalcogenide glass: Glass containing elements of group VI of the periodic table. It is transparent to **infrared light** and used to produce **infrared fibers** to transport **infrared laser beams**.

characteristic diffusion time: The reciprocal of the **diffusion coefficient** D_a of an agent diffusing in a **tissue** and characterizing the time interval of increase of applied agent concentration in a sample of ≈ 0.6 of concentration of this agent in the surrounding medium. When an agent is administrated through only one surface, which is typical for *in vivo* **topical**-agent application, the **characteristic-diffusion time**, $\tau = d^2/D_a$, where d is the thickness of the **tissue** layer of interest.

charge-coupled device (CCD): A solid-state-array electronic device that serves as an imaging chip and is used in digital photographic and video cameras, digital microscopes, and fast spectrometers for medical use. See also **back-illuminated charge-coupled device (CCD)**, **cooled charge-coupled device (CCD)**, **frame-transfer charge-coupled device (CCD)**, and **intensified charge-coupled device (ICCD)**.

chemical potential: In thermodynamics, the amount by which the **energy** of the system would change if an additional particle were introduced, with the **entropy** and volume held fixed. If a system contains more than one species of particle, there is a separate **chemical potential** associated with each species, defined as the change in **energy** when the number of particles of that species is increased by one. The **chemical potential** is a fundamental parameter in thermodynamics, and it is conjugate to the particle number.

chemiluminescence: A kind of **luminescence** or **bioluminescence** where the emission of **light** results from a chemical reaction without emission of heat.

chemotherapy: In its most general sense, the treatment of disease by chemicals, especially by killing microorganisms or **cancerous cells**. The term often refers to antineoplastic drugs used to treat **cancer** or the combination of these drugs into a cytotoxic standardized-treatment regimen. Most commonly, **chemotherapy** acts by killing **cells** presenting a high degree of **proliferation**, a main property of most **cancer cells**. This means that the treatment also harms **cells** that divide rapidly under normal circumstances, such as **cells** in the **bone marrow**, digestive tract, and **hair follicles**. The most common side effects of **chemotherapy** include myelosuppression (decreased production of **blood cells**), mucositis (**inflammation** of the lining of the **digestive tract**), and alopecia (**hair** loss). Newer anticancer drugs act directly against abnormal **proteins** in **cancer cells** and thus have fewer side effects—this is termed targeted therapy. In its non-oncological use, the term may also refer to **antibiotics** (antibacterial **chemotherapy**). Other uses of cytostatic-**chemotherapy** agents are the treatment of autoimmune diseases such as multiple sclerosis, **erythematosus lupus**, **rheumatoid arthritis**, and the suppression of transplant rejections.

chest: The part of the trunk between the **neck** and the abdomen, containing the cavity, and enclosed by the ribs, sternum, and certain vertebrae, in which the **heart**, **lungs**, etc., are situated.

chirality: In an object, describes the mirror-equal "right" or "left" modification. **Optical activity** is one of the exhibitions of **chirality**, when the asymmetric structure of a molecule or crystal existing of two forms ("right" and "left") causes the substance (ensemble of these molecules or crystal) to rotate the plane of **polarization** of the incident linearly **polarized light**: pure "right" or "left" optically active substances have identical physical and chemical properties, but their biochemical and physiological properties can be quite different.

cholesterol: A sterol (a combination steroid and **alcohol**) and a **lipid** found in the **cell membranes** of all body **tissues**, and transported in the **blood plasma** of all animals.

choroid: The membraneous, pigmented middle layer of the **eyeball** between the **sclera** and the **retina**. It contains numerous **blood vessels**. Its function is to absorb **light** to prevent **internal reflection** in the **eyeball** and to provide nourishment for the **retina**. The **choroid** is continuous with the **iris** in the front of the eye.

chroma: Refers to the perceived **intensity** of a specific **color**—a related but distinct concept from **colorfulness** and saturation. The **colorfulness** is relative to the **brightness** of another **color**, which appears white under similar viewing conditions.

chromatic aberration: The variation of either the **focal length** or the magnification of a **lens** system of different **wavelengths** of **light**. It is characterized by prismatic coloring at the edges of the optical image and **color** distortion within it.

chromatic dispersion: Used to emphasize **wavelength**-dependent nature of **light dispersion**. For example, both material **dispersion** and **waveguide dispersion** in **fibers** belong to **chromatic dispersion** because both are **wavelength** dependent. See also **dispersion**.

chromaticity coordinates: In the study of the perception of **color**, one of the first mathematically defined **color** spaces was the **CIE XYZ color** space (also known as **CIE** 1931 **color** space), created by the International Commission on Illumination (**Commission Internationale de l'Éclairage**) in 1931. The human eye has receptors for short (S), middle (M), and long (L) **wavelengths**, also known as blue, green, and red receptors. That means that one, in principle, needs three parameters to describe a **color** sensation. A specific method for associating three numbers (or tristimulus values) with each **color** is called a **color** space: **CIE** XYZ **color** space is one of many such spaces. However, the **CIE** XYZ **color** space is special because it is based on direct measurements of the human eye, and it serves as the basis from which many other **color** spaces are defined. The **CIE** 1964 standard observer is based on the mean 10-deg **color**-matching functions.

chromatin: The complex of **DNA** and **protein** found inside the nuclei of eukaryotic **cells**. The **nucleic acids** are in the form of double-stranded **DNA** (a double **helix**). The major **proteins** involved in **chromatin** are histone **proteins**, although many other chromosomal **proteins** have prominent roles too. Functions of **chromatin** are to package **DNA** into a smaller volume to fit in the **cell**, to strengthen the **DNA** to allow **mitosis** and **meiosis**, and to serve as a mechanism to control expression.

chromatin filament: Condensed **chromatin fibers** of 30 nm consisting of nucleosome arrays in their most-compact form.

chromophore: A molecule (or part of a molecule) where the **energy** difference between electrons in two different molecular orbitals falls within the **energy** possesed by **photons**

in the **visible/near-infrared spectrum**. It absorbs **light** with a characteristic spectral pattern. There are many kinds of **chromophores** in **tissues**; however, a few major **chromophores** predominantly determine, for example, the optical **absorption** within each **skin** layer. **Proteins** found in the **epidermis** contain the aromatic **amino acids tryptophan** and **tyrosine**, which have a characteristic **absorption band** near 270–280 nm. **Urocanic acid** and the **nucleic acids** also contribute to this **absorption band** with a maximum near 260–270 nm. Epidermal **melanin** plays an important role in limiting the **penetration depth** of **light** in the **skin**, effectively absorbing at all **wavelengths** from 300 to 1000 nm. But the strongest **absorption** occurs at shorter **wavelengths**, in the near-UV spectral range. Some of the major dermal **chromophores** are **oxyhemoglobin**, **deoxyhemoglobin**, **bilirubin**, carotenoids, and **porphyrins**. In the **infrared** spectral range, the **tissue-absorption spectrum** is essentially determined by the **absorption** of **water** and **lipids**.

chromophore-assisted light inactivation (CALI): A targeted inactivation of **proteins** to generate a **protein** loss of function at the time of **light** excitation. Light **energy** is targeted to destroy a **protein** of interest by binding it with a specific **antibody** labeled with the **chromophore malachite green**. Short-lived **free radicals** are generated when the dye is excited by **laser light** at 620 nm, a **wavelength** not well-absorbed by cellular components, resulting in photochemical damage to the bound **antigen** with minimal collateral damage to nearest neighbors. The technique has been useful in ascribing *in situ* function of a large number of **proteins** in **cells** and **embryos**. For example, it was applied to address the *in vivo* role of a **cell-adhesion molecule**, **Fasciclin I**, in the stereotyped **axon** growth of pioneer **neurons** during grasshopper limb development. **Chromophore-assisted light inactivation** has generated a number of related technologies based on different **chromophores**, localization strategies, and molecular-encoded **photosensitizers**, e.g., **fluorophore-assisted light inactivation**. Some technologies use the expression of a tetracysteine domain that can bind tightly to the **chromophore** DS Red. Its efficiency in **chromophore**-assisted **light**-inactivation-mediated damage and the **power** of molecular **genetics** by expressing the encoded binding domain are the major advantages. The novel, molecularly encoded **photosensitizer KillerRed** has high **efficacy** and has been used for both targeted phototoxicity and **chromophore-assisted light inactivation**. Other **photosensitizers**, such as **ruthenium red** and **gold nanoparticles**, are in use, and novel means of targeting the damage have been developed, including small-molecule binders and **RNA aptamers**.

chromosome: An organized structure of **DNA** and **proteins** found in **cells**. It is a single piece of coiled **DNA** containing many **genes**, regulatory elements, and other **nucleotide** sequences. **DNA**-bound **proteins** serve to package the **DNA** and control its functions. **Chromosomes** vary widely between different organisms. The **DNA** molecule may be circular or linear, and can be composed of 10^4 to 10^9 **nucleotides** in a long chain. Typically, **eukaryotes** have large, linear **chromosomes** and **prokaryotes** have smaller, circular **chromosomes**. **Cells** may contain more than one type of **chromosome**. For example, **mitochondria** in most **eukaryotes** have their own small **chromosomes**. In **eukaryotes**, nuclear **chromosomes** are packaged by **proteins** into a condensed structure called **chromatin**, which allows the very long **DNA** molecules to fit into the **cell nucleus**. The structure of **chromosomes** and **chromatin** varies through the **cell** cycle. **Chromosomes** are the essential unit for cellular division and must be replicated, divided, and passed successfully to their daughter **cells** so as to ensure the genetic diversity and survival of their progeny. Compaction of the duplicated **chromosomes** during **mitosis** and **meiosis** results in the classic four-arm structure. Chromosomal recombination plays a vital role in genetic diversity. If these structures are manipulated incorrectly, through processes known as chromosomal instability and translocation, the **cell** may undergo mitotic catastrophe and die, or it may aberrantly evade **apoptosis**, leading to the progression of **cancer**.

chyme: The semifluid mass of partly digested food expelled by the **stomach** into the **duodenum**.

cicatrix: New **tissue** that forms over a **wound** and later contracts into a **scar**.

cilia: A cilium is an organelle found in **eukaryotes**. Cilia are slender protuberances that project from the much larger **cell** body. There are two types of **cilia**: motile **cilia** and nonmotile (or primary) **cilia**, which typically serve as sensory organelles. Eukaryotic **cilia** are structurally identical to eukaryotic flagella, although distinctions are sometimes made according to function and/or length. In humans, primary **cilia** are found on nearly every **cell** in the body. Motile **cilia** are usually present on a cell's surface in large numbers and beat in coordinated waves. In humans, motile **cilia** are found in the lining of the **trachea**, where they sweep **mucus** and dirt out of the **lungs**. In female mammals, the beating of **cilia** in the fallopian tubes moves the ovum from the ovary to the **uterus**. In comparison to motile **cilia**, nonmotile **cilia** usually occur at the rate of one per **cell**. Nearly all mammalian **cells** have a single nonmotile primary cilium. Examples of specialized primary **cilia** can be found in human-sensory organs such as the eye and the nose. The outer segment of the rod photoreceptor **cell** in the human eye is connected to its **cell** body with a specialized nonmotile cilium. **Cilia** are important in **cell** functioning, and their physiological roles in chemical sensation, signal transduction, and control of **cell** growth are well established. The dysgenesis and **dysfunction** of **cilia** may lead to polycystic **kidney** disease, congenital **heart** disease, and some others.

ciliary body: A thickened circular structure at the edge of the **choroid** and at the border of the **cornea**. The **iris** and the suspensory **ligaments** are attached to it. It contains the **ciliary muscle** used in accommodation, and it secretes **aqueous humor**.

ciliary muscle: A smooth **muscle** that affects zonular **fibers** in the eye (**fibers** that suspend the **lens** in position during accommodation), enabling changes in **lens** shape for **light** focusing.

ciliary pigmented epithelium: Darkly colored **melanin-pigmented epithelial cell** layer of a **ciliary body**.

clinical trial (*Related terms*: clinical studies, research protocols, medical research): The application of the scientific method to human health. Researchers use **clinical trials** to test hypotheses about the effect of a particular intervention upon a **pathological** disease condition. Well-run **clinical trials** use defined techniques and rigorous definitions to answer researchers' questions as accurately as possible. The most common **clinical trials** evaluate new drugs, medical devices, biologics, or other interventions on patients in strictly scientifically controlled settings. **Clinical trials** are required for regulatory-authority approval of new therapies. Trials may be designed to assess the safety and **efficacy** of an experimental therapy, to assess whether the new intervention is better than standard therapy, or to compare the **efficacy** of two standard or marketed interventions. The trial **objectives** and design are usually documented in a clinical-trial protocol.

clock frequency: In electronics and especially in synchronous digital circuits, a signal used to coordinate the actions of two or more circuits. For example, the clock rate (**frequency**) of a computer **central processing unit** is normally determined by the **frequency** of an oscillator crystal.

C-mount: Type of **lens** mount commonly found on 16-mm movie cameras, closed-circuit television cameras, and trinocular-microscope phototubes. The letter "C" is said to stand for "cine," the original application being movie-camera **lenses**. The flange focal distance is 17.526 mm (0.6900 in.) for a **C-mount**. A **C-mount** adapter is used to connect **charge-coupled device (CCD)/complemantary metal-oxide semiconductor (CMOS) cameras** with trinocular microscopes. The CS-mount has a flange focal distance of 12.52 mm (0.493 in.), but is otherwise identical to the **C-mount**. Modern cameras and **lenses** are generally CS-mount rather than **C-mount**. With CS-mount cameras, both types of **lenses** can be used, but the **C-mount lens** requires a 5-mm ring

(VM400) to be fitted between the camera and **lens** to achieve a focused image.

coagulation: To cause particles (components) to collect together in a compact mass, e.g., the **coagulation** (**denaturation**) of egg white is brought about by heat. Denaturation of cellular and **tissue proteins** is the basis for thermal damage and **tissue laser welding**.

coenzyme: Small organic nonprotein molecules that carry chemical groups between **enzymes**. Many **coenzymes** are phosphorylated **water**-soluble vitamins; however, nonvitamins may also be **coenzymes**, such as **adenosine triphosphate (ATP)**. **Coenzymes** are consumed in the reactions in which they are substrates. For example, the **coenzyme** nicotinamide adenine dinucleotide is converted to **NAD+** by oxidoreductases. **Coenzymes** are, however, regenerated and their concentration maintained at a steady level in the **cell**.

coherence length: Characterizes the degree of temporal coherence of **light** emitted by a **light** source. $l_c = c\tau_c$, where c is the **speed of light** and τ_c is the **coherence time**, which is approximately equal to the pulse duration of the pulsed-**light** source or inversely proportional to the **wavelength bandwidth** $\Delta\lambda$ of a continuous-**wave light** source, $\tau_c \sim \lambda^2/(c\Delta\lambda)$. A **laser** with a narrow **bandwidth** $\Delta\lambda = 10^{-4}$ nm and **wavelength** $\lambda = 800$ nm has a **coherence length** $l_c \approx 6.4$ m. A **multimode diode laser** with $\Delta\lambda = 30$ nm and $\lambda = 830$ nm has $l_c \approx +23$ μm. For a **titanium–sapphire laser** with $\lambda = 820$ nm, the **bandwidth** may be as big as 140 nm, therefore the **coherence length** is very short: $l_c \approx 2$ μm. The shortest $l_c \approx 0.9$ μm is for a white-**light** source ($\Delta\lambda = 400$ nm). **Coherence length** is a fundamental parameter for **optical coherence tomography**, the smaller l_c, the better image resolution could be achieved. Optical coherence tomography systems based on a **titanium–sapphire laser** or a white-**light** source allows one to image **tissue** with a subcellular resolution of 1–2 μm.

coherence time: The quantity that characterizes the ability of a **light beam** to produce an **interference pattern** being mixed with a part of itself that was delayed for some time interval τ_c. **Coherence time** is approximately equal to the pulse duration of the pulsed-**light** source or inversely proportional to the **wavelength bandwidth** $\Delta\lambda$ of a continuous-**wave light** source, $\tau_c \sim \lambda^2/(c\Delta\lambda)$, where c is the **speed of light**.

coherent anti-Stokes Raman scattering (CARS): A nonlinear variant of **Raman spectroscopy** that combines, besides signal enhancement by more than four orders of magnitude, further advantages such as directional emission, narrow-spectral **bandwidth**, and no disturbing **interference** with **autofluorescence** because the **coherent anti-Stokes Raman scattering** signal is detected on the short-**wavelength** side of the excitation **radiation**. A **coherent anti-Stokes Raman scattering** signal is usually weaker than **Stokes–Raman scattering** because an excited vibrational state has to be populated before the **scattering** process. The excitation scheme of **coherent anti-Stokes Raman scattering** involving a pump **laser**, a Stokes **laser**, and probe **laser** allows generation of a strongly amplified anti-Stokes signal. The **macroscopic polarization** P, which is induced by an electric field E : $P = \chi^{(1)} \cdot \vec{E} + \chi^{(2)} \cdot \vec{E}\vec{E} + \chi^{(3)} \cdot \vec{E}\vec{E}\vec{E}, \chi^{(n)}$ is the susceptibility tensor of rank n, which is a property of matter. For most bulk samples, $\chi^{(2)}$ is close to zero due to the symmetry requirement and $\chi^{(3)}$ becomes the dominant **nonlinear-susceptibility** contribution. As **coherent anti-Stokes Raman scattering** depends on $\chi^{(3)}$ and $\chi^{(1)} \gg \chi^{(3)}$, the nonlinear effect can only be detected using extraordinarily intense electric fields in the megawatt range that are produced by **nanosecond** to **femtosecond laser** pulses.

coherent backscattering: The use of ultrafast **laser** pulses gives rise to a local peak of **intensity** backscattered within a narrow solid angle owing to scattered-**light interference**. In the exact backward direction, the **intensity** of the scattered **light** is normally twice the diffuse **intensity**. Such coherence **interference** arises from the time-reversal symmetry among various scattered **light** paths in the **backscattering** direction. This phenomenon is known as weak localization. The profile of the angular distribution of the coherent peak depends on the transport mean free path l_t and the **absorption coefficient** μ_a. The angular width of the peak is directly related to l_t, $\Delta\theta \approx \lambda/(2\pi l_t)$. In many hard and **soft tissues**, such as human-**fat tissue**, **lung-cancer tissue**, normal- and cataractous-eye **lens**, and myocardial, mammary, and dental **tissues**, the backscattered-coherent peak occurs when the probing-**laser** pulse is shorter than 20 ps.

coherent light: Light in which the **electromagnetic waves** maintain a fixed-phase relationship over a period of time, in which the phase relationship remains constant for various points that are perpendicular to the direction of propagation. It is typically produced by **lasers**.

coherent photons: See **ballistic photons**.

coherent-detection imaging (CDI): Method based on the optical heterodyne-detection technique: It is a coherence-gating method that discriminates the forward multiply **scattering** beam, preserving the direct geometrical **correlation** with the incident **light beam** against the diffuse component of transmitted **light**, which generally loses the properties of the incident beam, such as coherence, direction, and **polarization** due to **multiple scattering**. The optical heterodyne-detection method operates on the principle of mixing of two optical waves at different frequencies [$(\omega_0 + \omega_1)$ and $(\omega_0 + \omega_2)$, where ω_0 is the optical **frequency**, and ω_1 and ω_2 are radio-**modulation** frequencies], on a square-law detector such as a **photodiode**. The signal generated by the **photodetector** is the cross product of the two optical fields, signal I_1 and local oscillator I_2, $\sim \sqrt{I_1(t, x, y)} \cdot \sqrt{I_2} \cdot \sin[(\omega_1 - \omega_2)t + \phi(t, x, y)]$, where t, x, and y are the temporal and spatial coordinates. $\phi(t, x, y)$ is the spatial and time-dependent **phase shift** caused by the spatial and temporal fluctuations of **refraction** of the **tissue** under investigation. The signal amplitude is subject to temporal and spatial fluctuations caused by time- and spatial-dependent **attenuation** of **light** by

73

the **tissue**. The typical scheme of a coherent-detection-imaging system uses a well-**collimated** optical beam of a **continuous-wave**, **single-frequency laser** [**Ar laser** (514.5 nm), **He:Ne laser** (633 nm), **Kr laser** (647.1 nm), **titanium–sapphire (Ti: Al$_2$O$_3$)** laser (tuned in the range 700–1000 nm), or a diode-pumped **Nd:YAG laser** (1064 and 1319 nm)] with a **power** of a few dozen milliwatts that is split into signal and local oscillator beams. The local oscillator beam and the signal beam are **frequency** shifted (modulated) by a pair of acousto-optic modulators to 80 and 80.05 MHz, respectively. The signal beam (about 0.8 mm in diameter), after passing through the object, is mixed with the local oscillator beam at a silicon **photodiode** generating a signal at the intermediate **frequency** (IF) (the **beat signal**). The IF signal is then fed to a fast Fourier-transform **analyzer** that is interfaced to a personal computer. The dynamic range of the system, defined as P_{sat}/P_{min}, where P_{sat} is the optical power at which the detector is saturated and P_{min} is the minimal detected optical power, is about 140 **dB**. It should be noted that the signal **power** is proportional to the amplitude of the IF signal over the entire dynamic range of the heterodyne system. Very low optical power to the order of 10^{-17} W at a **wavelength** of 800 nm and a detection **bandwidth** limited to a few **hertz** could be detected. Using the **coherent-detection imaging** system, 2D (projection) imaging was successfully performed for various *in vitro* and *in vivo* biological objects such as chicken legs and eggs, human-**tumor** specimens, human teeth, animal **bones**, the **head** of an infant mouse, and a human finger. The **spatial resolution** of the system is in the range 0.3–0.5 mm, depending on the optical and scanning arrangement.

coherent-heterodyne optical detection: An indirect-detection method that offers a number of advantages over direct-detection methods: it has the highest sensitivity of any detection technique with signal-to-noise ratio (it is several orders of magnitude better than that achieved by incoherent methods); extraordinary dynamic range, about 15 orders or more magnitude of signal **power** for Hz-order **bandwidths**; excellent selectivity or filtering capability in **frequency-domain** and **polarization**, and high

spatial resolution, up to 60–80 lines per mm (with a confocal optical arrangement); substantial spatial selectivity or filtering capability due to highly directional **antenna properties of the optical heterodyne system**; and it allows for quantification of new **tissue** parameters by detecting the wavefront degradation within a given **tissue**. The quantum limit of optical detection corresponds to the signal-limited **shot noise** (when one employs a conventional photoelectronic detector) with the minimal detectable signal **power** $P_{min} = hvB_d/\eta_q$, where hv is the photon **energy**, B_d is the detection **bandwidth**, and η_q is the **quantum efficiency** of the detector. In the case of the direct-detection technique, this limit is impossible to reach. Only the optical heterodyning detection and **photon**-counting methods allow one to realize this standard **quantum detection limit**. The **field of view** of an optical-heterodyne system having an effective aperture A for signals at **wavelength** λ arriving within a single main antenna **lobe** expressed as a solid angle is defined by $\Omega \cong \lambda^2/A$. The antenna properties afford high **spatial resolution** for detection and ranging of various bio-objects and their image formation, and excellent directionality to distinguish one specific direction from another. These important features make it possible to detect and image very weak signals embedded in or hidden by appreciably large optical noise or background. The optical-heterodyning technique shows good potential for applications in **tissue spectroscopy** and imaging.

cohesion: The **adhesion** between similar molecules.

cold cataract: Temperature-induced reversible **cataract**.

collagen: A tough, inelastic, **fibrous protein**. On boiling, it forms **gelatin**. After adding **acetic acid**, it swells up and dissolves. **Collagen** is formed and maintained in **tissues** by **fibroblasts**. It forms **white fibers** in **connective tissue**. The tropocollagen or "**collagen** molecule" subunit is a rod of about 300 nm long and 1.5 nm in diameter, composed of three polypeptide strands. Subunits spontaneously self-assemble, with regularly staggered ends, into even larger arrays in the **extracellular** spaces of **tissues**. There is some covalent **crosslinking** within the triple helices, and a variable amount of covalent **crosslinking** between tropocollagen helices, to form the different types of **collagen** found in different mature **tissues**. This is similar to the situation found with the α-keratins in **hair**. A distinctive feature of **collagen** is the regular arrangement of **amino acids** in each of the three chains of the **collagen** subunits. In **bone**, entire **collagen** triple helices lie in a parallel, staggered array. 40-nm gaps between the ends of the tropocollagen subunits probably serve as nucleation sites for the deposition of long, hard, fine crystals of the mineral component, which is (approximately) **hydroxyapatite** with some phosphate. This is how certain kinds of **cartilage** turn into **bone**. **Collagen** gives **bone** its elasticity and contributes to fracture resistance. There are many **collagen** types that are different in their composition and structure, types I to V are the most abundant. Types I, II, III, V, VII, and XI are capable of **fibril** formation. Their distribution in **tissues** are as follows: Type I, **dermis**, **bone**, **cornea**, **tendon**, **cartilage**, **vessel** wall, **intestine**, **dentin**, **uterine** wall, **fat** mashwork; Type II, **cartilage**, notochord, **vitreous humor**, **nucleus** pulposus; Type III, **dermis**, **intestine**, **gingiva**, **heart valve**, **uterine** wall, **vessel** wall; Type IV and VII, **basement membranes**; Type V, **cornea**, placental **membranes**, **bone**, **vessel** wall, **cartilage**, **gingiva**; Type XI, **cartilage**, intervertebral disk, **vitreous humor**. In optical measurements, **collagen index of refraction** is of importance. For example, for type I it is $n = 1.43$ (fully **hydrated**) and 1.53 (dry) at 850 nm.

collagen fiber: Bundles of **collagen fibrils** (see **white fibers**, **white fibrous tissue**).

collagen fibril: **Collagen** molecules packed into an organized, overlapping bundle.

collagen secondary structure: **Collagen** molecule subunit that is a rod composed of three polypeptide strands, each of which is a left-handed **helix**. These three left-handed helices are twisted together into a right-handed coil, a triple **helix**, and a cooperative quaternary structure stabilized by numerous hydrogen bonds.

collapse: Catastrophic compression.

collimated: Term related to **light** or a particle beam whose rays or trajectories are nearly parallel, and therefore will spread slowly as it propagates. A perfectly **collimated** beam with no divergence cannot be created (due to **diffraction**), but **light** and particle beams can be approximately **collimated** by a number of processes and instruments, e.g., by means of a collimator. **Collimated light** is sometimes said to be focused at infinity. Thus as the distance from a point source increases, the spherical wavefronts become flatter and closer to plane waves, which are perfectly **collimated**.

collimated light beam: Beam of **light** in which all rays are parallel to each other.

collimated transmittance: The optical **transmittance** T_c measured using the incident-**collimated light beam** and distant **photodetector** behind one or a few distant **pinholes**.

collisional-quenching rate: Nonradiative relaxation of the excited molecular-**energy** state (level) by collisions with surrounding molecules. In a condensed medium, the rate of collisional relaxation is significantly higher than the radiative one.

colloid isoelectric point: The **pH** value of the **dispersion** medium of a colloidal suspension at which the colloidal particles do not move in an electric field.

colloid: Solutions containing particles with large molecular weights (nominally MW > 30,000). In normal **blood plasma**, **plasma proteins** are such particles. As solutes, **colloids** contribute to the total **osmotic pressure** of the solution, referred to as **colloid osmotic pressure** or as **oncotic pressure**.

colloid structure: Dispersion of colloidal particles in a continuous phase (the **dispersion** medium) of a different composition or state. True solutions of materials have dimensions within the colloidal range (1 nm to 100 nm), e.g., molecules of relatively large molecular mass such as polymers and **proteins**, or aggregates of small molecules, as in soaps and detergents under certain conditions (association colloids).

colon: The first or anterior part of the **large intestine**, having sacculated walls lined with a smooth **mucous membrane**. In the lining are **glands** secreting **mucus** but no digestive **enzymes**. **Water** is absorbed from the unassimilated liquid material, leaving feces. The **colon** leads directly into the rectum.

colonic: Related to the **colon**.

color: Term sometimes used to define **wavelength** or spectral interval (see **light** and **light-wavelength** range, **chromaticity coordinates**, red/green/blue), as in two-**color** radiometry (meaning a method that measures in two spectral intervals). Also used conventionally (visual **color**) as a means of displaying a **thermal image**, as in **color** thermogram. See also **false color map**.

color temperature: A characteristic of **visible light** that has important applications in lighting, photography, videography, **biomedical optics**, **biophotonics** and other fields. The **color temperature** of a **light** source is the temperature of an ideal **blackbody radiator** that radiates **light** of comparable **hue** to that **light** source (see correlated-**color temperature**). The temperature is conventionally stated in units of absolute temperature, kelvin (K). Color temperature is related to **Planck's law** and to **Wien's displacement law**. For thermal **light** sources such as **arc lamps**, higher **color temperatures** (5000 K or more) are called cool **colors** (blueish-white). Lower **color temperatures** (2700–3000 K) are called warm **colors** (yellowish-white through red).

color theory: See **colorimetry**.

colored body: See **nongraybody**.

colorfulness: Refers to the perceived **intensity** of a specific **color**. Related but distinct concept from **chroma** and saturation. The difference between a **color** against gray.

colorimetry: The science and technology used to quantify and physically describe the human **color** perception. Similar to **spectrophotometry** but distinguished by its interest in reducing spectra to the physical correlates of **color** perception, most often the 1931 **CIE** XYZ **color**-space tristimulus values and related quantities (see **chromaticity coordinates, luminous intensity, luminosity function**). With three attributes [**colorfulness** (**chroma** or saturation), **lightness** (or **brightness**), and **hue**], any **color** can be described.

colposcope: An endoscopic instrument providing *in vivo* examination of the vaginal and cervical **mucosa** with a high magnification.

colposcopy: The *in situ* examination of the vaginal and cervical **mucosa** using the **colposcope**.

columnar epithelium: These **cells** are taller than they are wide. Simple **columnar epithelium** is made up of a single layer of **cells** that are longer than they are wide. The **nucleus** is also closer to the base of the **cell**. The **small intestine** is a tubular organ lined with this type of **tissue**. Unicellular **glands** called goblet **cells** secrete **mucus** and are scattered throughout the simple columnar-**epithelial cells**. The free surface of the columnar **cell** has tiny hairlike projections called microvilli, which increase the surface area for **absorption**.

Commission Internationale de l'Eclairage (CIE): The French title of the International Commission on Illumination.

complementary metal-oxide semiconductor (CMOS) camera: Operates at lower voltages than a **charge-coupled-device (CCD)** camera, reducing **power** consumption for portable applications. Analog- and digital-processing functions can be integrated readily onto the **CMOS** chip, reducing system package size and overall cost.

complementary metal-oxide semiconductor (CMOS) image sensors: The sensors in which each active **pixel**-sensor cell has its own buffer **amplifier**, and can be addressed and read individually. A commonly used cell has four transistors and a photoelement. All **pixels** on a column connect to a commonsense **amplifier**. These devices are the basis for the **CMOS camera**.

complex conjugation: The number corresponding to a given complex number that represents the given number's **reflection** with respect to the real axis.

computed tomography (CT): A medical imaging method employing tomography created by computer processing. Digital geometry processing is used to generate a 3D image of the inside of an object from a large series of 2D x-ray images taken around a single axis of rotation. Computed tomography produces a volume of data that can be manipulated, through a process known as "windowing," in order to demonstrate various bodily structures based on their ability to block the **x-ray** beam. Modern scanners allow the volume of data to be reformatted in various planes or even as volumetric (3D) representations of structures. See also **computer tomography**.

computer tomography: The imaging of a selected plane (slice) in the body and 3D computer reconstruction of the image of a whole object on the basis of many individual images (slices) using one of the following methods: **x-ray computed tomography (CT)**, **magnetic resonance imaging (MRI)**, **positron emission tomography (PET)**, or **optical imaging**.

confocal microscopy (CM): Microscopy that employs the confocal principle [two optically conjugate diaphragms (**pinholes**) or small-sized slits in the object and image planes] for the selection of scattered (**ballistic**) **photons** coming from a given volume. Provides 3D imaging of living **tissues** with a subcellular resolution and in-depth **tissue** optical slicing (sectioning). It works in two modes, **reflection** scanning and **fluorescence**. A powerful tool for **noninvasive** 3D microvascular imaging, thanks to the development of fluorescent-**labeling** techniques. Confocal microscopes provide clear images in "optically thick" biological **tissues**. Instead of a **pinhole**, a **single-mode optical fiber** can be placed in between the **objective lens** and the detector to allow only the **light** that originates from within a tiny focal volume below the **tissue** surface to be collected. Sources of **light** from all other depths become spatially filtered by the **fiber** (**pinhole**). Significant progress has been made with **endoscope**-compatible confocal instruments for visualizing inside the human body. These methods are being developed for clinical use as an adjunct to **endoscopy** to guide **tissue biopsy** for surveillance of **cancer**, improve diagnostic yield, and reduce pathology investigation costs. These efforts are technically challenged by demanding performance/parameter requirements, including small instrument size, high axial resolution, large **penetration depth**, and fast frame rate. An imaging depth of ~500 μm is sufficient to evaluate most early disease processes in the **epithelium**. Premalignant **cells** are frequently defined by abnormal morphology of the **cell nucleus**, and diagnosis requires both an axial- and transverse-subcellular resolution on the order of <5 μm. Motion **artifacts** can be introduced by organ peristalsis, heartbeats, and respiratory displacement, requiring a frame rate of >4 per sec. Dual-axes **confocal microscopy** performs off-axis illumination and collection of **light** to further overcome **tissue scattering**.

confocal-light absorption and scattering-spectroscopic (CLASS) microscopy: Combines the principles of **confocal microscopy** with **light-scattering spectroscopy**, an optical technique that relates the spectroscopic properties of **light** elastically scattered by small particles to their size, **refractive index**, and shape. The multispectral nature of **light-scattering spectroscopy** enables it to measure internal **cell** structures, which are much smaller than the **diffraction limit**, without damaging the **cell** or requiring **exogenous** markers that could affect **cell** function. **CLASS microscopy** approaches the accuracy of electron **microscopy** but is nondestructive and does not require the **contrast agents** common to optical **microscopy**. When imaging the **cell**, the origin of the confocal-**light-absorption** and **scattering**-spectroscopic signal is **light scattering** from the subcellular compartments. Although there are hundreds of **cell** types, the subcellular compartments in different **cells** are rather similar and are limited in number with sometimes well-described **scattering**-amplitude/**wavelength/scattering**-angle signatures that allows one to reconstruct scatter size, **refractive index**, and shape from measurements of **light-scattering** properties by solution of the inverse-**scattering** problem. **CLASS microscopy** is applicable in such diverse areas as obstetrics, neuroscience, ophthalmology, cellular and **tissue** imaging with nanoparticulate markers, and drug discovery.

confocal-microscopy time-lapse fluorescence imaging: This time-dependent confocal-**microscopy** measurement combined with fluorescent-**protein**-reporter lines is a powerful tool for studying **cell** migration and organ development, as well as for investigation of cellular consequences of genetic manipulations. Several genetic strands have been engineered that express fluorescent **proteins** in specific **tissues** of the **embryo**, e.g., ε-globin-EGFP expressing **green fluorescent protein (GFP)** in primitive erythroblasts; Flk1–H2B–EYFP expressing nuclear yellow fluorescent **protein** (YFP) in the endothelial **cells**; and Oct4-GFP expressing GFP in primordial germ **cells**. Fuorescent imaging has been used in different models to visualize and analyze the cellular dynamics during development *in vivo*. The use of tagged fluorescent **proteins** under control of specific regulatory elements has significantly increased the ability to track individual **cells**, characterize **tissue** dynamics, and understand the formation of complex cytoarchitectures. Using the ε-globin-EGFP transgenic-mouse line expressing **GFP** in embryonic **blood cells**, early circulation events were quantified in studying the initiation of **blood** formation. There is a transgenic model in which mCherry fluorescent **protein** is expressed in the embryonic **endothelium** and **endocardium** that allows for **membrane** localization of the fluorescent **protein**, and therefore, outlines the structure of the **vasculature** and reveals cellular morphology and **cell–cell** boundaries between the endothelial **cells**. As mCherry has an emission peak at 610 nm, it is easily separated from blue, green, or yellow fluorescent **proteins**.

conjunctiva: A delicate **mucous membrane** covering the **cornea**, the front part of the **sclera**, and lining the eyelids. It protects the **cornea**.

connective tissue: Various body **tissues** that bind together and support organs and other **tissues**, e.g., **connective tissue** surrounds **muscles** and **nerves**, connects **bones** and **muscles**, and underlies the **skin**. Cartilage and **bone** are also **connective tissues**. Typical **connective tissue** consists of **cells** scattered in an amorphous **mucopolysaccharide** matrix in which there are varying amounts of **connective-tissue fibers** (mainly **collagen**, but also **elastin** and **reticulin**).

constant-fraction discriminator (CFD): Electronic signal-processing device, designed to mimic the mathematical operation of finding a maximum of a pulse by finding the zero of its slope. Some signals do not have a sharp maximum but short rise times.

constructive interference: Interference of two or more waves of equal **frequency** and phase, resulting in their mutual reinforcement and producing a single amplitude equal to the sum of the amplitudes of the individual waves.

continuous wave (CW): **Waves** that are not intermittent or broken up into damped-**wave** trains, but unless intentionally interrupted, follow one another without any interval of time between them. Light–**tissue** interaction depends significantly on temporal parameters of the **light**, whether it is **continuous wave** or pulsed.

continuous-wave (CW) laser: Laser producing **continuous wave (CW)** radiation or light.

continuous-wave radiation-transfer theory (CW RTT): The stationary **radiation**-transfer theory that describes the **intensity** distribution of **continuous-wave light** in a **scattering** medium. Based on the stationary integro-differential equation for the **radiance** (or specific **intensity**), which is the average **power**-flux density at a point r in a given direction s.

contrast: The difference in visual properties that makes an object (or its representation in an image) distinguishable from other objects and the background. In visual perception, **contrast** is determined by the difference in the **color** and **brightness** of the object and other objects within the same **field of view**. A large **contrast** is a big difference, and contrasting objects are boldly different. It can refer to **contrast** (visibility) of regular **interference** or **speckle** patterns, the difference in **color** and **light intensity** between parts of an image [see **imaging (image) contrast**]. The Weber **contrast** is defined as $C_W = (I - I_b)/I_b$ with I and I_b representing the **intensity** of the features and the background **intensity**, respectively. It is commonly used in cases where small features are present on a large uniform background, i.e., the average **intensity** is approximately equal to the background **intensity**. Michelson **contrast**, $C_M = (I_{max} - I_{min})/(I_{max} - I_{min})$, with I_{max} and I_{min} representing the highest and lowest **intensity**, is commonly used for patterns where both bright and dark features are equivalent and take up similar fractions of the area (such as **interference fringes**). In **root-mean-square contrast**, intensities I_{ij} are the ith and jth element of the 2D image of size M by N, and $\bar{I}$ is the average **intensity** of all **pixel** values in the image. It does not depend on the spatial-**frequency** content or the spatial distribution of **contrast** in the image (defined as the **standard deviation** of the **pixel** intensities). The image is assumed to have its **pixel** intensities normalized in the range (0, 1).

$$K = \sqrt{\frac{1}{MN} \sum_{i=0}^{N-1} \sum_{j=0}^{M-1} \left(I_{ij} - \bar{I}\right)^2}$$

contrast agents: Chemical compounds used to improve the quality of **x-ray**, magnetic-resonance imaging, positron-emission tomography, or optical-tomography images. **X-ray** agents (also called radiocontrast agents) are a type of medical **contrast** medium used to improve the visibility of internal body structures in x-ray-based imaging techniques such as **computed tomography**. **X-ray contrast agents** are typically iodine or barium compounds. Examples are verografin, **trazograph**-60 and -76, and **hypaque**-60 and -76. Magnetic-resonance imaging functions through different principles and thus utilizes different **contrast agents**. There, the most commonly used compounds for **contrast** enhancement are gadolinium-based. The so-called dynamic **contrast**-enhanced magnetic-resonance images have had success in the characterization of multiple sclerosis, retinal disease, and human **breast cancer**. **Optical imaging** encompasses many different techniques that use UV to **near-infrared light** to visualize **tissue** abnormalities imparted through **absorption** and **scattering** of **light**, as well as emission of **fluorescence**. Different **biocompatible contrast agents** (probes) for optical detection of diseases have been synthesized and characterized for their potential to engender disease-specific optical signals within the **tissue**, including **cyanine dyes**, tetrapyrroles, lanthanide chelates, and some others. Chemical, optical, and pharmocological properties were exploited to provide **extracellular** dyes, target-specific conjugates, activatable probes, or prodrugs. Optical **contrast agents** such as **indocyanine green** and **methylene blue** have traditionally been employed to measure cardiac output, detect retinal disease, diagnose renal failure, and assess hepatic function. Advances in the development of quantitative **near-infrared** diagnostic technologies and molecular-probe design stimulate increased interest in the use of optical **contrast agents** for new medical applications, including **cancer**

detection, measurement of cerebral **blood flow**, burn-depth assessment, monitoring **muscle** function, and monitoring of **photosensitizer** concentration for photodynamic therapy. For example, **fluorescence** of **toluidine blue O** dye in combination with **polarization** measurements is used for *in vivo cancer-lesion* demarcation; **albumin blue** is used for **albumin**-related **functional imaging**; functionalized **near-infrared** dye **IRDye 800CW carboxylate** is much more effective than indocyanine green; **green fluorescent protein** allows for selective **contrast** images of internal **lesions**; and δ-aminolevulenic acid as a prodrug endogenously synthesizes in the **cells** and **tissues** the metabolic **contrast agent protoporphyrin IX**. Different kinds of **nanoparticles**, including golden **nanoparticles**, are used both for x-ray and optical-image contrasting. The major advantage of golden **nanoparticles** applied to **optical imaging** is the absence of **photobleaching**. See also **quantum dot**.

contrast of the intensity fluctuations: The relative difference between **light** and dark areas of a **speckle** pattern.

controlling of tissue optical properties: Reflection, absorption, scattering, and **fluorescence** in living **tissues** and **blood** can be effectively controlled by various methods. Staining (sensitization) of biological materials is used extensively to study mechanisms of interaction between their constituent components and **light** and for diagnostic purposes and selective **photodestruction** of individual components of living **tissues**. This approach underlies the diagnosis and photodynamic therapy of **malignant neoplasm**, **UV**-A photochemotherapy of **psoriasis** and other **proliferative disorders**, angiography in ophthalmology, and many other applications in medicine. In the **visible** and **near-infrared**, **tissues** and bioliquids are low-absorbing but highly **scattering media**. **Scattering** defines spectral and angular characteristics of **light** interacting with living objects, as well as its **penetration depth**, thus **optical properties** of **tissues** and **blood** may be effectively controlled by changes of **scattering** properties. The living **tissue** allows one to control its optical (**scattering**) properties using various physical and chemical actions, such as compression, stretching, dehydration, **coagulation**, **UV light** irradiation, exposure to low temperature, and impregnation by chemical solutions, **gels**, and **oils**. All these phenomena can be understood if **tissue** is considered as a **scattering** medium that shows all optical effects that are characteristic to turbid physical systems. It is well known that **turbidity** of a dispersive physical system can be effectively controlled by providing matching of refractive indices of the **scatterers** and the ground material by addition of an agent with a **refractive index** higher than that of the ground material. This is a so-called **optical immersion technique**. Another possibility to control **optical properties** of a dispersed system is to change its packing parameter and/or scatter sizing. In many practical cases, such as long-pulse **laser heating**, reversible and irreversible changes in the **optical properties** of **tissue** are induced. **UV** irradiation causes **erythema** (**skin** reddening), stimulates **melanin** synthesis, and can induce **edema** and **tissue proliferation** if the **radiation** dose is sufficiently large. All these photobiological effects may be responsible for variations in the **optical properties** of **skin** and need to be taken into consideration when prescribing **phototherapy**. Also, **UV** treatment is known to cause **color** development in the human **lens**. Natural physiological changes in **cells** and **tissues** are also responsible for their altered **optical properties**, which may be detectable and thus used as a measure of these changes. For example, measurements of the **scattering coefficient** allow one to monitor **glucose** or **edema** in the human body, as well as **blood** parameters. Optical characteristics of **blood** are functions of **hemoglobin saturation** with **oxygen**, changes of **hematocrit** value, temperature, and parameters of flow.

cooled charge-coupled device (CCD): Highly sensitive charge-coupled device with the thermal noise suppressed by cooling of the photosensitive chip.

copolymer (*Synonym*: heteropolymer): A polymer derived from two (or more) monomeric species, as opposed to a homopolymer, where only one **monomer** is used.

copper-vapor laser: An atomic metal-vapor **laser** with a pulse mode of generation, a high mean **power** up to ~40 W, a high-pulse-repetition rate up to ~30 kHz, and a short-pulse duration of 3–50 ns. Pulse **power** is up to ~200 kW, and pulse **energy** is around $2 \cdot 10^{-3}$ J. Its efficiency is around 1%. It is the most powerful **laser** in the **visible** range. Around 70% of total **energy** is concentrated on the green line at 510.5 nm, and the remaining 30% on the yellow line at 578.2 nm. It is widely used in dermatology for birthmark treatment, including **port-wine stains**.

coproporphyrin: A **porphyrin** occurring as several isomers. The III isomer, an intermediate *in heme* biosynthesis, is excreted in the feces and urine in such diseases as hereditary coproporphyria and variegate porphyria. The I isomer, a side product, is excreted in congenital erythropoietic porphyria disease. **Coproporphyrin** is used as a test to measure red-**blood cell porphyrin** levels in evaluating of **porphyrin** disorders.

cornea: The transparent covering at the front of the **eyeball**, it is the modified continuation of the **sclera**. Refracts **light** and is the most important element in the refractive system of the eye.

corneocyte [*Synonyms*: horny cell; keratinised cell (keratinocyte)]: The dead, **keratin**-filled **squamous cell** of the **stratum corneum**.

cornification: Conversion of **epithelium** to the stratified **squamous** type. For instance, the conversion of **skin cells** into **keratin** or other horny material such as nails or scales.

coronary arteries: Right and left **coronary arteries** both originate from the beginning (root) of the **aorta**, immediately above the aortic **valve**. The left **coronary artery** originates from the left aortic sinus, while the right **coronary artery** originates from the right aortic sinus.

correlated color temperature (CCT): Measure of the quality of white **light** emitted from a **light** source, expressed as the temperature of a **blackbody** of the same **color**.

correlation: The degree of co-relation between two or more attributes or measurements on the same group of elements. In **probability** theory and statistics, **correlation** indicates the strength and direction of a linear relationship between two random variables. In general statistical usage, **correlation** refers to the departure of two variables from independence, although **correlation** does not imply causation.

correlation coefficient: A number of different coefficients are used to characterize **correlation** between two random variables for different situations. Best known is the Pearson product-moment **correlation coefficient**, which is obtained by dividing the covariance of the two variables by the product of their **standard deviations**.

correlation length: Length within which the degree of **correlation** between two measurements of a spatially dependent quantity is high (close to unity)—for example, the **correlation length** of the **scattering** surface of the spatial inhomogeneities (random relief).

correlation-diffusion equation: Describes the transport of temporal field **correlation** function in a system that multiplies scattered **laser radiation**. It may be valid for turbid samples with the dynamics of **scattering** particles governed by **Brownian motion**, and random and shear flow.

cortex (*Synonym*: cerebral cortex): Outer layer of the cerebral hemisphere, consisting of **gray matter** and rich in synapses. It is extensive in mammals, with **fissures** and folds.

cosmetics: Substances used to enhance or protect the appearance or odor of the human body. **Cosmetics** include skincare creams, lotions, powders, perfumes, lipsticks, fingernail polishes, eye and facial makeup, permanent waves, **hair colors**, deodorants, baby products, bath **oils**, bubble baths, and many other types of products. The **Food and Drug Administration** defines cosmetic purpose as "intended to be applied to the human body for cleansing, beautifying, promoting attractiveness, or altering the appearance without affecting the body's structure or functions."

coupler: Optical or acoustical device that interconnects optical or acoustical components with less loss of **energy**.

coupling gel: A **gel** that matches the optical or acoustical properties of different elements of a device and minimizes amplitude of **light** or acoustic reflecting signals (or both) from boundaries of the elements.

craniocaudal projection: Projection showing the direction from the **cranium** to the posterior end of the body.

cranium: A domed, bony case composed of several **bones** joined by sutures. It encloses and protects the **brain**.

cross talk: The interrelation between measured signals induced by originally independent parameters (for example, by changes in **blood volume** and oxygenation). This factor is determined by **calibration** on a model (e.g., a **blood** model).

cross-correlation frequency (*Synonym*: cross-correlation signal): A difference in the **frequency** of **intensity**-modulated **light** at a certain **wavelength** and **photodetector-gain modulation**. It carries the same phase and amplitude information as the original optical signal.

cross-correlation measurement device: A system that down-converts **radio frequency** prior to phase measurements.

cross-correlation signal: See **cross-correlation frequency**.

crosslinking: To attach by a cross-link—a bond, atom, or group linking the chains of atoms in a polymer, **protein**, or other complex organic molecule.

cross-polarization imaging: Belongs to **polarization**-imaging methods. A much simpler version of this technique is realized by placing a **polarization** filter in front of the detector with **polarization** orientation perpendicular to that of the filter in front of the **light** source. It allows one to detect events in the **skin** microvascular network. The **algorithms** are based on orthogonal-**polarization spectroscopy** and **tissue**-viability imaging. See also **cross-polarization orthogonal-polarization spectroscopy (CP OCT).**

cross-polarization orthogonal-polarization spectroscopy (CP OCT): Belongs to **polarization spectroscopy**/orthogonal-**polarization spectroscopy** methods. This is a much simpler version of **polarization spectroscopy**/orthogonal-**polarization spectroscopy**, that provides pathology imaging for deeper layers (up to 1.5 mm). Light **depolarization** caused by **light scattering** and **tissue birefringence** both lead to the appearance of a CP component in the backscattered **light**, which is detected. **Pathological** processes are characterized by the changes in the amount of **collagen fibers** and their spatial organization; therefore, a comparative analysis of CP **backscattering** properties of normal and **pathological tissues** may be used for early diagnosis of **neoplastic** processes.

cryogenic: Related to treatments using very low temperatures (below $-150\,°C$, $-238\,°F$ or 123 K) and the behavior of materials at those temperatures.

cryosection: A frozen-sectioning procedure that is used to perform rapid microscopic analysis of a **tissue** specimen. Used most often in oncological surgery and **tissue** research.

cryosurgery (*Related term*: cryotherapy): Application of extreme cold to destroy abnormal or diseased **tissue**. Used to treat a number of diseases and disorders, especially **skin** conditions. Warts, **moles**, **skin** tags, solar keratoses, and small **skin cancers** are candidates for cryosurgical treatment. Some internal disorders are also treated with **cryosurgery**, including **liver cancer**, **prostate cancer**, and cervical disorders.

crystal violet: Other names are gentian violet, methyl violet 10B, ahexamethyl pararosaniline chloride. It is an organic compound having bactericidal and antifungal properties. It is the primary agent used in the **Gram's stain** test, perhaps the single most important bacterial identification test in use today, and it is also used by hospitals for the treatment of serious heat **burns** and other injuries to the **skin** and **gums**. Typically prepared as a weak (e.g., 1%) solution in **water**, it is painted on **skin** or **gums** to treat or prevent fungal infections.

crystalline: A **crystalline** material has a regular crystal lattice. It does not necessarily form a single, regular crystal, e.g., all metals are **crystalline** because the atoms have a regular arrangement.

crystalline lens: Transparent structure surrounded by a thin capsule and situated immediately behind the **pupil** of the eye. It has the shape of a biconvex **lens** and is attached to the **eyeball** by suspensory **ligaments**. It refracts **light** onto the **retina**.

C-scan: Made from many **T-scans** along either Cartesian (X, Y) or polar coordinates (ρ, θ), repeated for different values of the other transverse coordinates, Y, X, θ, or ρ, respectively, in the transverse plane. The repetition of **T-scans** along the other transverse coordinate is performed at a slower rate than that of the **T-scans**, called the frame rate. In this way, a complete raster is generated. This is a so-called *en-face* image. Different transversal slices are collected for different depths Z, either by advancing the optical path difference in the **optical coherence tomography** in steps after each complete transverse (X, Y) or (ρ, θ) scan, or continuously at a much slower speed than the frame rate.

cutaneous: Relating to the **skin**.

cyanine dye: Synthetic dye family belonging to polymethine group. Cyanines have many uses as fluorescent dyes, particularly in biomedical imaging. Depending on the structure, they cover the **spectrum** from **IR** to **UV**. Cy3 and Cy5 are reactive **water**-soluble fluorescent dyes. Cy3 dye has ~550 nm excitation and ~570 nm fluorescent-mean **wavelengths**, while Cy5 absorbs in the ~649 nm and is fluorescent in the range ~650/670 nm. They are usually synthesized with reactive groups on either one or both of the nitrogen side chains so that they can be chemically linked to either **nucleic acids** or **protein** molecules. Labeling is done for visualization and quantification purposes. The dyes are used in a wide variety of biological applications in **genomics** and **proteomics**. Merocyanines are a class of fluorescent dyes typified by merocyanine I. Merocyanine 540 was the first fluorescent dye used for measuring **membrane** potential.

cyclophotocoagulation: A **transscleral laser** procedure for **glaucoma** treatment. In this procedure, the **ciliary body** is treated with a **laser** to decrease its production of aqueous, which in turn reduces **pressure** inside the eye. Usually about 20 to 40 **laser** delivery applications are completed.

cyst: A closed, bladderlike sac formed in **tissues**. It contains fluid or semifluid matter.

cystitis: An infection of the **bladder**, but the term is often used indiscriminately and covers a range of infections and irritations in the lower urinary system.

cytochrome: Iron-containing **proteins** that take part, mainly as **coenzymes**, in cellular respiration. It is found abundantly in aerobic organisms: they are oxidized by dissolved **oxygen** in a **cell**, and reduced by oxidizable substances in the **cell**. It is the main vehicle for the use of **oxygen** in **metabolism**.

cytochrome c oxidase (Cox): A large transmembrane **protein** complex found in **bacteria** and the **mitochondrion**. It is the last **protein** in the electron-transport chain, and it receives an electron from each of four **cytochrome c** molecules, and transfers them to one **oxygen** molecule, converting molecular **oxygen** to two molecules of **water**. In the process, it translocates four protons, helping to establish a chemiosmotic potential that the **adenosine triphosphate (ATP)** synthase then uses to synthesize **ATP**. **Absorption** spectra obtained for **cytochrome c oxidase** in different oxidation states were found to be very similar to the action spectra for biological responses to **light**. Therefore, it was proposed that **cytochrome c oxidase** is the primary photoacceptor for the red/**near-infrared** range in mammalian **cells** (see **low-level laser therapy**).

cytometry: The methods and instruments for the structural and functional study of **cells** and **bacteria**, e.g., **flow cytometry** is a technique for automatic measurement and analysis of **cells** and other small particles suspended in a medium. See **flow cytometry, image cytometry**, *in vivo* **flow cytometry, laser flow cytometry, opto-acoustic flow cytometry, photothermal flow cytometry, scanning cytometry**.

cytoplasm: All the protoplasm of a **cell** exclusive of the **nucleus**. It is not just a simple, slightly viscous, fluid. In it are situated various structures, called organelles, each concerned with different functions of the **cell**. The **plasma membrane** is part of the **cytoplasm**.

cytoskeleton: Made of **fibrous proteins** (e.g., **microfilaments, microtubules**, and intermediate filaments). In many organisms it maintains the shape of the **cell**, anchors organelles, and controls internal movement of structures.

cytosol: The internal fluid of the **cell** wherein a portion of **cell metabolism** occurs. **Proteins** within the **cytosol** play an important role in signal-transduction pathways and glycolysis. In **prokaryotes**, all chemical reactions take place in the **cytosol**. In **eukaryotes** the portion of **cytosol** in the **nucleus** is called nucleohyaloplasm. Cytosol also surrounds the **cytoskeleton**; the **cytosol** is a "soup" with free-floating particles, but it is highly organized on the molecular level (compare to **cytoplasm**, which also includes the organelles).

Dale–Gladstone law: One of the **refractive index** mixture rules stating that the mean value of **refractive index** $\bar{n}$ of a composition represents an average of the refractive indices of its noninteracting components related to their **volume fractions**. n_i and f_i are the **refractive index** and **volume fraction** of the individual components, respectively, and N is the number of components when volume additivity is assumed, i.e., $\sum_i f_i = 1$.

$$\bar{n} = \sum_{i=1}^{N} n_i f_i$$

dalton (Da):   Unit of mass used to express atomic and molecular masses. Also, it is the approximate mass of a hydrogen atom, a proton, or a neutron. The atomic mass unit is one-twelfth of the mass of an isolated atom of carbon-12 (^{12}C) at rest and in its ground state. In biochemistry and molecular biology the term **dalton** is referenced with the symbol Da. The **Avogadro constant** (N_A) and the **mole** are defined so that one **mole** (1 mol) of a substance with atomic or molecular mass of 1 Da will have a mass of precisely 1 g, thus 1 Da = 1 g/mol (for isotopically pure substances). Because **proteins** are large molecules, their masses are often in kilodaltons, where one kilodalton is 1000 Da. The unified atomic mass unit, or **dalton**, is not an SI unit of mass, but it is accepted for use with SI. The one-to-one relationship between **daltons** and g/mol is true, but to be used accurately for practical purposes, any calculations must be with isotopically pure substances or involve much more complicated statistical averaging of multiple isotopic compositions.

dark noise: An accumulation of heat-generated electrons in the **photodetector** with no incident **light**. In **charge-coupled-device (CCD) sensors** these electrons end up in the photosites and contribute a snowlike appearance to the image. A related concept, dark current, refers to the rate of generation of these electrons, most of which come from boundaries between silicon and silicon dioxide in the **charge-coupled-device (CCD) sensor**.

dark-field illumination: Used in dark-field **microscopy** for imaging of optically transparent nonabsorbing specimens, where illuminating **light** does not enter into the ocular and only **light** scattered by microparticles of the specimen creates the image. In the **field of view** of the microscope on the dark background, bright images of the specimen particles (which differ by their **refractive index** from the surrounding medium) are seen.

dark-field photoacoustic microscopy (PAM): Special system that uses a pulsed **laser beam** delivered by a **multimode optical fiber** passed through a conical **lens** to form a ring-shaped illumination. This is weakly focused into biological **tissues**, where the optical focus coaxially overlaps with the ultrasonic focus. The **dark-field illumination** is combined with the acousto-optical confocal configuration. The **laser**-pulse **energy** deposited into the **tissue** is partially absorbed and converted into heat, which induces a local **pressure** rise via transient thermoelastic expansion. The **pressure** rise travels through the **tissue** in the form of a wideband ultrasonic **wave** referred to as a **photoacoustic wave**, and it is detected by an **ultrasonic transducer**. The system provides a high **signal-to-noise ratio (SNR)** because the **photoacoustic** signal in the detectable surface area is greatly minimized.

DC measurements: Measurements done using direct current (DC) electronics.

decibel (dB): The engineering unit for the ratio of the input **power** P_{in}, in a given device to the output **power** P_{out}. It is convenient to measure the logarithm of the ratio log (P_{out}/P_{in}), and the decibel is a standard unit that is equal to 10 times that log: 10 log (P_{out}/P_{in}) **dB**.

deconvolution microscopy: Microscopy technique based on the knowledge of the **point spread function** of the microscope-imaging system and its reversing by computer-based methods using various 2D or 3D **algorithms**. This can be an advantage over other types of 3D **microscopy** such as **confocal microscopy**, because **light** is not thrown away but reused. For 3D deconvolution, one typically provides a series of images derived from different **focal planes** (called a Z-stack) plus the knowledge of the **point spread function**, which can be either derived experimentally or theoretically from knowing all contributing parameters of the microscope.

decorrelation of speckle: Relates to statistics of the second order that characterize the size and distribution of **speckle** sizes and show how fast the **intensity** changes from point to point in the **speckle** pattern: decorrelation means that such changes of **intensity** tend to be faster.

decylmethylsulfoxide: N-decylmethylsulfoxide (nDMSO) is a **tissue**-penetrating agent, such as **dimethyl sulfoxide**.

deep random-phase screen (RPS): A random-phase screen that induces phase fluctuations in a scattered field with a **variance** that is much more than unity.

deflectometry: A **photorefractive technique** based on detection of refractive-index gradients above and inside the sample using a **laser probe** beam.

deformation: In biomechanics, **deformation** is a change in shape due to an applied force. It can be a result of tensile (pulling) forces, compressive (pushing) forces, shear, bending, or torsion (twisting). **Deformation** is often described in terms of strain.

degree of circular polarization (DOCP): From the **Stokes vector**, the **DOCP** is derived as DOCP $= \sqrt{V^2}/I$. See **light polarization**, **degree of polarization (DOP)**, and **Stokes parameters**.

97

degree of linear polarization (DOLP): From the **Stokes vector,** the **DOLP** is derived as DOLP $= \sqrt{Q^2 + U^2}/I$ or experimentally $P_L = (I_\parallel - I_\perp)/(I_\parallel + I_\perp)$, where $I_\parallel$ and $I_\perp$ are the **intensity** of **light** polarized in parallel and perpendicular to **polarization** plane, respectively. See **light polarization, degree of polarization (DOP),** and **Stokes parameters.**

degree of polarization (DOP): The ratio of the **intensity** of **polarized light** to the total **intensity** of **light.** From the **Stokes vector,** the **DOP** is derived as DOP $= \sqrt{Q^2 + U^2 + V^2}/I$. If the DOP of a light field remains at unity after transformation by an optical system, this system is nondepolarizing; otherwise, the system is depolarizing. See **light polarization, Stokes parameters, depolarization,** and **depolarization length.**

dehydration: Removal or loss of **water** by a **tissue** or a **cell.** It may be induced by heating or by action of **hyperosmotic** agents.

deionized water (DIW) (*Synonym*: demineralized water): **Water** that has had its mineral ions removed—such as cations from sodium, calcium, iron, and copper, and anions such as chloride and bromide. Deionization is a physical process that uses specially manufactured ion-exchange resins that bind to and filter out the mineral salts from **water.** Because the majority of **water** impurities are dissolved salts, deionization produces high-purity **water** that is generally similar to **distilled water,** and the process is quick and low cost. However, deionization does not significantly remove uncharged organic molecules, **viruses,** or **bacteria,** nor does it remove the hydroxide or hydronium ions from **water,** because these are the products of the self-ionization of **water** to equilibrium and therefore impossible to remove. Only specially made strong-base anion resins can remove **Gram-negative bacteria.** Deionization can be done continuously and inexpensively using electrodeionization.

delay generator (DG): An electronic device that is used in many types of experiments, controls, and processes where electronic timing of a single event or multiple events using a common timing reference is needed. The delay generator may initiate a sequence of events or be triggered by an event. The digital-delay generator differs from ordinary electronic timing because of the high synchronicity of its outputs to each other and to the initiating event.

delta (δ)-aminolevulinic acid (ALA) (*Synonym*: 5-aminolevulinic acid): A prodrug that leads to the **endogenous** synthesis of **protoporphyrin IX** in the **cells** and **tissues** when applied either systematically or topically. **Photodynamic therapy** drugs, such as Levulan®, Metvix®, Alasens®, and **Hexvix®**, are efficient for the treatment of actinic keratoses, **squamous-cell carcinomas**, and basal-**cell carcinomas**. With **photodynamic therapy**, a typical irradiation **wavelength** is 630–635 nm with the typical **laser** dose of 150 J/cm^2.

delta (δ)-Eddington approximation: A simple yet accurate method that was proposed for determining monochromatic radiative fluxes in an absorbing–**scattering** atmosphere. In this method the governing **phase function** is approximated by a Dirac delta function forward-scatter peak and a two-term expansion of the **phase function**. The fraction of **scattering** into the truncated forward peak is taken proportional to the square of the phase-function asymmetry factor, which distinguishes the delta-Eddington approximation from others of similar nature. It is one of the approximations of the actual **phase function** for **tissue**. In the **diffusion approximation** of **radiation-transfer theory**, it is the best function for simulating **light** transport in **tissues** characterized by an **isotropic scattering**.

delta T (ΔT): The temperature difference between two targets, usually comparable targets under comparable conditions.

demineralization: Loss of mineral from mineralized **tissues**. In **tooth tissue**, **demineralization** may lead to **caries**. In **bone tissue**, **demineralization** causes **osteoporosis**. **Bacteria** in

tooth plaque use simple **carbohydrates** such as **sucrose** and **glucose** in our diet for their metabolic needs and produce **lactic acid**. During the breakdown of these substrates, this acid can demineralize the **tooth**. **Demineralization** of outermost **tooth** layers, **enamel** and **cementum**, is the starting point of **tooth** destruction. Small amounts of **tooth demineralization** occur daily; **remineralization** can occur as mineral is replaced with calcium and phosphate from **saliva**.

demineralized water: See **deionized water (DIW)**.

demodulation: The separation and extraction of modulating low-**frequency** waves from a modulated carrier **wave** (high-**frequency** or optical **wave**). The device or circuit used for **demodulation** is called a detector or demodulator.

denaturation: The alteration of a **protein** shape through some form of external stress (e.g., applying heat, acid, or alkali), in such a way that it will no longer be able to carry out its cellular function. Denatured **proteins** can exhibit a wide range of characteristics, ranging from loss of solubility to communal **aggregation**.

dendrite: Filaments that arise from the **neuron-cell** body, often extending for hundreds of microns and branching multiple times, giving rise to a complex "dendritic tree."

dendritic cell: **Immune cells** that form part of the immune system. Their main function is to process **antigen** material and present it on the surface to other **cells** of the immune system, thus functioning as **antigen**-presenting **cells**. They act as messengers between the innate and adaptive immunities. Present in small quantities in **tissues** that are in contact with the external environment, mainly the **skin** (where there is a specialized dendritic **cell** type called Langerhans **cells**) and the inner lining of the nose, **lungs**, **stomach**, and **intestines**. It is also found in an immature state in the **blood**. Once activated, they migrate to the **lymph node** where they interact with T and B

lymphocytes to initiate and shape the adaptive-**immune response**. At certain development stages they grow branched projections, the **dendrites**, which give the **cell** its name.

dental plaque: A **biofilm** (usually of a pale yellow to white in **color**) that builds up on the teeth. If not removed regularly, it can lead to dental cavities (**caries**) or **periodontal** problems (such as **gingivitis**). Its clinical appearance is a soft, sticky, whitish film. It accumulates on teeth and other hard structures in the **mouth**, e.g., fillings, crowns, dentures, as well as **soft tissue**. On the microscopic level it is **bacterial biofilm**. 80–90% of plaque is microorganisms, mostly **bacteria**. It occasionally contains some nonbacterial organisms like **yeasts** and **viruses**. The remaining 10–20% are substances from **bacteria** as well as the host: sugars, **proteins**, **fats**, and minerals, e.g., calcium, phosphate, and traces of fluoride, host **epithelial cells**, and **immune cells**. **Dextran** is the most important bacterial by-product, formed from the breakdown of **sucrose**, it provides adhesive properties that influences plaque deposition. Three major steps of plaque formation are as follows: (1) soon after the **tooth** is cleaned, a thin layer of **proteins** from **saliva** (**pellicle**) deposit on **tooth** surface; (2) in spite of some antimicrobial action of the **pellicle**, **bacteria** can bind to certain components in the **pellicle** (the earliest colonizers tend to be **Gram-positive bacteria**, followed by **Gram-negative** and **anaerobic bacteria**); and (3) secondary-bacterial colonization and plaque maturation. It is estimated that more than 325 species of **bacteria** have been found in plaque out of the total potential of the over 500 **oral** bacterial species recorded. The late colonizers, which are typically found in the **oral cavity**, tend be main groups found in subgingival plaque. Eventually there occurs a microecosystem on the **tooth** surface, which is represented by gross plaque. This complex environment is also protective in that it helps prevent invasion by **exogenous bacteria**. As mineral content of plaque increases, it calcifies to form calculus/tartar. **Calcification** of plaque can occur just hours after plaque deposition, but calculus is usually seen two days later. Supragingival calculus is most commonly seen on the backs of lower-anterior teeth. The mineral in supragingival calculus comes from **saliva**. The mineral in subgingival calculus comes from **gingival crevicular fluid**. Plaque can further accumulate on calculus and act as a **tissue** irritant that causes an inflammatory response.

dentin: A hard, middle-calcified, elastic, yellowish material of the same substance as **bone**. It is the main structural part of a **tooth** extending from crown to root. **Dentin** is composed of base material that is pierced by mineralized dentinal tubules 1–5 μm in diameter, which makes it porous. Tubule density is in the range of $3–7.5 \times 10^6$ cm^{-2}. Dentin contains organic components and natural **hydroxyapatite** (**apatite**) crystals 2–3.5 nm in diameter and up to 100 nm in length, which intensively scatter **light**. On average, it contains 70% **hydroxyapatite** crystals, 20% **proteins** (e.g., **collagen**), and 10% **water**. Softer than **enamel** (but slightly harder than **bone**), but unlike **enamel**, **dentin** is living **tissue**. The **cells** that form **dentin** (odontoblasts) lie at the border of **dentin** and **pulp** during the life of a **tooth**, which gives **dentin** the ability to grow and repair.

dentinal hypersensitivity: Short, sharp **pain** that arises from exposed **dentin** in response to stimuli. **Pain** cannot be ascribed to any other dental defect or pathology. Stimuli are generally non-noxious, e.g., thermal, tactile. It is important to exclude other causes of short, sharp **pain** such as **caries**, fractured **tooth**, and leaky restorations. The "hydrodynamic theory" is the most accepted theory to date. Dentinal tubules contain fluid, and stimuli cause movement of this fluid, which is thought to trigger **nerves** in the **pulp**. Two events are required for **dentin** hypersensitivity: exposure of **dentin** and access to **pulp** through the **dentin** tubular system. Root exposure due to **gingival** recession is the most common situation in which **dentinal hypersensitivity** is found, when the **cementum** layer is lost and **dentin** becomes exposed to the **oral** environment. Natural **pulp**-protective mechanisms with continuous **irritation** include the formation of reparative **dentin** at the **dentin–pulp** interface, which creates a longer path for stimuli to travel and the formation of **sclerotic dentin** in which tubules are obliterated. The majority of sufferers are in the 20–40 age group.

Incidence decline in older age groups may be due to the lower permeability of **dentin** with age resulting from the formation of **sclerotic** and reparative **dentin**.

deoxyhemoglobin: Hemoglobin disintegrated with **oxygen**. It has a primary **absorption band** at 430 nm, and it has a single secondary **absorption band** at 555 nm. It exhibits the lowest **absorption** at **wavelengths** longer than 620 nm.

depolarization: Deprivation (destruction) of **light polarization**. When **polarized light** traces a **tissue** its **depolarization** (destruction of **light polarization**) occurs because of the complex character of **light** interaction with an inhomogeneous (**scattering**) medium (**tissue**).

depolarization length: Length of **light**-beam transport in a **scattering**-depolarizing medium at which the **degree of polarization** decays to the definite level compared to the totally polarized incident **light**. It is characteristic of interaction of **polarized light** with a **scattering** medium or a **tissue**.

depth of field (DOF): The portion of a scene that appears acceptably sharp in the image. Although a **lens** can precisely focus at only one distance (see **focal depth**), the decrease in sharpness is gradual on either side of the focused distance, so that within the depth of focus, the lack of sharpness is imperceptible under normal viewing conditions. In some specific cases, it may be desirable to have the entire image sharp, and a large **depth of field** is appropriate. At other times, a small **DOF** may be more effective. For example, for **optical coherence tomography**, a large **DOF**, and for **confocal microscopy**, a smaller one, are typical. The **DOF** is determined by the subject distance (the distance to the plane that is perfectly in focus), the **lens**-effective **focal length**, the **lens** F-**number**, and the format size. For a given format size, at moderate subject distances, **DOF** is approximately determined by the subject magnification and the **lens** F-**number**. For a given F-**number**, increasing the magnification, either by moving closer to the subject or using a **lens** of greater **focal length**, decreases the **DOF** (**microscopy** case). Decreasing magnification increases **DOF** (in the case of **optical coherence tomography**). For a given subject magnification, increasing the F**-number** (decreasing the aperture diameter) increases the **DOF**. Decreasing F**-number** decreases **DOF**. Digital technology provides additional means of controlling the extent of image sharpness even after the image is made.

depth of modulation: For amplitude **modulation**, this is the ratio of the amplitude of the alternating component of a signal to its mean value.

dermal papilla: Extensions of the **dermis** into the **epidermis**. They sometimes can be perceived at the surface of the **skin**.

dermatitis: Inflammation of the **skin**.

dermatosis: Any disease of the **skin**.

dermis: The inner layer of the **skin**. It is composed of **connective tissue**, **blood** and **lymph vessels**, **muscles**, and **nerves**. **Collagen fibers** are abundant in the **dermis** and run parallel to the surface of the **skin**, giving the **skin** elasticity. **Sweat glands** and **hair follicles** are scattered throughout the **dermis**. The **dermis** is much thicker than the **epidermis** and develops from mesoderm.

desorption: Phenomenon and process opposite of sorption (that is, adsorption or **absorption**), whereby some of a sorbed substance is released. This occurs in a system that is in the state of sorption equilibrium between bulk phase (fluid, i.e., a gas or liquid solution) and an adsorbing surface (a solid or a boundary separating two fluids). When the concentration (or **pressure**) of the substance in the bulk phase is lowered, some of the sorbed substance changes to the bulk state. In chemistry, especially chromatography, **desorption** is the ability of a chemical to move with the mobile phase; the more a chemical desorbs, the less likely it will adsorb. Thus, instead of sticking to the stationary phase, the chemical moves up with the solvent front.

desquamation: Shedding of the outer layers of **skin**, e.g., once the rash of measles fades, there is **desquamation**.

destructive interference: Interference of two waves of equal **frequency** and opposite phase, resulting in their cancellation where the negative displacement of one always coincides with the positive displacement of the other.

detectivity star (D*): Sensitivity figure of merit of an **infrared detector**. It is equal to the reciprocal of noise-equivalent power, which is normalized to the unit area and **bandwidth** of a **photodetector** so that higher D* values indicate better performance. It is taken at specific test conditions of chopping **frequency** and information **bandwidth** and displayed as a function of **wavelength**.

developed speckle: **Speckles** that are characterized by **Gaussian statistics** of the complex amplitude, the unity **contrast** of **intensity** fluctuations, and a negative exponential function of the **intensity probability** distribution (the most-probable **intensity** value in the corresponding **speckle** pattern is equal to zero, i.e., **destructive interference** occurs with the highest **probability**).

dextran: A complex, branched **polysaccharide** made of many **glucose** molecules joined into chains of varying lengths.

diabetes (*Synonym*: diabetes mellitus): Metabolic disorder characterized by **hyperglycemia** (high **blood** sugar). The World Health Organization recognizes three main forms of diabetes: Type 1, type 2, and gestational diabetes (occurring during pregnancy). These forms have similar signs, symptoms, and consequences, but different causes and population distributions. Type 1 is usually due to autoimmune destruction of the pancreatic beta **cells**, which produce **insulin**. Type 2 is characterized by **tissue**-wide **insulin** resistance and varies widely; it sometimes progresses to loss of beta-**cell** function.

diabetes mellitus: See **diabetes**.

diabetic retinopathy: Retinopathy (damage to the **retina**) caused by complications of **diabetes**, which can eventually lead to blindness. It is an ocular manifestation of systemic disease that affects up to 80% of all diabetics who have had **diabetes** for 15 years or more.

diagnostic window: See **therapeutic window**.

diaphanography: A **noninvasive** method of examining the **breast** or other human organ by transillumination using **visible** or **infrared light**.

diaphragm: A dome-shaped sheet of **tissue**, part **muscle** and part **tendon**, separating the thoracic and abdominal cavities.

diastolic: Related to diastole, that is, the period of time when the **heart** relaxes after contraction. Ventricular diastole is when the ventricles are relaxing, while atrial diastole is when the atria are relaxing.

diattenuation: See **dichroism**.

dichroic (dichromatic) filter (*Synonyms*: reflective, thin-film, and interference filters): Can be made by coating a glass substrate with a series of optical coatings using the principle of **interference**. They usually reflect the unwanted portion of the **light** and transmit the remainder. Their layers form a sequential series of reflective cavities that resonate with the desired **wavelengths**. Other **wavelengths** destructively cancel or reflect as the peaks and troughs of the waves overlap. They are widely used in **biophotonics**, because many **interference filters** with different central **wavelengths** and passbands are available on the market. Which **color** range and sharpness is used is determined by the thickness and sequence of the coatings. They can be used in devices such as the **dichroic (dichromatic) prism** and **dichroic (dichromatic) mirror (beamsplitter)** to separate a beam of **light** into different color components. The basic scientific instrument of this type is a **Fabry–Pérot interferometer (etalon)**.

dichroic (dichromatic) mirror (beamsplitter): A mirror made on the basis of thin-film technology by coating a glass substrate with a series of interferential optical coatings and used to split **light beams** into different color components.

dichroic (dichromatic) prism: An optical **prism** made on the basis of thin-film technology by coating the prism side with a series of interferential optical coatings. It is used to split **light beams** into different color components.

dichroism (*Synonym*: diattenuation): Phenomenon related to pleochroism of a **uniaxial crystal** so that it exhibits two different **colors** when viewed from two different directions under transmitted **light**. Pleochroism is the property possessed by certain crystals that exhibit a variety of **colors** when viewed from different directions under transmitted **light**: this is one exhibition of the optical anisotropy caused by the anisotropy of **absorption**. The types of pleochroism are circular **dichroism** (different **absorption** for **light** with right- and left-circular **polarization**) and linear **dichroism** (different **absorption** for ordinary and extraordinary rays). In **tissue** models, linear **dichroism**, i.e., different **wave attenuation** for two orthogonal **polarizations**, in systems formed by long cylinders or plates is defined by the difference between the imaginary parts of the effective indices of **refraction**. Depending on the relationship between the sizes and the optical constants of the cylinders or plates, this difference can take both positive and negative values. The magnitude of **diattenuation** is related to the density and other properties of the **collagen fibers**, whereas the orientation of the fast axis indicates the orientation of the **collagen fibers**.

dielectric polarization density (*Synonym*: macroscopic polarization): The quantity P that characterizes a dielectric material's response to electric field $\vec{E}$, i.e., $P = \chi \cdot \vec{E}$, where χ is the **electric susceptibility** of a material.

differential interference contrast (DIC) microscopy: A system that consists of a special **prism** (see **Nomarski polarizing interference microscope**, **Wollaston prism**) in the condenser that splits **light** into two beams with orthogonal **polarization** states— ordinary and extraordinary. The spatial difference between the two beams is minimal (less than the maximum resolution of the **objective**). After passing through the specimen, the beams are reunited by a similar **prism** in the **objective**. In a homogeneous specimen, there is no difference between the two beams, and no **contrast** is being generated. However, near a refractive boundary (say a **nucleus** within the **cytoplasm**), the difference between the ordinary and the extraordinary beams will generate a relief in the image. Differential **interference contrast** requires a **polarized light** source to function. Two polarizing filters have to be fitted in the **light** path, one below the condenser (the **polarizer**), and the other above the **objective** (the **analyzer**). Differences in **optical density** will show up as differences in relief. **Contrast** is very good and the condenser **aperture** can be used fully open, thereby reducing the **depth of field** and maximizing resolution. In cases where the optical design of a microscope produces an appreciable lateral separation of the two beams (classical **interference microscopy**), the result is not a relief image, but it can nevertheless be used for the quantitative determination of mass-thicknesses of microscopic objects.

differential optical-absorption spectroscopy (DOAS): A technique for measuring trace amounts of polluting molecules in the atmosphere or metabolic molecules in the human respiratory tract.

differential phase-sensitive optical coherence tomography (DPS OCT): This technique detects phase **contrast** in the direction of beam separation. Refractive-index variations cause phase variations in the sample beam. The **probe** beam is split by **birefringent wedges** and **collimated** by the sample **lens**. Two orthogonally polarized beams separated by a small distance x illuminate the sample. The backscattered beams are combined by the **birefringent wedges** and separated by the polarizing beamsplitter (**Wollaston prism**) in the detection **arm**. From the **photodetector** signals three interferograms and the corresponding three images are obtained: two **intensity** images, and a phase-difference image. Measurements of **Angstrom–nanometer**-scale pathlength change between the beams $[(\lambda/4\pi)\Delta\varphi]$ in clear and **scattering media** can be provided. **Differential phase-sensitive optical coherence tomography** was demonstrated to be suitable for **noninvasive**, sensitive, and accurate monitoring of analyte concentration, including **glucose**. It provides quantitative **dispersion** data that are important in predicting the propagation of **light** through **tissues**, in **photorefractive surgery**, and in **tissue** and **blood refractive index** measurements. It detects phase gradients caused by transversal variations of the **refractive index** and/or the phase change on **reflection** at interfaces.

diffraction: A phenomenon associated with a **wave** motion when a **wave** train (optical, acoustical, thermal, **photon**-density, etc.) passes the edge of an obstacle opaque to the **wave** motion. The phenomenon is a particular case of **interference**. The waves are bent at the edge of the obstacle, which acts as a source of secondary waves, all coherent. Interference between a primary **wave** and a secondary **wave** produces **diffraction** bands, which are, in fact, **interference** bands.

diffraction limited: When the resolution of an **optical imaging** system, namely, a microscope, telescope, or camera is fundamentally limited by **light diffraction**. An optical system with the ability to produce images with angular resolution as good as the instrument's theoretical **diffraction limit**. The resolution of a given instrument is proportional to the size of its **objective**, and inversely proportional to the **wavelength** of the **light** being observed. For optical systems with a circular aperture, the size of the smallest feature in an image that is **diffraction limited** is the size of the **Airy disk**. An empirical **diffraction limit** based on the assumption of a human observer is given by the Rayleigh criterion [see **Rayleigh (resolution) limit**]. The resolution R (measured as a distance) is $R = 1.22\lambda/(2n\sin\theta)$, where θ is the **lens** collecting angle, which depends on the width of **objective lens** and its focal distance from the specimen, n is the **refractive index** of the medium in which the **lens** operates, λ is the **light wavelength**, and the quantity $n\sin\theta$ is known as the **numerical aperture**. Light is illuminating or emitting (**fluorescence microscopy**) by the sample. For **visible light**, the best R is about 200 nm. Modern microscopes with video sensors may be slightly better than the human eye in their ability to discern overlap of **Airy disks**. For specialized imaging, foreknowledge of some characteristics of the image can also improve on technical resolution limits through computerized image processing. However, resolution below this theoretical limit can be achieved using **diffraction** techniques such as **4Pi-microscopy** and **STED microscopy** or their combination. Combined application of these two techniques by destructively focusing two beams on a point source allows one to resolve objects as small as 30 nm.

diffraction of photon-density wave (intensity wave): The bending of **photon density waves** around obstacles in their path. The phenomenon exhibited by wavefronts that are modulated when passing the edge of an opaque body, thereby causing a redistribution of **photon density wave** amplitude within the front. They are detectable by the presence of minute bands with high and low amplitudes at the edge of a shadow. The phenomenon is a particular case of **interference** between primary and secondary **photon density waves**.

diffractometry: Measuring techniques based on the phenomenon of **wave diffraction**.

diffuse optical imaging: **Optical imaging** based on selective detection of diffusing **photons** that carry information about macro-inhomogeneities within a **scattering** medium when used at various gating techniques for diffuse **photon** pathlengths. The reconstructed local **absorption** and **scattering** properties of the object are used for imaging of **tissue** pathology [see **diffuse optical tomography (DOS)**].

diffuse optical spectroscopy (DOS): Optical **spectroscopy** of highly **scattering media** (**tissues**) where measured spectra depend not only on **absorption** and **fluorescence** spectra of **chromophores** and **fluorophores** contained in the medium under study, but also on **scattering** properties of the object. Typically, **collimated transmittance** T_c, **total transmittance** T_t, and **diffuse reflectance** R_d are measured. Spatially resolved measurements with one or more irradiating and one or more detecting **fibers** separated by distances r_{sd} and orientated normally, or under some angle to the **tissue** surface, are often used. This last technique is more suitable for *in vivo* measurements. Time-resolved measurements with pulse or **intensity**-modulated probing **light beams** are also often used, especially in *in vivo* measurements (see **time-resolved spectroscopy** and **frequency-domain spectrometer**).

diffuse optical tomography (DOT): Optical tomography that is based on the measurements of **continuous-wave**, pulsed, or modulated **light**-beam **transmittance** or spatially resolved **reflectance** of **scattering media** with an object (i.e., **tumor**) hidden in it. Synchronous **light beam** detector scanning devices or systems with multiple fixed-position **light** sources and **photodetectors** are used to provide 3D images. The **backprojection algorithm** is used to provide image reconstruction along the paths of **ballistic photons** and/or least-**scattering photon** propagation. The method is used for tomography of thick **tissues** (**breast**, **brain**, **arm**).

diffuse photons: The **photons** that undertake multiple scattering with a broad variety of angles.

diffuse reflectance: **Optical reflectance** of a turbid sample R_d measured using the **integrating sphere**, which collects all **light** scattered in the backward direction.

diffuse reflection: Light scattered from the **scattering** sample (**tissue**) in the backward direction. This usually accounts for all reflected **light** with the exception of **Fresnel reflection (specular reflection)** from the object surface.

diffuse reflector: Surface that reflects a portion of the incident **radiation** in such a manner that the reflected **radiation** is equal in all directions. A mirror is not a **diffuse reflector**, but many **tissues** are.

diffusion: The process by which one gas mixes with another by the movement of the molecules of one gas into another and vice versa. The term is also used to characterize the action of two miscible liquids or a solid in contact with a solvent, the passage of molecules through a porous **membrane**, and the migration of any kind of particles within the **media** with collisions, including **photons**.

diffusion approximation (*Synonym*: diffusion theory): Approximated **diffusion**-type solution of the **radiative-transfer equation** that is accurate for describing **photon** migration in infinite, homogeneous, highly **scattering media**. **The diffusion approximation** criterion is that the **reduced scattering coefficient** be much bigger than the **absorption coefficient**, $\mu'_s \gg \mu_a$, typically $\mu'_s \sim 10$ cm^{-1} and $\mu_a \sim 0.1$ cm^{-1}.

diffusion coefficient: The proportionality coefficient between mean-square displacement of a particle within a time interval τ : $\langle \Delta r^2 \rangle \sim D\tau$. It may be related to molecular or **photon diffusion**.

diffusion theory: See **diffusion approximation**.

diffusion-wave spectroscopy (DWS): **Spectroscopy** based on the study of **dynamic light scattering** in dense **media** with **multiple scattering** and related to the investigation of the dynamics of particles within very short time intervals. Used for **blood-flow measurements** in highly **scattering tissues**, especially in **brain** and **cancerous breast tissue**.

digestive tract: See **gastrointestinal tract**.

digital electronic autocorrelator: A device that reconstructs with a high accuracy the time-domain **autocorrelation function** of **intensity** fluctuations.

digital holography: The technology of acquiring and processing holographic measurement data, typically via a **charge-coupled device (CCD)** camera or a similar device. In particular, this includes the numerical reconstruction of object data from the recorded measurement data, in contrast to an optical reconstruction that reproduces an aspect of the object. This method typically delivers 3D surface or **optical-thickness** data.

digital micromirror device (DMD): Every **pixel** on a DMD chip is a reflective mirror. A video image is displayed on the DMD chip. The micromirrors then tilt very rapidly as the image changes. This process produces the grayscale foundation for the image. In a single chip projection system, **color** is added as **light** passes through a high-speed **color** wheel and is reflected off of the micromirrors on the digital **light**-processing chip as they rapidly tilt toward or away from the **light** source. In more advanced projection systems that use a three-chip design (separate chips for red, green, and blue), the spinning **color** wheel is not required.

digital microscopy: The use of an optical microscope with a digital imaging system such as a **charge-coupled device (CCD)** or **complementary metal-oxide semiconductor (CMOS) camera**. See **transillumination digital microscopy (TDM)**.

113

digital oscilloscope: Device that analyzes with a high accuracy the waveform of alternating-current signals.

dimethyl sulfoxide (DMSO): Dimethyl sulfoxide is the chemical compound $(CH_3)_2SO$. This colorless liquid is an important polar-aprotic solvent. It is readily miscible in a wide range of organic solvents, as well as in **water**, and it can penetrate **skin** very readily, allowing the handler to taste it. This unique capability to penetrate living **tissues** without causing significant damage is probably related to its relatively polar nature, its capacity to accept hydrogen bonds, and its small and compact structure. This combination of properties results in its ability to associate with **water**, **proteins**, **carbohydrates**, **nucleic acid**, ionic substances, and other constituents of living systems.

diode laser: **Semiconductor** injection **laser**. This **laser** is pumped by electrical current through a multilayered **semiconductor** structure (**heterostructure**). One of the most widely used **diode lasers** is the **GaAs laser** with emission in the near infrared, at about 830 nm. More-complex compositions allowing one to have a desired **wavelength** and output **power** are also designed: GaP_xAs_{1-x} **lasers** [emit **light** from 640 nm (x = 0.4) to 830 nm (x = 0)], $Ga_xIn_{1-x}As_yP_{1-y}$ **lasers** at y = 2.2x and for different values of x, emit in the range from 920 to 1500 nm. The main **diode-laser radiation wavelengths** are 670, 780, 830, 1300, and 1550 nm, and their output **power** is from a few milliwatts to a few watts. Indium gallium nitride ($In_xGa_{1-x}N$) quantum-well structures are efficient **light** emitters. In **UV**, blue, and green **light-emitting diodes** and **diode lasers**, the emission **wavelength** depends on the material bandgap and can be controlled by the GaN/InN ratio [from near **UV** (390 nm) for 0.02 In/0.98 Ga and violet-blue (420 nm) for 0.1 In/0.9 Ga to blue (440 nm) for 0.3 In/0.7 Ga]. A series of powerful **lasers** from blue to **near-infrared** with **power** up to 50 W in the **near-infrared** are available on the market: 405 nm violet-blue **laser** (150 mW); 442 nm (50 mW), 447 nm (400 mW) blue **lasers**; 635 nm (5 W), 640 nm (300 mW), 655 nm (2.5 W), 685 nm (20 mW), 690 nm (800 mW), 705 nm (25 mW), 730 nm (30 mW) red **lasers**; and 785 nm (1.2 W),

114

808 nm (10 W), 830 nm (30 mW), 845 nm (30 mW), 885 nm (5 W), 915 nm (50 W), 940 nm (50 W), 965 nm (2 W), 975 nm (50 W), 980 nm (50 W), 1450 nm (500 mW), 1550 (600 mW), and 1560 nm (1 W) **near-infrared lasers**. Pb_xS_{1-x}, $Sn_xPb_{1-x}Te$, and $Sn_xPb_{1-x}Se$ **lasers**, for different values of x, emit in the range from 2.5 to 49 µm. **Diode-laser power** can vary greatly. A single diode irradiator may have a few watts in the output, and diode arrays and matrices may have up to 100 W. A **quantum-well laser** has a quantum-dimension **heterostructure** as a lasing medium, and owing to a high **gain**, it has a high slope of the **watt**/ampere characteristic and lower threshold currents. A single **diode-laser** emitter has a typical size of **laser aperture** of 1.5–100 µm and cavity length of 0.5–3 mm, with the maximal output **power** in the range of 0.5 to 10 W. High-**power** diode lasing is usually a plate planar array of **laser** bar with a **laser aperture** up to 10 mm; one **laser** bar comprises 10–90 single **laser** emitters with maximal output **power** in the range of 20 to several hundred watts. **Diode lasers** are the most efficient **lasers**, with efficiency up to 70%. They have a very high beam divergence of 50–90 deg in a fast axis and 5–20 deg in a slow axis; however, special micro-optics allow one to form a low-divergence beam and/or to provide coupling-diode **laser power** into the **fiber**. **Diode lasers** can work in the **continuous-wave** mode or in pulse mode by pulse-pumping electrical current. They are prospective **light** sources for photomedicine because of their high efficiency (conversion of electrical to **light energy**), their long life (often more than 10^5 h), and their ability to emit many different **wavelengths** from **UV** to **IR** with a high **power**. **Diode lasers** are also used for pumping other **lasers**, which allows the production of very robust and compact totally solid-state systems, such as a **diode-pumped solid-state (DPSS) laser** or a **fiber laser**.

diode-pumped solid-state (DPSS) laser: An integrated **solid-state laser** with a crystal lasing medium and optical pumping provided by a single **laser** diode or by a **laser** (**light**) diode array or matrix. For example, a diode-pumped **Nd:YAG laser**.

diole(o)ylphosphatidylethanolamine (DOPE): Neutral **lipid**, used as a carrier system.

115

dipole moment: Defined by the mutual displacement and charges of the system of two charged particles (model of molecule). It defines the electrical field of the electrically neutral system for the distances larger than its size and action of external fields on the system. At changes of **dipole moment**, the system is emitting **electromagnetic waves**.

dipropylene glycol: $HOC_3H_6OC_3H_6OH$, molecular weight 134.18, **refractive index** 1.438–1.442. It is a colorless, viscous, practically nontoxic, and slightly **hygroscopic** liquid with a melting point of 78 °C and a boiling point of 231 °C. The substance is miscible in **water**, **alcohols**, esters, and most organic solvents and various vegetable oils, and it is used as a solvent, coupling agent, and chemical intermediate in many fields, including **cosmetics**.

direct thermography: Thermal imaging and measurement of a surface whose thermal signature is, or is directly affected by, the target of concern, i.e., the target of concern has little or no thermal insulation between it and the surface measured.

disaggregation: The separation of an aggregate body into its component parts.

Discosomared (DS red): Red fluorescent **protein** of *Discosoma spp*.

disk laser: A high-**power**, **solid-state laser** based on a very thin lasing medium (typically 100–300 μm), which is integrated with one of the **laser mirrors** and thus can be efficiently cooled. Allows for high **power** generation at **diode-laser** pumping (see **diode-pumped solid-state (DPSS) laser**). Diameter of active (pumped) area is from 1 mm (for low-**power lasers**) up to 10 mm (for high-**power lasers**). **Yb:YAG lasers** and **Nd:YAG lasers** are commercially available. **Disk lasers** can work in single mode (TEM_{00}) regime with a high output **power** and high efficiency. The total efficiency including **laser** pumping and cooling is more than

25%. **Laser** working time can be up to 50,000 h. For example, a typical **Q-switched Yb:YAG disk laser** (1030 nm) has pulse duration of 300 ns, pulse **frequency** of 10 kHz, maximal pulse **energy** of 100 mJ, **peak power** above 200 kW, and can couple a **laser beam** coupled to **optical fiber** with a core diameter of 400 µm.

dispersion: In general, the state of being dispersed, for instance, such as a **photon** trajectory. Specifically in optics, it is the variation of the **index of refraction** of a transparent substance, such as a glass, with the **wavelength** of **light**. The **index of refraction** increases as the **wavelength** decreases, thus the separation of white or compound **light** into its respective **colors** is possible, as in the formation of a **spectrum** by a **prism** and other optical elements (see **chromatic dispersion**, **group-velocity dispersion**, **material dispersion**, **optical-fiber dispersion**, **phase-velocity dispersion**). In statistics, the **scattering** of values of a variable around the mean or median of a distribution. In chemistry, a system of dispersed particles suspended in a solid, liquid, or gas.

dispersion compensation: For example in **fibers**, all three types of **fiber dispersion** can be modified by the type and concentration of dopants used to control the **fiber** material **dispersion**. Designing the **fiber** parameters allows one to adjust the **waveguide dispersion** and the **modal dispersion**. A finite amount of positive **group-velocity dispersion** is needed in the application of **fiber**-grating compression of optical pulses, whereas finite negative **group-velocity dispersion** is needed for the generation and propagation of soliton pulses in a **fiber**. In most applications that use **fibers** to transmit optical signals, **dispersion** in a **fiber** causes undesirable spreading of the signal, limiting the **bandwidth** of transmission. Thus it is important to reduce the **dispersion** to close to zero. **Single-mode fibers** are the choice in that case because they have no **modal dispersion**. The zero-**dispersion** point of pure silica is near the window of a local minimum of **attenuation** at 1.3 µm (see **fiber near-infrared (NIR) transmission window**). Transmission systems based on this **wavelength** have the combined advantage of low **fiber attenuation** and low **dispersion**. The real minimum of **attenuation** appears at 1.55 μm. Therefore, it is important to shift the point of zero **dispersion** to this **wavelength**, which could be provided by a proper combination of used dopants and **waveguide** parameters (these are the so-called **dispersion**-shifted **fibers**). The close-to-zero **dispersion** in both 1.3- and 1.55-μm windows can also be accomplished by special profiling of the **fiber**, resulting in what is called "**dispersion**-flattened **fibers**," which have low **dispersion** in the region between 1.3–1.55 μm with zero crossings at both **wavelengths**. For **multimode fibers**, it is important to minimize the **modal dispersion**, which is minimal for $\alpha = 2 + \delta$ (see **modal dispersion**). In its turn, the value of δ depends on the dopants and the optical **wavelength**; in the **near-infrared** it is usually within the range of ±0.3 for most dopants. Therefore, the optimum profile for a low-**dispersion multimode fiber** is one close to a quadratic profile of a **graded-index fiber** ($\alpha \cong 2$). A **graded-index fiber** that has a minimum **modal dispersion** also has a minimum **waveguide** contribution to the intramode **dispersion** for each individual mode. There are multilayer **Bragg mirror** designs that have properties of chirped mirrors for **dispersion compensation**.

dissector: Transmitting television tube. It can be used as a coordinate-sensitive **photodetector**.

dissociation: General process in which ionic compounds (complexes, molecules, or salts) separate or split into smaller molecules, ions, or **radicals**, usually in a reversible manner. For instance, reversible **dissociation** of **collagen fibers**. **Dissociation** is the opposite of association and recombination.

distilled water: Produced by a process of distillation, having an **electrical conductivity** of not more than 10 μS/cm, and total dissolved solids of less than 10 mg/L. Distillation involves boiling the **water** and then condensing the steam into a clean container. The procedure kills **bacteria** and leaves most solid contaminants behind. For many applications, cheaper alternatives such as **deionized water** are used.

distribution-size function: Function that describes the distribution of **probability** of particle-size value over the size values in the system.

deoxyribonucleic acid (DNA): A long-chain compound formed from many **nucleotides** bonded together as units in the chain. A strand of **DNA** is formed from molecules of deoxyribose (a sugar) and molecules of phosphoric acid attached alternatively in a chain. It is found only in the **chromosomes** of animals and plants and in the corresponding structures in **bacteria** and **viruses**. The **DNA** chain is 2.2 to 2.6 nm, and one **nucleotide** unit is 0.33 nm long. Although each individual repeating unit is quite small, **DNA** polymers can be very large molecules containing millions of **nucleotides**. For instance, the largest human **chromosome** is approximately 220 million base pairs long. In living organisms, **DNA** usually exists as as a pair of molecules that are held tightly together. These two long strands are shaped as a double **helix**. **DNA** is made up of four building blocks, the **nucleotides** A, C, G, and T. Their molecular weights are not identical, however; to estimate **DNA** molecular weight, an average molecular weight of 342 Da (**daltons**) per **nucleotide** can be accepted. Because **DNA** is double stranded, a pair of **nucleotides** is 684 Da. For example, a bacterial **cell** has a million (10^6) **nucleotide** pairs per **cell**, thus its **DNA** molecular weight is 6.84×10^8 Da. Mammal **cells** have about 10^3 times more.

Doppler effect: The apparent change in the **frequency** of a **wave**, such as a **light wave** or **sound wave**, resulting from a change in the distance between the source of the **wave** and the receiver. In the limit where the speed of the **wave** is much greater than the relative speed of the source and observer (as is often the case with **electromagnetic waves**, e.g., **light**), the **Doppler-frequency shift** f_D between incident **wave** and **wave** scattered (reflected) by a movable object under angle θ is given by the relation: $f_D = (2n/\lambda_0) \cdot \sin(\theta/2) \cdot v \cdot \cos\phi$, where n is the **refractive index** of a **medium** where **light** propagates, λ_0 is the **wavelength** of the incident **light** in vacuum, v is the velocity of the movable object that scatters (reflects) **light**, and ϕ is the angle between directions of the incident **light** and motion of the object. The **Doppler effect** is the basis for a number of spectroscopies such as **Doppler spectroscopy, quasi-elastic light scattering (QELS) spectroscopy, spectroscopy** of **intensity fluctuations, photon-correlation spectroscopy**, and **diffusion-wave spectroscopy**, as well as a key phenomenon in **Doppler interferometry, optical coherence tomography**, and **Doppler optical coherence tomography**.

Doppler frequency shift: See **Doppler effect**.

Doppler interferometry: Dynamic dual-beam interferometry when the reference beam pathlength is scanned with a constant speed. The Doppler signal induced is the measuring signal for depth profiling of an object placed in the measuring beam. This method is used in partially coherent interferometry or **optical coherence tomography** of **tissues**. The technique is conventionally implemented with the use of a dual-beam **Michelson interferometer**. If the pathlength of **light** in the reference arm is changed with a constant linear speed v, then the signal arising from the **interference** between the **light** scattered in a backward direction (reflected) from a sample and **light** in the reference arm is modulated at the Doppler **frequency** (see **Doppler effect**) $\Delta f_D = (2n/\lambda_0) \cdot v$. Owing to the small **coherence length** of a **light** source l_c, the Doppler signal is produced by backscattered **light** only within a very small region (on the order of the **coherence length** l_c) that corresponds to the current optical pathlength in the reference arm. The **interference** signal at the Doppler **frequency**, which is determined by the scanning rate v of a mirror in the reference arm, is proportional to the coefficient of **reflection** of the nonscattered component from an optical inhomogeneity inside the examined **scattering** object, i.e., **tissue**. One can localize an inhomogeneity in the longitudinal direction by equalizing the lengths of the signal and reference arms of the

interferometer within the limits of the **coherence length** of the **light** source (typically ~1–10 μm).

Doppler microscopy: **Doppler spectroscopy** of a medium at a microscopic scale.

Doppler optical coherence tomography (Doppler OCT): Combines the Doppler principle with **optical coherence tomography** to obtain high-resolution tomographic images of static and moving constituents in highly **scattering tissues**. When **light** backscattered from a moving particle interferes with the reference beam, a **Doppler frequency shift** occurs in the **interference fringe**, $f_{Ds} = (2V_s n \cos \varphi)/\lambda_0$, where V_s is the velocity of a moving particle, n is the **refractive index** of the medium surrounding the particles, φ is the angle between particle flow and sampling beam, and λ_0 is the vacuum-center **wavelength** of the **light** source. Longitudinal-flow velocity (velocity parallel to the probing beam) can be determined at discrete user-specified locations in a turbid sample by measurement of the **Doppler frequency shift**. Transverse-flow velocity can also be determined from the broadening of the spectral **bandwidth** due to the finite numerical aperture of the probing beam. Scanning of the reference mirror of the optical coherence tomography system at velocity v produces a Doppler signal at **frequency** f_D. **Blood** or **lymph** flow with velocity V_s produces another Doppler signal on the **frequency** f_{Ds}, therefore, the signal of **Doppler optical coherence tomography** is proportional to $A(t) \cos[2\pi(f_D - f_{Ds})t + \varphi(t)]$, where $A(t)$ is the reflectivity and $\varphi(t)$ is the **phase shift** defined by a **scatterer** position. Fiber optic **Doppler optical coherence tomography** is widely used for measurements of directed **blood flow** in subsurface **vessels** under a layer of **tissue**. Electronic data processing allows for the separation of the signal characterizing the amplitude of backward **scattering** (which is necessary for the generation of a stationary tomogram of an object), from the Doppler signal (which characterizes the velocity of **scatterers** at a given point of an object). Optical microangiography is built on the basis of Doppler and **Fourier-domain optical coherence tomography (OCT)**.

Doppler spectroscopy: **Spectroscopy** based on the study of **dynamic light scattering** (**Doppler effect**) in **media** with **single scattering**, and related to investigation of the dynamics (velocity) of particles in measurements of the **Doppler frequency shifts** in the **frequency** of the waves scattered by the moving particles. It is used for **blood-flow measurements**.

dorsal: Term refers to anatomical structures that are either situated toward or grow from the top side of an animal or human. In humans, the top of the **hand** and foot are considered **dorsal**.

double-integrating sphere (DIS) technique: Technique for *in vitro* evaluation of the **optical parameters** of **tissue** samples (**absorption coefficient** μ_a, **scattering coefficient** μ_s, and **scattering anisotropy factor** g). Often combined with **collimated-transmittance** measurements, it implies either sequential or simultaneous measurement of three parameters: **Total transmittance** T_t (using the **integrating sphere**), **diffuse reflectance** R_d (using the **integrating sphere**), and **collimated transmittance** T_c (using a distant detector behind the **pinhole** at the top of the **integrating sphere**).

double-balanced mixer (DBM): An electronic device that serves for mixing two optically detected signals having the same modulation **radio frequency** but different amplitudes and phases.

double-distilled water: Abbreviated as ddH$_2$O, Bidest. water, or DDW, it is prepared by the double distillation of **water**. It was standard technology for production of highly purified laboratory **water** for biochemistry and trace analysis until combination methods of purification became widespread.

dry mouth (*Synonym*: xerostomia): A pathology characterized by lack of **saliva** production due to loss of **salivary gland tissue** or a problem with **saliva** secretion as a side effect of certain medications, **radiation** therapy, and **Sjögren's syndrome**. Other causes are **dehydration**, poorly controlled **diabetes**,

HIV, and sarcoidosis. Hundreds of medications are reported to cause **salivary gland dysfunction**. These medications include antidepressants, sedatives, antihistamines, and antihypertensives. Many of these medications interfere with **nerve** stimulation of **salivary glands** (anticholinergic effect). Others can impact the secretion of **water** into the ducts. As **radiation** of the **head** and **neck** is a therapy for **head** and **neck cancers**, the **salivary-gland tissue** that lies in the path of **radiation** can be destroyed as a therapy side effect. Hyposalivation is the clinical sign, and **dry mouth** is the symptom. Hyposalivation occurs when stimulated **salivary**-flow rate falls below 0.7 ml/min (normal values are around 1.5 ml/min). Symptoms of **dry mouth** are experienced when **glandular** fluid production falls by about 50%. In some rare cases the symptom of **dry mouth** can occur without lowered **salivary** flow, such as for **mouth** breathers and somatoform disorders. The following symptoms may be present in varying degrees depending on severity of **dry mouth**: difficulty chewing and swallowing, retention of food debris in the **mouth**, alterations in taste, burning sensation, sticky **tongue**, difficulty with speech, bad breath (**halitosis**), poor denture fit, loss of the antimicrobial benefit of **saliva**. A key aspect of "morning breath" is the minimal **salivary** flow at night. The following signs may be present in varying degrees depending on severity of **dry mouth**: dry **lips** and **mucosa**, fissured **tongue**, denture sores, **caries**, **oral** candidiasis (**yeast** infection), and malnutrition.

dual-axes confocal microscopy: The dual-axes architecture of **confocal microscopy** performs off-axis illumination and collection of **light** to overcome **tissue scattering**. As a result, greater dynamic range and **tissue penetration depth** can be achieved, allowing for the collection of vertical cross-sectional images in the plane perpendicular to the **tissue** surface. This view allows for greater sensitivity to subtle changes that alter the normal **tissue**-growth patterns and reveals early signs of disease processes compared to that provided by horizontal cross-sectional images.

dual-beam coherent interferometry: See **Doppler interferometry**.

duct: A tube with an outlet that discharges fluids from one system to another, e.g., the **bile duct** discharges **bile** from the **liver** into the alimentary canal, or milk drains through **ducts** into a cistern in the mammary **gland**.

ductal-carcinoma *in situ*: See **duct** and **carcinoma**.

duodenum: The first section of the **small intestine**, where most chemical digestion takes place. In humans it is a hollow, jointed tube about 25–30 cm long connecting the **stomach** to the **jejunum**.

dura mater (*Synonym*: pachymeninx): The tough and inflexible outermost of the three layers of the meninges surrounding the **brain** and **spinal cord**. The *dura mater* itself has two layers: a superficial layer, which is actually the skull's inner periosteum, and a deep layer, the *dura mater* proper.

dye laser: A **laser** in which the **laser** medium is a liquid dye. **Dye lasers** emit in a broad spectral range (e.g., in the **visible**) and are tunable. **Wavelength** range is from 340–960 nm [with usage of such dyes as stilbene (390–435 nm), coumarin 102 (460–515 nm), **rhodamine** 6G (570–640 nm), and many others]— at **optical frequency doubling**, from 217 to 380 nm, and at optical-parametric conversion, from 1060 to 3100 nm. Emitted **energy** is from 1 mJ to 50 J in periodic-pulse mode. Mean **power** is from 0.06–20 W. Pulse duration is from 0.007 to 8 μs. Pulse **frequency** is from a single pulse to 1 kHz. Used in **spectroscopy** and photochemistry of biological molecules, it is a good universal tool for different areas of photomedicine and is one of the best **lasers** for **blood-vessel coagulation**.

dynamic light scattering: Light **scattering** by a moving object that causes a **Doppler-frequency shift** of the scattered **wave** relative to the **frequency** of the incident **light**. It is a fundamental basis for **Doppler spectroscopy** or **quasi-elastic light scattering (QELS) spectroscopy**, **spectroscopy**

of **intensity** fluctuations, **photon-correlation spectroscopy**, and **diffusion-wave spectroscopy**.

dynode chain of the PMT: A system of electrodes, each of which serves for emission of secondary electrons in a vacuum tube.

dysfunction: Any disturbance in the function of an organ or body part.

dysplasia: An abnormality in the appearance of **cells** indicative of an early step toward transformation into a **neoplasia**. It is therefore a preneoplastic or **precancerous** change. This abnormal growth is restricted to the originating system or location, e.g., a displasia in the **epithelial cell** layer will not invade into the deeper **tissue**, and a displasia solely in a **red-blood-cell** line (refractory anaemia) will stay within the **bone marrow** and cardiovascular systems. The best-known form of displasia is **cervical-intraepithelial neoplasia**, the precursor **lesions** to **cervical cancer**. This **lesion** is usually caused by an infection with the **human papilloma virus**.

dysplastic: Related to **dysplasia**.

ear: The sense organ that detects sound. The vertebrate **ear** shows a common biology from fish to humans, with variations in structure according to order and species. It not only acts as a receiver for sound, but plays a major role in the sense of balance and body position. The word **ear** may be used correctly to describe the whole vertebrate **ear** or just the **visible** portion. In most animals, the **visible ear** is a flap of **tissue** that is also called the pinna, although in humans, the pinna is more often called the auricle. In **biomedical optics** the **lobe** of the human **ear** is used as convenient model for **noninvasive blood oxygenation** and **microcirculation** studies. In animals such as rats, mice, and rabbits, the pinna is used as an *in vivo* model for **noninvasive blood** studies.

ectodermal dysplasia: A hereditary condition characterized by abnormal development of the **skin**, **hair**, nails, teeth, and **sweat glands**.

edema: Effusion of serous fluid into the interstices of **cells** in **tissue** spaces or into body cavities.

effective emissivity: Also called **emittance**, it is the measured emissive value of a particular surface under existing measurement conditions (rather than the generic tabulated value for the surface material) that can be used to correct a specific measuring instrument to provide a correct temperature measurement.

effective-attenuation coefficient: The exponential decay rate of **fluence** far from the **light** source, $\mu_{eff} = [3\mu_a(\mu'_s + \mu_a)]^{1/2}$, where μ_a is the **absorption coefficient** and μ_s is the **scattering coefficient**. Also referred to as inverse-**diffusion** length, $\mu_{eff} = 1/l_d$, 1/cm.

efficacy: A measure of the effectiveness of a lamp (see **halogen lamp**, **krypton-arc lamp**, **mercury-arc lamp**, **xenon-arc lamp**) in converting electrical **power** to **light**. Measured in **lumens** per **watt** (lm/W).

elastic (static) light scattering: Light **scattering** by static (motionless) objects that occurs elastically, without changes in **photon energy** or **light frequency**.

elastin: An elastic, **fibrous protein** resistant to boiling and to **acetic acid**. It forms highly elastic **yellow fibers** in **connective tissue**. **Elastin** is formed and maintained in **tissues** by **fibroblasts**.

elastography: A **noninvasive** method in which stiffness or strain images of **soft tissue** are used to detect or classify its mechanical properties and therefore to investigate **lesions** and pathologies. For example, a **tumor** or a suspicious **cancerous** growth is normally 5–30 times stiffer than the background of normal **soft tissue**, thus, applied mechanical compression or vibration deforms the **tumor** less than the surrounding **tissue**. A strain image may, under particular simplifying assumptions, be interpreted as representative of the underlying Young's modulus distribution. Ultrasonic imaging (see **ultrasonography**) is the most common medical-imaging technique for producing elastograms. For example, transient **ultrasound elastography** is applied to *in vivo* monitoring of **liver** elasticity and its **correlation** with the fibrosis score (or cirrhosis). Other techniques, such as **magnetic-resonance-imaging (MRI) elastography** and **computed tomography** are also used. However, **ultrasound** has the advantages of being cheaper, faster, and more portable than these techniques. Optical **elastography** based on **speckle**, **optical coherence tomography**, and **holographic interferometry** is a promising approach for clinical studies, but before it can be employed as a reliable diagnostic tool, more fundamental work remains.

elastosis: Breakdown of elastic **tissue**, e.g., the loss of elasticity in the **skin** of elderly people that results from degeneration of **connective tissue**.

electrical conductance: Measures how easily electricity flows along a certain path through an electrical element. The **SI**-derived unit of conductance is the **siemens**. For purely resistive circuits, **electrical conductance** is related to **electrical resistance** by: $G = 1/R$, where R is the **electrical resistance**. This is true for the real impedances only.

electrical conductivity: (*Synonym*: specific conductance) A measure of a material's ability to conduct an electric current. When an electrical potential difference is placed across a conductor or **semiconductor**, its movable charges flow, giving rise to an electric current. The conductivity σ is defined as the ratio of the current density j to the electric field strength $E : j = \sigma E$. For anisotropic materials the conductivity is a 3×3 matrix (a rank-2 tensor), which is generally symmetric. The conductivity is the inverse of

127

electrical resistivity ρ and has the **SI** units of **siemens** per meter (S/m): $\sum = 1/\rho$, where ρ is in ohm/m.

electrical resistance: A measure of opposition of an object to the passage of a steady electric current through it. An object of uniform cross section A will have an **electrical resistance** R proportional to its length l, inversely proportional to its cross-sectional area, and proportional to the resistivity of the material: $R = \rho l/A$ (measured in **SI** units as ohms, Ω), where ρ is the static **electrical resistivity** [measured in ohm × meters (Ω × m)]. R is the inverse of **electrical conductance** measured in **siemens**. For a wide variety of materials and conditions, R does not depend on the amount of current through or the potential difference (voltage) across the object, meaning that the **resistance** R is constant for the given temperature and material. Therefore, the **resistance** of an object can be defined as the ratio of voltage (V) to current (I), in accordance with Ohm's law: $R = V/I$.

electrical resistivity: Specific **electrical resistance** or volumetric resistivity. It is a measure of how strongly a material opposes the flow of electric current. Low resistivity indicates a material that readily allows the movement of electrical charge. **Electrical resistivity** is defined as $\rho = E/j$, where ρ is the static resistivity (in **SI** units measured in volt × meters per ampere, V × m/A). E is the magnitude of the electric field (volts per meter, V/m) and j is the magnitude of the current density (amperes per square meter, A/m^2). The **electrical resistivity** ρ can also be given as $\rho = R(A/l)$, where ρ is the static resistivity [ohm × meters (Ω×m)]. R is the **electrical resistance** of a uniform specimen of the material (ohms, Ω) and l is the length of the piece of material (meters, m). A is the cross-sectional area of the specimen (square meters, m^2).

electric susceptibility: A measure of how easily dielectric material polarizes in response to an electric field, which, in turn, determines the electric **permittivity** of the material and thus influences many phenomena in that medium, such as the **speed of light**. Linear susceptibility is defined as the constant of proportionality (which may be a tensor) relating an electric field $\vec{E}$ to the induced **dielectric-polarization density** P, i.e., the **macroscopic polarization**.

electroendosmosis: See **electro-osmosis**.

electromagnetic radiation (EMR) (*Synonym*: electromagnetic wave (EMW)): Has the form of self-propagating waves in a vacuum or in matter and consists of electric- and magnetic-field components that oscillate in phase perpendicular to each other and perpendicular to the direction of **energy** propagation. **Electromagnetic radiation** is classified in order of increasing **frequency** and decreasing **wavelength** as radio waves, microwaves, **terahertz radiation**, **infrared radiation**, **visible light**, **UV radiation**, **x-rays**, and gamma rays. A small window of frequencies is sensed by the human eye and called the **visible spectrum**, or **light**. **Electromagnetic radiation** carries **energy** and momentum that may be imparted to matter with which it interacts.

electromagnetic resonance: Appears at interaction of the incident **radiation** with molecules attached to a rough metallic surface. Induced due to collective excitation of conduction electrons in small metallic structures. Also called **surface-plasmon resonance**. **Surface-enhanced Raman scattering (SERS)** is based on such electromagnetic effect.

electromagnetic wave (EMW): See **electromagnetic radiation (EMR)**.

electromagnetic-interference (EMI) noise (*Synonym*: radio-frequency interference (RFI)): Disturbances to electrical signals caused by electromagnetic **interference** or radio-frequency interference. In thermography, this may cause noise patterns to appear on the display.

electron-multiplying charge-coupled device (EMCCD): Also known as an L3Vision charge-coupled device (L3CCD or Impactron CCD), is a **charge-coupled device (CCD)** in which a **gain** register is placed between the shift register and the output **amplifier**. The **gain** register is split up into a large number of stages, in each stage the electrons are multiplied by impact ionization in a similar way to an **avalanche diode**. The **gain probability** at every stage of the register is small ($P < 2\%$) but because the number of elements is large ($N > 500$), the overall **gain** can be very high [$g = (1 + P)^N$], with single-input electrons giving many thousands of output electrons. Reading a signal from a charge-coupled device gives a noise background, typically a few electrons. In an **electron-multiplying charge-coupled device**, this noise is superimposed on many thousands of electrons rather than a single electron. The devices thus have negligible readout noise. **Electron-multiplying charge-coupled devices** show a similar sensitivity to intensified **charge-coupled devices**, between 10^{-11} and 10^{-14} W· cm^{-2}. **Electron-multiplying charge-coupled-device** cameras need a cooling system to cool the device chip down to temperatures around 170 K.

electronic energy transfer (EET): See **Förster resonance energy transfer (FRET)**.

electronic excitation: An **electronic transition** for which an electron in an atom is activated (given more **energy**). The electron moves to an **energy** level farther from the atom nucleus.

electronic micrograph: Micrographs of **tissue** and/or **cell** components received with the help of the **electronic microscope**.

electronic microscope: A parallel beam of electrons from an electron gun is passed through a very thin slice of **tissue**. Differential **scattering** of the electron beam takes place, and an image of **tissue** microstructure is carried forward in the electron beam. The electron **lens** is used to focus the electron beam on a fluorescent screen, where a magnified image is formed. The image is registered using an optical camera. The resolving power of the **electronic microscope** is very much greater than that of a **light microscope**.

electronic noise: A noise that is caused by random fluctuations in an electrical signal and is characteristic of all electronic circuits. Noise generated by electronic devices varies greatly, as it can be produced by several different effects. **Thermal noise** and **shot noise** refer to a **white noise** and are inherent to all devices and define fundamental limitations of signal processing. Other types of noise depend mostly on manufacturing quality and material defects, such as **pink noise (flicker noise), burst noise**, or **radio-frequency** noise generated by an **avalanche photodiode**. A **dark noise** of a **photodetector** is also an **electronic noise**. Noise **power** is measured in **watts** or **decibels (dB)** relative to a standard **power**. The spectral distribution of noise can vary with **frequency**, so its **power density** is measured in watts per **hertz** (W/Hz). Because the **power** in a resistive element is proportional to the square of the voltage across it, noise voltage (density) can be described by taking the square root of the noise **power density**, resulting in volts per root **hertz** ($V/Hz^{1/2}$).

electronic transition: When an electron in an atom is activated (given more **energy**) the electron moves to an **energy** level farther from the atom nucleus. When an electron moves back to a lower level, **energy** is given out as **electromagnetic radiation**.

electronic wave function: The magnitude of the **wave** function (ψ) represents the varying amplitude of the stationary-**wave** system, in 3D it represents an electron situated around a nucleus. Associated with the stationary **wave** is a **frequency**, ν; ψ^2 is the density of electron per unit volume; $\psi^2 dV$ is the **probability** of finding the electron, when it is considered as a particle, in a volume dV. The total volume of the orbital gives a **probability** of unity. The effective electrical charge associated with a volume dV is $-e\psi^2 dV$, where e is the charge of an electron. The four quantum numbers define possible states of the stationary waves.

electro-osmosis (*Synonym*: electroendosmosis): The motion of polar liquid through a **membrane** or other porous structure (generally, along charged surfaces of any shape and also through nonmacroporous materials, which have ionic sites and allow for **water** uptake. The latter is sometimes referred to as "chemical **porosity**") under the influence of an applied electric field.

electrophoresis: Movement of colloidal particles in an electric field. When two platinum electrodes connected to a direct-current supply are placed in a lyophobic solution (the disperse phase has no attraction for the continuous phase), the colloidal particles will move either to **cathode** or anode depending on the charge on the particle. Used for drug delivery in medicine.

electroporation: A short pulse of voltage in the range 5–200 V · cm^{-2} applied to a biological **membrane** induces its **porosity**, which enhances **membrane** permeation for big molecules.

embryo: A multicellular diploid **eukaryote** in its earliest stage of development, from the time of first **cell** division until birth. In humans, it is called an **embryo** until about eight weeks after fertilization, and from then it is instead called a fetus. The development of the **embryo** is called embryogenesis. In organisms that reproduce sexually, once a sperm fertilizes an egg **cell**, the result is a **cell** called the zygote that has half of the **DNA** of each of the two parents. See also **pre-embryos**.

emission spectroscopy: Based on measurement of the **emission spectrum** of a chemical element or chemical compound. The relative **intensity** at each **wavelength** of **electromagnetic radiation** emitted by the preliminary excited element's atoms or the compound's molecules when they are returned to a ground state. Each element's **emission spectrum** is unique and characterizes element concentration. Thus, **spectroscopy** can be used to identify the elements and determine their concentration in matter of unknown composition. Similarly, the emission spectra of molecules can be used in chemical analysis of substances. In **emission spectroscopy**, different techniques for sample atomization and ionization are used, such as for flame, arc/spark dischargers, microwave heating, electron beam, and **laser evaporation**. For example, the sample containing the relevant substance to be analyzed is drawn into the burner and dispersed into the flame as a fine spray. The solvent evaporates first, leaving finely divided solid particles that move to the hottest region of the flame where gaseous atoms and ions are produced. Here electrons in atoms are excited effectively and emit **light**, which is commonly detected by a **spectrometer**. **Emission spectroscopy** is a well-developed, routine technique widely used for the investigation of different biological materials in medicine and criminology to identify extremely small amounts of metabolic products, drugs, or foreign molecules in human **tissues** and **blood**. See also **laser-induced-breakdown spectroscopy (LIBS)** and **laser microspectral analysis (LMA)**.

emission spectrum: The emission obtained from a luminescent material at different **wavelengths** when it is excited by a narrow range of shorter **wavelengths**.

emissivity: Ratio of a target-surface's **radiance** to that of a **blackbody** at the same temperature, viewed from the same angle and over the same spectral interval. It is a generic look-up value for a material with values ranging from 0 to 1.0. Alternatively, the ratio of a flat, optically polished, opaque target surface **radiance** to that of a **blackbody** at the same temperature, viewed from the same angle and over the same spectral interval. The latter definition characterizes the property of the material. When defined this way, **emittance** is used to characterize the material when it is other than flat, optically polished, and opaque.

emittance: The ratio of a target surface's **radiance** to that of a **blackbody** at the same temperature, viewed from the same angle over the same spectral interval. A generic look-up value for a material. Values range from 0 to 1.0.

enamel: A hard (hardest **tissue** in a body), elastic, white material that contains no **cells** and that is almost a completely inorganic substance. **Enamel** covers the crown of a **tooth**. Dental **enamel** consists of 87–95% natural **hydroxyapatite** (**apatite**) crystals and the rest are **water** and **proteins**. Crystals are organized in keyhole-shaped interlocking rods and prisms. These rods are formed as **enamel**-forming ameloblasts migrate toward the outer layer of **tooth**. Once **enamel** is formed, ameloblasts die. Thus if **enamel** is destroyed, it cannot be regenerated. These rods/prisms are 4–6 µm wide and extend from the dentine-**enamel** junction to the outer surface of the **tooth**. Because of their size, number, and **refractive index**, the prisms are the main **light scatterers** in **enamel**. It is translucent and grayish white in **color**, it has yellow **hue** due to underlying **dentin**.

encapsulated drugs: Encapsulation of some drugs significantly reduce their toxicity (gastrointestinal, **cutaneous**, etc.) especially at the higher-dose level and often increases drug efficiency. Various encapsulation technologies are used, including **liposomes**.

endocard (endocardium): The serous **membrane** that lines the cavities of the **heart**.

endogenous: "Arising from within." **Endogenous** substances are those that originate from within an organism, **tissue**, or **cell**. In biological systems, endogeneity refers to the recipient of **DNA** (usually in **prokaryotes**). However, due to homeostasis, discerning between internal and external influences is often difficult.

endoplasmic reticulum (ER): An elaborate series of membranous sacs that communicate with each other in a 3D network and occur in the endoplasm of a **cell**. The connection between two sacs is an anastomosis. **Endoplasmic reticulum** is either rough surfaced or smooth surfaced. Rough **endoplasmic reticulum** carries **ribosomes** on the outside surface of the sacs. Smooth **endoplasmic reticulum** carries no **ribosomes**. The functions of **endoplas-**

mic reticulum include the transfer of materials in **cells** by providing a circulatory system of channels, the formation of **lysosomes**, and **lipid metabolism**.

endoscope: A rigid or flexible tube that contains a **light**-delivery system to illuminate the organ or object under inspection (the **light** source is normally outside the body and the **light** is typically directed via an optical-**fiber** system). It includes a **lens** system transmitting the image to the viewer from the fiberscope, and an additional channel to allow entry of medical instruments or manipulators. There are a number of different **endoscopes** equipped with diagnostic **lasers** as **light** sources for quantitative imaging and **spectroscopy** using **light reflectance**, **fluorescence**, or **Raman scattering**. Endoscopic **optical coherence tomography** and **confocal microscopy** systems, as well as **endoscopic nonlinear optical imaging** systems are also available. **Endoscopes** are used to deliver optical **radiation** from high-**power lasers** to provide a minimally **invasive laser** surgery of internal organs.

endoscopic nonlinear optical imaging: Advances in **fiber optics**, micro-optics, and miniaturized optical and/or mechanical scanners have promoted rapid development and clinical translation of nonlinear optical (e.g., **two-photon fluorescence** and **second harmonic generation**) **microscopy** enabling depth-resolved endomicroscopic imaging of internal organs with unprecedented resolution. An all-**fiber**-optic rapid-scanning nonlinear optical-imaging endomicroscope for basic laboratory research, translational early disease detection, and image-guided interventions has been designed.

endoscopic optical coherence tomography: Application of the **fiber** optical **light**-delivering and **light**-collecting cables allows one to build the flexible low-coherent imaging system providing the possibility of endoscopic analysis of human **tissue**s and organs. The typical **optical coherence tomography** system developed for endoscopic applications (high-speed *in* *vivo* intra-arterial imaging) uses a solid-state Cr^{+4}:Forsterite **laser** with Kerr **lens mode-locking** as an illumination source with a median **wavelength** of 1280 nm and a **bandwidth** of 75 nm. It provides actual depth resolution with a **pixel** size equal to 9.2 μm, a lateral resolution of 30 μm, and confocal parameter of 1.74 mm. Electronics allow one to capture 4 frames per second for 512 transverse image **pixels**. The reference-arm phase-delay scanning device consists of an oscillating galvanometer mirror, **lens**, and grating. A whole family of diagnostic **endoscopic optical coherence tomography** devices suitable for studying the internal organs has been created on the basis of a miniaturized electromechanical unit (optical probe) for controlling and performing lateral scanning. This probe is located at the distal end of the sample arm, and its size fits the diameter and the curvature radius of standard **biopsy** channels of **endoscopes**. The probing beam is swung along the **tissue** surface with amplitude of 2 mm. The distance between the output **lens** and a sample varies from 5 to 7 mm. The focal-spot diameter is 20 μm. Implementation of an extended flexible arm of the **OCT interferometer** became feasible through the use of **polarization-maintaining fibers** as a means for transportation of the low-coherence probing **light**. This eliminates **polarization** fading caused by **polarization** distortions at the bending of the **endoscope** arm. The device features high-quality **fiber polarizers** and **couplers**. The "single-frame" dynamic range of the **optical coherence tomography** scheme determined as the maximum variation of the reflected signal **power** within a single image frame attains 35–40 dB with the scanning rate of 45 cm/s and the image depth of 3 mm (in free-space units). An **optical coherence tomography** image with 200×200 **pixels** is acquired for approximately 1 s. This **acquisition rate** is sufficient to eliminate influence of movement of internal organs (moving **artifacts**) on the image quality. A high-resolution **optical coherence tomography** balloon-imaging catheter and an ultrathin **optical coherence tomography** imaging needle have also been designed.

endoscopy: Minimally **invasive** diagnostic and/or surgery medical procedures that are used to assess the interior surfaces of an organ by inserting an **endoscope** into the body. The instrument may have a rigid or flexible tube and not only provide an image for visual inspection and photography but also enable taking biopsies and retrieving foreign objects.

endothelium: A single layer of **squamous cells** lining the **heart**, **blood vessels**, and **lymph vessels**. The **cells** are tessellated, i.e., have wavy boundaries that interdigitate, or fit together. **Endothelium** is morphologically similar to **epithelium**, but is derived from mesoderm.

energy: The ability of **light** (as well as other forms of **energy**, such as mechanical, thermal, electrical, chemical, and nuclear) to produce some work. **Energy** E is measured in **joules** (J), it is the product of **power** (**watts**) (W) and time (sec or s). The smaller and bigger energetic units are in use in **biomedical optics** and photomedicine to characterize **light** sources and delivery optics, such as the microjoule (μJ), 10^{-6} J; the millijoule (mJ), 10^{-3} J; and the kilojoule (kJ), 10^{3} J.

energy density (*Synonym*: **fluence**): The photophysical, photochemical, or photobiological effects produced by light's interaction with **tissues** are dependent on **energy density** and/or **power density** that is provided within the target area. **Energy density** or **fluence** is the **energy** of the **light wave** that propagates through a unit area that is perpendicular to the direction of propagation of the **light wave**. **Fluence** is measured in J·cm^{-2} or J·m^{-2}. The relationship between **fluence** (F) and **intensity** (I) is given by: $F = I \times \tau_p$, where τ_p is the length of pulse (**pulsewidth**) or exposure time. In inhomogeneous **light-scattering media** to which **tissues** belong, the **fluence rate** parameter is often used.

en face **image:** See **C-scan**.

enteric nervous system: A subsystem of the peripheral **nervous system**, which has the capacity, even when severed from the

137

rest of the **nervous system** through its primary connection by the vagus **nerve**, to function independently in controlling the **gastrointestinal tract**.

entropy: A measure of the amount of disorder in a system. The more disordered the system, the higher the **entropy**. An **entropy** change occurs when a system absorbs or evolves heat. The change in **entropy** ΔS is measured as the heat change ΔQ divided by the temperature T at which the change takes place, $\Delta S = \Delta Q / T$.

environmental rating: A rating applied to an operating unit (typically an electrical or mechanical enclosure) to indicate the limits of the environmental conditions under which the unit will function reliably and within published performance specifications.

enzyme: A **protein** produced by a living **cell** that acts as a catalyst in biochemical changes. There are many different types of **enzymes**, some of which promote a narrow range of chemical reactions on chemically related substances. Most others promote a single chemical reaction. Most metabolic chemical reactions are dependent on **enzymes** to promote them at the rate required for an organism to function properly. A very small quantity of an **enzyme** is sufficient to convert a large quantity of a substance. Each **enzyme** has optimum conditions for its action, e.g., temperature about 35–40 °C, a specific pH, the presence of a **coenzyme** for some reactions, and the absence of inhibiting substances.

eosin: A fluorescent red dye resulting from the action of bromine on **fluorescein**, used to stain **cytoplasm**, **collagen**, and **muscle fibers** for examination under the microscope. Structures that stain readily with **eosin** are termed *eosinophilic*. There are actually two very closely related compounds both commonly referred to as **eosin**. One is **eosin** Y, a tetrabromo derivate of **fluorescein** (also known as **eosin** Y ws, **eosin** yellowish, Acid Red 87, C.I. 45380, bromoeosine, bromofluoresceic acid, D&C Red No. 22), which is very slightly yellowish. The other is **eosin** B, a dibromo dinitro derivate of **fluorescein** (also known as **eosin** bluish, Acid Red 91,

C.I. 45400, Saffrosine, **Eosin** Scarlet, or imperial red), which is very slightly bluish. The two dyes are interchangeable. **Eosin** is most often used as a counterstain to **hematoxylin** in **H&E stain**.

epicard (epicardium): The inner serous layer of the pericardium, lying directly upon the **heart**.

epidermal-stripping sample: A thin slice of **epidermis** obtained with the use of medical glue and a quartz (glass) or metal plate.

epidermis: The outer layer of the **skin**. It is a stratified **epithelium** that varies relatively little in thickness over most of the human body (between 75–150 μm), except on the palms and soles, where its thickness may be 0.4–0.6 mm. The **epidermis** is conventionally subdivided into (1) *stratum basale*, a basal-**cell** layer of **keratinocytes**, which is the germinative layer of the **epidermis**; (2) the *stratum spinosum*, which consists of several layers of polyhedral **cells** lying above the germinal layer; (3) the *stratum granulosum*, which is a layer of flattened **cells** containing distinctive cytoplasmic inclusions (**keratohyalin granules**); and (4) the overlying **stratum corneum**, consisting of lamellae of anucleate thin, flat squames that are terminally differentiated **keratinocytes**. Besides the body site, epidermal thickness is related to age, gender, **skin** type, pigmentation, and **blood** content. The mean thickness of the *stratum corneum* is ~18 μm at the **dorsal** aspect of the **forearm**, ~11 μm at the shoulder, and ~15 μm at the buttock. Corresponding values for the cellular **epidermis** (*stratum granulosum*, *stratum spinosum*, and *stratum basale*) are ~57 μm, 70 μm, and 81 μm, respectively. For the whole **epidermis** thickness of ~81 μm, its layers are typically ranged from top to bottom as the following: 0–11 μm is occupied by the **stratum corneum**, 11–34 μm by the *stratum granulosum*, 34–64 μm by the *stratum spinosum*, and 64–81 μm by the *stratum basale*.

epidural: Related to the *dura mater*.

epi-fluorescence interference and absorption-filter combinations: Typically include an excitation filter, **dichroic (dichromatic) mirror (beamsplitter)**, and a barrier (or emission) filter that are housed in a filter cube (or optical block). The appropriate filter set is selected to match the spectral excitation and emission characteristics of **chromophores**, e.g., used in widefield **fluorescence-microscopy** investigations. Nikon **fluorescence**-filter combinations are provided in narrow-, medium-, and wide-passband excitation versions with corresponding emission filters available with either band-pass or long-pass spectral characteristics.

Epi-LASIK: Refers to **laser** refractive surgery and can be considered as superficial **laser-assisted** *in situ* **keratomileusis (LASIK)**. However, it is more similar to **laser**-assisted subepithelial **keratectomy** or **laser-assisted epithelial keratomileusis (LASEK)**, where instead of chemical **epithelial cell** layer thickening by **alcohol**, a mechanical procedure is explored. Unlike with **alcohol** there is no chance of damaging the limbal stem **cells**, and it is also relatively less painful than **LASEK**.

episclera: The layer of the eye **sclera**.

epithelial cells: Cells that cover or line the body surface and cavities. Keratinized **epithelium** is structured to withstand abrasion. Keratin is a **protein** produced by mature **epithelial cells** called **keratinocytes**.

epithelial tissue: Tissue consisting of a sheet of **epithelial cells** held together by a minimal amount of cementlike material between the **cells**. It covers exposed surfaces and lines the cavities and tubes of the body. Beneath most **epithelial tissue** is a thin sheet of **connective tissue**, the **basement membrane**, which separates epithelia from **tissues** below. Besides its protective function, **epithelial tissue** frequently has a secretory function, in which case it is sometimes known as **glandular tissue**.

epithelium: A sheet of **epithelial tissue. Epithelium** is derived from ectoderm and endoderm. Epithelia of multiple layers are called stratified epithelia. Stratified **squamous epithelium** is found in the **skin, cervix,** and **oral cavity.** In healthy **tissues,** the **epithelium** often consists of a single, well-organized layer of **cells** with *en face* diameter of 10–20 μm and height of 25 μm.

erbium:yttrium aluminium garnet (Er:YAG) laser (*Synonym*: erbium laser): A **solid-state laser** whose lasing medium is the crystal Er:YAG with emission in **mid-infrared** at 2.79–2.94 μm. It is one of the most prospective **lasers** for **ablation** of different **tissues,** including **skin** and **hard tissues,** because of its unique **wavelength** that coincides with the strongest **water-absorption band** (normal oscillatory modes of **water** molecules, λ = 2.91 μm). The **power** ranges from a few **watts** to a few tenths of **watts.** For miniature systems (a crystal 4 mm in diameter and 75-mm long), the pulse duration in the free-run regime is in the **microsecond** range with the pulse-repetition rate of 25 Hz, pulse **energy** of a few **joules,** and **average power** of a few **watts.** In the **Q-switching** regime the pulse duration is in the **nanosecond** range with pulse **energy** of ~100 mJ.

erythema (*Synonym*: skin reddening): Abnormal redness of the **skin** due to local congestion, as in **inflammation.** For instance,the skin's response to **UV** irradiation.

erythematosus lupus: An usually chronic disease of unknown cause, occasionally affecting internal organs, characterized by red, scaly patches on the **skin.**

erythematous: Relating to, or causing, **erythema.**

erythrocyte [*Synonym*: red blood cell (RBC)]: A flattened, disk-shaped **cell** that circulates in the **blood** stream and contains respiratory **pigment, hemoglobin.** Red **blood cells** carry **oxygen** and carbon dioxide, away from and toward the **lung.** The **cell** is readily distorted, elastic, and immotile. Mammalian **erythrocytes**

have no nuclei, but the **erythrocytes** of **embryos** have nuclei. Erythrocytes are formed in red **bone marrow**, are destroyed by erythrophages, and have a relatively short life (average 120 days in humans). There are approximately 5 million per cubic millimeter in normal human **blood**. A normal human **erythrocyte** in **plasma** has the shape of a concave–concave disk with a diameter varying from 7.1 to 9.2 μm, a thickness of 0.9–1.2 μm in the center and 1.7–2.4 μm on the periphery, and a volume of 90 μm^3. Its **index of refraction** is 1.4 in the **wavelength** range 600–1100 nm.

erythrodermia: General name of the expressed and usually widespread **skin** redness (**erythema**), often accompanied by scales on the **skin**.

esophagus: A tube connecting the **pharynx** with the **stomach**, usually about 25-cm long in adults. It is divided into three parts: jugular, **chest**, and **abdominal**.

etalon: See **Fabry–Pérot interferometer**.

ethanol: See **alcohol**.

ether: General name for a class of chemical compounds that contain an **ether** group, an **oxygen** atom connected to two (substituted) alkyl groups. A typical example is the solvent and anesthetic diethyl **ether**, commonly referred to simply as "**ether**" (ethoxyethane, CH_3–CH_2–O–CH_2–CH_3).

ethylene glycol: A colorless, sweet liquid (see **alcohol**) used chiefly as a solvent.

ethylenediaminetetraacetic acid (EDTA): EDTA is used extensively as an anticoagulant in the analysis of **blood** samples. It is also used for preventing clumping of **cells** grown in liquid suspension in **cell culture**, as a decalcifying agent in **histology** to make it possible to cut sections using a microtome, for treatment of eye corneal ulcers in animals, and some other biomedical applications.

eukaryote: Animals, plants, **fungi cells**, and protists are **eukaryotes**, organisms with a complex **cell** or **cells**, in which the genetic material is organized into a **membrane**-bound **nucleus** or nuclei. Animals, plants, and **fungi cells** are mostly multicellular.

evanescent wave: A nearfield standing **wave** with an **intensity** that exhibits exponential decay with distance from the boundary at which the **wave** was formed. **Evanescent waves** are a general property of **wave** equations, and can, in principle, occur in any context to which a **wave** equation applies. They are formed at the boundary between two **media** with different **wave**-motion properties, and are most intense within one-third of a **wavelength** from the surface of formation. In optics and acoustics particularly, **evanescent waves** are formed when waves traveling in a medium undergo **total internal reflection** at a boundary because they strike it at an angle greater than the so-called critical angle. The physical explanation for the existence of the **evanescent wave** is that the electric and magnetic fields (or **pressure** gradients, in the case of acoustic waves) cannot be discontinuous at a boundary, as would be the case if there were no **evanescent wave** field.

evanescent-wave sensor: Light of a fixed **wavelength** is reflected off the working optical interface (glass plate, **prism**, **fiber tip**, **fiber** core/cladding interface, etc.) of the chip at the angle of **total internal reflection**, and detected inside the instrument. This induces the **evanescent wave** to penetrate through the optical interface and some distance into the liquid or **tissue** connected with the working surface of the sensor. The **refractive index** at the working side of the chip surface has a direct influence on the behavior of the **light** reflected off the interface. In this way biological interactions can be measured to a high degree of sensitivity. **Fiber (waveguide) evanescent-wave** biosensors where the propagation constant through the **waveguide** is changed by the **absorption** of molecules to the **waveguide** surface are designed. Highly integrated miniature interferometric devices are used for signal detection in such sensors. Many optical biosensors based on the phenomenon of **surface-plasmon resonance** use **evanescent-wave** techniques. The **light** is projected from the glass, and an **evanescent wave** penetrates through the metal film. **Plasmons** are excited at the outer side of the film. This configuration is used in most practical applications, where binding of a target analyte to a receptor on the gold surface produces a measurable signal.

Evans blue: A biological dye (stain).

evaporation: The process whereby atoms or molecules in a liquid state gain sufficient **energy** to enter the gaseous state. It is the opposite process of condensation. **Evaporation** is exclusively a surface phenomena and should not be confused with boiling. Most notably, for a liquid to boil, its vapor **pressure** must equal the ambient **pressure**, but this is not necessary for **evaporation** to occur.

excimer laser: A **laser** whose lasing medium is an excited molecular complex, an excimer (molecule-dimer). The emission is in the **UV**. Examples include the ArF **laser**, 193 nm; KrF **laser**, 248 nm; XeCl **laser**, 308 nm; and XeF **laser**, 351 nm. **Lasers** are tunable in some limits (10–20 nm). Because of a high **absorption** of **tissues** in the **UV** range, **excimer lasers** are widely used for **tissue ablation**. They enable highly precise **tissue**-depth lasing as well as in the transverse direction. Eye-refractive surgery technologies are based on these **lasers**.

excision: "To remove as if by cutting." In surgery, an **excision** (or resection) is the complete removal of an organ or a **tumor**, as opposed to a **biopsy**. An excisional **biopsy** (sometimes called a tumorectomy) is the removal of a **tumor** along with a minimum of healthy **tissue**. It is therefore an **excision** rather than a **biopsy**.

excitation-emission map (EEM): See **fluorescence excitation-emission map**.

excitation spectrum: The **emission spectrum** at one **wavelength** is monitored and the **intensity** at this **wavelength** is measured as a function of the exciting **wavelength**.

excited state (*Synonym*: excited energy level):   Electrons possess **energy** according to their position in relation to the nucleus of an atom. The closer the electron is to the nucleus the lower the **energy**. When the **energy** of an electron changes, it must do so in certain definite steps and not in a continuous way. Electrons are positioned according to their **energy** state and these positions are called **energy** levels and sublevels. The levels are counted by their steps outward and the numbers allotted to them are their quantum numbers.

exogenous: Refers to an action or object coming from outside a system; the opposite of **endogenous**. For example, an **exogenous contrast agent** in medical imaging refers to a liquid injected into the patient that enhances visibility of a pathology, such as a **tumor**. An **exogenous** factor is any material that is present and active in an individual organism or living **cell** but that originated outside of that organism, as opposed to an **endogenous** factor, and includes both pathogens and therapeutics. **DNA** introduced to **cells** via transfection or viral infection (transduction) is an **exogenous** factor. Carcinogens are **exogenous** factors.

extinction coefficient: See **attenuation coefficient**.

extracellular: "Outside the **cell**." This space is usually taken to be outside the **plasma membranes** and is occupied by fluid.

extracellular matrix (ECM):   The **extracellular** part of **tissue** that usually provides structural support to the **cells** in addition to performing various other important functions. The **extracellular matrix** is the defining feature of **connective tissue**. It includes the interstitial matrix and the **basement membrane**. The interstitial matrix is present between various **cells** (i.e., in the intercellular spaces). **Gels** of **polysaccharides** and **fibrous proteins** fill the **interstitial space** and act as a compression buffer against the stress placed on the **extracellular matrix**.

ex vivo: Taken from a living organism. Pertaining to experiments on animal or human organs that are excised from the living body and kept in conditions very close to the natural ones. In **tissue** optics, it is one of the productive approaches toward standardization of optical-property measurements of freshly excised (not fixed) **tissue** at conditions kept close to that of the living **tissue**, i.e., temperature, **hydration**, **pH**, etc.

eyeball: A spherical structure composed of supporting **tissues** in which the photoreceptors (see **retina**) and refractive media (see **cornea** and **crystalline lens**) for concentrating **light** on the **nervous tissues** are situated. The **iris** divides the **eyeball** into the anterior and posterior chambers.

Fabry–Pérot interferometer (*Synonym*: etalon): An **interferometer** that is a combination of two parallel mirrors (reflecting planes) displaced from each other by a distant L (**interferometer** length). It is used as a precise **optical filter** in super-resolution **spectroscopy** and as a cavity in **lasers**.

facial tissue: Refers to a class of soft, absorbant, disposable paper that is suitable for use on the face.

Fahrenheit: Temperature scale based on 32 °F as the freezing point of **water** and 212 °F as the boiling point of **water** at standard atmospheric **pressure**. A temperature interval of 1 °F is equal to an interval of 5/9 degrees of **Celsius temperature scale (centigrade)**. The **Fahrenheit** and **Celsius temperature scales** converge at −40 degrees, i.e., −40 °F and −40 °C represent the same temperature. **Fahrenheit/Celsius temperature scale** conversion formulae: (°F) = (°C) × 9/5 + 32, and (°C) = [(°F) − 32] × 5/9. **Fahrenheit/Kelvin temperature scale** conversion formulae: (°F) = (K) × 9/5 − 459.67 and (K) = [(°F) + 459.67]× 5/9.

false-color map: A **color** map in which the measured parameter of each **color** is prescribed a specific value, e.g., the measured velocity of **blood flow** within the selected **skin** area. It is used for fast, qualitative estimation of parameter distribution and change.

far zone: See **far-field diffraction zone**.

Faraday rotator: An optical device that rotates the **polarization** of **light** using the Faraday effect, which in turn is based on a magneto-optic effect. This works because one **polarization** of the input **light** is in ferromagnetic resonance with the material, which causes its phase velocity to be higher than the other.

far-field diffraction zone (*Synonym*: far zone): The zone where Fraunhofer **diffraction** takes place. A type of **diffraction** in which the **light** source and the receiving screen are effectively at an infinite distance from the **diffraction** object, i.e., parallel beams of **wave** trains.

far-infrared (FIR): See **light wavelength range**.

fasciclin: Membrane-associated glycoprotein. **Fasciclin** I (70 kDa) appears to be an extrinsic **membrane protein**. **Fasciclin** II (95 kDa) is an integral **membrane protein**.

fast-Fourier transform (FFT) analysis: A fast **algorithm** for the expression of any periodic function as a sum of sine and cosine functions, as in an **electromagnetic wave** function.

fat: (1) Any substance that can be extracted from **tissues** by **ether**, hot **ethanol**, or gasoline (**fat** solvents). This is a broad definition covering neutral **fats**, sterols, steroids, carotenes, and terpens. In this sense, **lipids**, lipins, and lipoids are **fats**. (2) True **fat** or neutral **fat**, as considered in dietetics, an ester of **glycerol** with one, two, or three different **fatty acids** replacing the three hydroxyl groups of the trihydric **alcohol, glycerol**. (3) Any substance that is a true **fat** and solid below 20 °C. This is in contrast to an **oil**. (4) See **adipose tissue**.

fatty acid: A carboxylic acid, often having a long unbranched aliphatic tail (chain). Can be either saturated or unsaturated. **Fatty acids** derived from natural **fats** and **oils** may be assumed to have at least eight carbon atoms, e.g., caprylic acid (octanoic acid). Most of the natural **fatty acids** have an even number of carbon atoms, because their biosynthesis involves acetyl-CoA, a **coenzyme** carrying a two-carbon-atom group. **Fatty acids** are produced by the hydrolysis of the ester linkages in a **fat** or biological **oil** (both of which are triglycerides), with the removal of **glycerol**.

fat cell: See **adipocyte**.

fatty tissue: See **adipose tissue**.

female breast: See **breast**.

femoral biceps muscle: The **muscle** pertaining to the thigh or femur.

femtosecond (fsec) (fs): 10^{-15} sec (s).

fiber (optics): An optical **waveguide** that uses a phenomenon of **total internal reflection** for **light** transportation with low losses and is made from transparent silica (SiO_2) glass, polymer, or crystal, is cylindrical in form, and usually has a circular cross section. Typically it consists of two parts: An inner part or core, with a higher **refractive index** (RI) and through which **light** propagates; and an outer part or cladding, with a lower **refractive index** and which provides a totally reflecting interface between core and cladding. **Optical fibers** are often made of silica (SiO_2) glass. The refractive-index step and profile are controlled by the concentration and distribution of dopants, for example, the core can be doped with germania (GeO_2) or alumina (Al_2O_3) or other oxides, such as P_2O_5 or TiO_2, for a slightly higher **refractive index** than that of a silica cladding. Alternatively, to take advantage of low-loss pure silica, the cladding can be doped with fluorine for a slightly lower index while the core contains undoped pure silica. Silica **fibers** are ideal for **laser-light** delivery in the **visible** and **NIR** because of their low loss (see **fiber**

losses) and low **dispersion** (see **fiber dispersion**) in these spectral regions. Fibers made of other materials are also available and are broadly used in medicine and related applications, e.g., low-cost polymer (plastic) **fibers** can be used for short-distance **light** delivery of relatively low-**power radiation**, and **IR fibers**, transparent in the range from 2–20 µm, are applicable for chemical sensing, thermometry, and **IR laser power** delivery. Light-guiding properties of **fibers** are defined by their structure; there are step-index and graded-index **fibers**, **multimode**, **single-mode**, and **polarization-maintaining fibers**. The relative refractive-index difference of the core and cladding, $\Delta \cong (n_1 - n_2)/n_1$, for **single-mode fibers** is much less than 1%, for low-aperture **multimode fibers** it is 1–2%, and for wide-aperture silica-polymer or polymer **fibers** with the **numerical aperture** NA $=$ 0.25–0.75 it is 10–20%. The **fiber** core has a radius a; the core diameter, $2a$, typically ranges from a few (3–10) **micrometers** for a **single-mode fiber** to 50–1000 µm for a **multimode fiber**. It is designed for the **fiber** to support a desired number of guided modes. The outer diameter, $2b$, of a **fiber** is determined by the requirement that the cladding be thicker than the **penetration depth** of a guided-mode field to prevent the field from reaching the air-cladding boundary and by the consideration of easy handling. The standard outer-diameter size for **single-mode** and low-aperture **multimode fibers** is 125 µm. Medical **fibers** have a wider range of core and outer diameters. Typical wide-aperture silica-polymer **fibers** have core diameter $2a =$ 200–800 µm and cladding thickness of 30–70 µm. The total diameter of a **fiber** with a protective cover could be from few hundred microns to few millimeters.

fiber (biology): A long strand of scleroprotein. **Fibers** are either **collagen**-forming **white fibers**, **elastin**-forming **yellow fibers**, or **reticulin**-forming **reticular fibers**. **Fibers** form part of a noncellular matrix around and among **cells**. They are formed and maintained in a **tissue** by **fibroblasts**. A matrix may consist of an amorphous, jellylike **polysaccharide** together with the three types of **fibers**. **Cells** and a matrix form a **connective tissue**. Different forms of **connective tissue** possess varying proportions of the constituents of the matrix.

fiber acceptance angle: The largest incident angle, with respect to the normal of the end face of a **fiber**, that allows for an optical beam to be coupled into the **fiber** core. A **wave** entering the **fiber** at an incident angle smaller than the **acceptance angle**, θ_a, will be totally reflected at the core–cladding interface and thus will be guided in the **fiber** core. A **wave** entering at an incident angle larger than θ_a will be partially transmitted through the core–cladding interface after entering the **fiber** and will not be guided. $\theta_a = \sin^{-1}(NA/n) = \sin^{-1}\left[\left(\sqrt{n_1^2 - n_2^2}\right)/n\right]$, where *NA* is the **fiber numerical aperture**, and n_1, n_2, and n are the refractive indices of **fiber** core, cladding, and surrounding medium contacting the **fiber tip**, respectively.

fiber attenuation: Several factors contribute to **attenuation** of the **power** of an optical **wave** propagating in an **optical fiber**. When an optical **wave** propagates in a lossy medium with an **attenuation coefficient** α, its **intensity** decays exponentially with distance *L*. Because the **power** of an optical **wave** in a **fiber** is simply the integration of its **intensity** over the cross section of the **fiber**, the **attenuation** of optical power over a propagation distance is given by $P_{\text{out}} = P_{\text{in}}e^{-\alpha L}$, where P_{in} and P_{out} are the input and output **power**, respectively. **Fiber attenuation** is measured in **watts** or milliwatts/microwatts in low-**power** applications, or kilowatts/megawatts in high-**power** applications, while α is given per centimeter, meter, or kilometer when *L* is measured in centimeters, meters, or kilometers. In practical engineering applications, it is convenient to use **decibels (dB)** as a measure of relative changes of quantities. The **attenuation coefficient** α is then measured in **decibels** per meter or kilometer: $A = -(1/L) \times 10 \log(P_{\text{out}}/P_{\text{in}})$, where P_{in} and P_{out} are measured in **watts**, milliwatts, or microwatts. *A* is conventionally given in **decibels** per kilometer α (dB/km) $=$ 4.34α (1/km) and α (1/km) $=$ 0.23α (dB/km). **Power** can also be measured in **decibels** and has units of **decibel-watts** (dBW), **decibel**-milliwatts (dBm), or **decibel**-microwatts (dBμ) defined as follows: P (dBW) $=$ 10 $\log P$ (W), P (dBm) $=$ 10 $\log P$ (mW), and P (dBμ) $=$ 10 $\log P$ (μW). When **power**

is given in **decibel watts** and the **attenuation coefficient** is in **decibels** per kilometer, P_{out} (dBW) = P_{in} (dBW) − α (dB/km) L (km). Similar formulas can be written for **power** measured in **decibel**-milliwatts and **decibel**-microwatts and are very convenient and useful in practical applications as they relate the input **power**, output **power**, and **attenuation** in a simple arithmetic relation. **Attenuation** of **light** in a **fiber** is primarily caused by **absorption** and **scattering**. In addition, there are mechanical losses and losses due to nonlinear-optical effects. The effects of these loss mechanisms vary, but they add up to the total loss in a **fiber**. (See **fiber losses** and medical **fibers**.) At guiding of pulse-periodic **laser radiation** by a **fiber** of the length L, the **fiber**-output pulse **energy** E_2 is connected with the input (**laser**) pulse **energy** E_1 as $E_2 = \eta E_1 \exp\left(-\int_0^L \chi_0 dx\right)$, where **fiber** input- and output-coupling efficiency $\eta = \eta_1 \cdot \eta_2 \cdot \eta_3$, $1 - \eta_1$ and $1 - \eta_2$ are losses caused by **Fresnel reflection** for the input and output **fiber** endfaces; η_3 is the effective losses caused by **light**-beam divergence; χ_0 is the stationary distributed losses at the length $L > L_{st}$ along x direction. It follows that maximal transmitted **energy** E_{2max}, or **energy density** $W_{2max} \approx E_{2max}/\pi a^2$, at the **fiber** output are defined by its length L, coupling efficiency η, and **fiber radiation** resistance. For **UV radiation** of **excimer lasers** (λ = 308 and 351 nm) with the beam divergence of 3 **mrad** and pulse repetition rate of 5 Hz guided by a silica **fiber** with $L \geq L_{st}$ ($L_{st} \leq$ 20 cm) at mean-**energy density** of $W_1 \approx 3$ J$\cdot$cm^{-2}, the distributed losses are independent on W_1, i.e., only linear **attenuation** occurs. In contrast, for shorter **wavelength** (λ = 248 nm) the nonlinear losses are essential, $\chi_0 = \alpha + \beta W_2$ ($\alpha = 3 \cdot 10^3$ cm^{-1}, $\beta = 5.3 \cdot 10^{-2}$ cm/J), which considerably limit the output **energy density** W_2. Efficiency of coupling depends on the **fiber**-tip quality and could be of $\eta \approx 0.94 \pm 0.04$. In the **IR** from 2–13 μm, the total **attenuation** of Ag-halide (0.25 AgCl/0.75 AgBr) cladding-free **fiber** is described by the relation $\alpha = (0.5 + 16.2/\lambda^2)$, dB/m. Its high **index of refraction** causes essential **light attenuation** due to **Fresnel reflection** from the **fiber** face. For example, for **CO$_2$** laser only 70% of **power** is transmitted through the 0.9-mm **fiber** of 1-m length, 8% of **power** is lost due to **scattering** and **absorption**, and the remaining 22% by **reflection**.

fiber Bragg grating: See **Bragg mirror (reflector)**.

fiber bundle: A flexible bundle of individual **optical fibers** arranged in an ordered or disordered manner and correspondingly named regular and irregular bundles. Irregular-**fiber bundles** are used for illumination and collection of **light** from a **tissue**, and regular-**fiber bundles** provide transportation of the **tissue** image. Historically, **fiber bundles** were the first **light guides** and currently are widely used in medicine, particularly for **endoscopy**. Multicomponent glasses are the materials used in bundle manufacturing. Between the individual **fibers**, there are **light**-isolating glass layers with a low **refractive index**. Light-guiding **fibers** can be as small as 2 μm or smaller. However, bundles of **multimode fibers** with a core diameter of 5–9 μm typically are used. Modern flexible regular bundles have a total diameter of 0.3–3.0 mm (with the number of **fibers** up to 150,000), and a high numerical aperture, $NA \approx 0.5–1.0$. **Fiber-bundle transmittance** is not very high, usually between 30–70% per meter, and resolution is between 10–50 lines per 1 mm. The resolution is defined by a **pixel** size (individual **fiber** core diameter), which can be only a few **micrometers**.

fiber connector: Terminates the end of an **optical fiber**, and enables a quick connection and disconnection to other instrumentation. The connectors mechanically couple and align the cores of **fibers** so that **light** can pass. Most **optical-fiber connectors** are spring- loaded, and the **fiber** endfaces of the two connectors are pressed together, resulting in a direct glass-to-glass or plastic-to-plastic contact, avoiding any glass-to-air or plastic-to-air interfaces to minimize connector losses. Connectors for **multimode** and **single-mode fibers** are available.

fiber coupler: A fiber-optic device that interconnects optical components.

fiber divider: An optical-**power** divider built -on the basis of **multimode**, **single-mode**, or **polarization-maintaining optical fibers**. Typically two or more **fibers** are coupled together so that an appreciable proportion of the optical **energy** is guided by the **fibers**.

fiber group-velocity dispersion: When measuring the transmission delay or the broadening of optical pulses due to **optical-fiber dispersion**, the **group-velocity dispersion** coefficient defined as $D_\lambda = -D/c\lambda = -(2\pi c/\lambda^2)\,(d^2k/d\omega^2) = -(\lambda/c)(d^2n/d\lambda^2)$ is usually used. This coefficient is generally expressed as a function of **wavelength** in units of **picoseconds**/km/nm. It is a direct measure of the chromatic pulse-transmission delay over a unit transmission length.

fiber laser: Laser with an active medium in the form of glass or crystal **optical fiber** with core doped by active ions such as Nd (neodymium), Yb (ytterbium), Er (erbium), Tm (thulium). For a typical medical **fiber laser**, core diameter is 7–10 μm and cladding is 30–50 μm. Length is from a few centimeters to a few meters. **Multimode fibers** with activated core of 30–50 μm in diameter are also used. Effective pumping of activated **fibers** is provided by lamps and **LEDs** transversely. Most **diode lasers** are used to provide effective longitudinal pumping. Diode-**laser power** is injected through the cladding or directly in the core of such **fiber** for pumping of active ions. **Fiber lasers** are highly efficient and the best-quality **laser beams** have a wide range of **wavelengths** from **UV** to **IR** and an average output **power** from a few milliwatts to a few tenths of a **watt**. The following **lasers** are widely used in **laser** surgery and thermotherapy: Yb (970 nm), Nd (1060 nm), Er (1560 nm), Yb/Er (970/1560 nm), and Tm (1900 nm). **Laser cartilage** thermoplastics and surgery could optimally use **radiation** of 970 nm (10–20 W), 1560 nm (2.5–5 W), 970 nm/1560 nm (10/2.5 W), and 1900 nm (3 W). For laparoscopic surgery and treatments of **blood vessel** pathologies, a more intensive **light** is appropriate—970 nm (30 W), 1060 nm (30 W), and 1560 nm (15 W). Another type of **fiber laser** explores nonlinear properties of **fibers**, including **Raman scattering**, stimulated **Raman scattering (SRS)** with solitons, and four-**photon** mixing effects. In that case, no activation is needed but a very long **fiber** should be used, from a few meters up to a few kilometers. Generated discrete **wavelengths** are in the range from 400–1600 nm with a continuum up to 2000 nm. Output-pulse **power** is up to a few tenths of a kilowatt is typical. A **fiber laser** is a robust instrument for biomedical applications because it combines active media with **light** transportation to a target **tissue** or **cell**.

fiber loss: Optical-loss mechanisms include electronic **absorption** (for example, the **bandgap** of fused silica is about 8.9 eV), which corresponds to the **photon energy** of **light** at the **UV wavelength** of approximately 140 nm. This causes strong **absorption** of **light** in the **ultraviolet** region due to **electronic transitions** across the **bandgap**. Light in the **visible**- and **infrared** regions has **photon** energies less than the **bandgap energy** and is not expected to be absorbed through direct **electronic transition** across the **bandgap**. However, in practice, the **bandgap** of a material is not sharply defined but usually has bandtails extending from the conduction- and valence bands into the **bandgap**. This is due to a variety of reasons, e.g., thermal vibrations of the lattice ions and microscopic imperfections of the material structure. In particular, an amorphous material such as fused silica generally has very long bandtails. These bandtails lead to an **absorption** tail extending into the **visible** and **infrared** regions. Empirically, it is found that the **absorption** tail at **photon** energies below the **bandgap** fall off exponentially with **photon energy**. Molecular **absorption** is also an important loss mechanism in the **infrared** region because the **absorption** of **photons** is accompanied by transitions between different vibrational modes of molecules. For example, the fundamental **vibrational transition** of fused silica causes a very strong **absorption** peak at about 9 μm. Nonlinear effects contribute to important harmonics and combination frequencies corresponding to minor **absorption** peaks at 4.4, 3.8, and 3.2 μm. The result is a long **absorption** tail extending into the **NIR**, causing a sharp rise in **absorption** at optical **wavelengths** longer than 1600 nm. Molecular **absorption** is the major cause of **attenuation** in the

IR spectral region for a silica **fiber.** Impurity **absorption** could be very important in the **NIR** because most impurity ions such as OH^-, Fe^{2+}, and Cu^{2+} form **absorption bands** in this region where both electronic and molecular **absorption** losses (for example, in the host silica glass) are very low. Near the peaks of the impurity **absorption bands,** an impurity concentration as low as one part per billion can contribute to an **absorption** loss as high as 1 dB/km. Impurities in silica **fibers** have been reduced to levels where losses associated with their **absorption** are negligible, with the exception of the OH^- radical. The OH^- radical results from the presence of **water,** which can enter a **fiber** through the manufacturing process or as **humidity** in the environment. Therefore, **fibers** are protected from **water** by plastic coating to reduce the loss caused by OH^- **absorption.** The **absorption** peak due to the fundamental vibration of the OH^- ions appears at 2.73 μm where intrinsic molecular **absorption** of silica is strong. The most important **absorption** peaks are those at the harmonics and combination frequencies of 1390, 1250, and 950 nm. **Rayleigh scattering** is the intrinsic **scattering** in a **fiber** caused by variations in density and composition that are built into the **fiber** during the manufacturing process. These variations are primarily the result of thermal fluctuations in the density of glass material and variations in the concentration of dopants before material passes its glass transition point to become a solid, and so are a fundamental thermodynamic phenomenon that cannot be completely removed. They create microscopic fluctuations in the **index of refraction.** The loss due to **Rayleigh scattering** is very important in the short-**wavelength** region but falls off rapidly as the **wavelength** increases. **Waveguide scattering** (resulting from imperfections in the **waveguide** structure of a **fiber,** such as nonuniformity in the size and shape of the core, perturbations in the core–cladding boundary, and defects in the core or cladding), can be generated in the manufacturing process. In addition, environmentally induced effects, such as stress and temperature variations, also cause imperfections. The imperfections in a **fiber waveguide** result in additional **scattering** losses, which sometimes induces coupling between different guided modes. Nonlinear losses occur because **light** is confined over long distances. Nonlinear optical effects can become important even at a relatively moderate optical power. Nonlinear optical processes such as **stimulated Brillouin–Mandelshtam scattering (SBMS)** and **stimulated Raman scattering (SRS)** can cause significant **attenuation** in the **power** of an optical signal. Other nonlinear processes can induce mode mixing or **frequency** shift, all contributing to the loss of a particular guided mode at a particular **frequency**. Because nonlinear effects are **intensity** dependent, they can become very important at high optical powers. The limiting effect at short **wavelengths** is **Rayleigh scattering**, which dominates the electronic **absorption**, e.g., fused silica in this spectral region. In the **IR** region beyond 1600 nm, **attenuation** is completely dominated by intrinsic **absorption** due to molecular vibrations of silica. In the **NIR** region, **attenuation** strongly depends on the concentration of the OH^- impurity. Also in this low-loss region, any amount of loss caused by **waveguide scattering** would be relatively significant. Therefore, **attenuation** in this spectral region varies with the quality of the **fiber**. The **attenuation coefficient** is also mode dependent; the fundamental mode generally has lower **attenuation** than high-order modes because its **power** is more confined to the core. As such, **single-mode fibers** usually have lower **attenuation** than **multimode fibers**. Among **multimode fibers** of a fixed outer diameter, such as the standard 125-μm size, those with larger cores, and simultaneously thinner claddings, typically have higher **attenuation** because the **intensity** distribution spreads farther out. A graded-index **fiber** usually has lower **attenuation** than does a comparable step-index **multimode fiber** because the **intensity** in a **graded-index fiber** is more concentrated at the center of the **fiber**. There are also bending losses caused by **fiber** macrobends that are encountered in the looping or routing of **fibers**, and by microbends, which are typically created by **mechanical stresses** associated with bundling, packaging, and handling, and at connection losses incurred at the junctions of **fibers**. Bending loss can be understood from the viewpoint of ray optics or **wave** optics. Losses caused by controlled bending can be quantified and used for the design of **fiber** sensors for biomedical applications. For **IR fibers**, the losses are a result of impurities and imperfections, which give rise to a large **absorption** and **scatter-**

ing with the **fiber attenuation** of a few **decibels** per meter (dB/m) only.

fiber material dispersion: **Dispersion** of the materials of interest in **optical fibers**, in particular pure and doped silica. The parameters of interest are the **refractive index** n the **group refractive index** n_g = $n - \lambda(dn/d\lambda)$, and the **group-velocity dispersion** D_λ = $-(\lambda/c)(d^2n/d\lambda^2)$. These parameters are commonly given as a function of the free-space **wavelength** λ. The **index of refraction** of pure silica in the **wavelength** range between 0.2–4 μm is given by the following empirically fitted **Sellmeier equation**: n^2 = $1 + (0.6961663\lambda^2)/[\lambda^2 - (0.0684043)^2] + (0.4079426\lambda^2)/[\lambda^2 - (0.1162414)^2] + (0.8974794\lambda^2)/[\lambda^2 - (9.896161)^2]$, where λ is in **micrometers**. The **index of refraction** can be changed by adding dopants to silica, thus facilitating the means to control the index profile of a **fiber**. Specifically, doping with germania increases the **index of refraction** and also increases material **dispersion**. As a result, the point of zero material **group-velocity dispersion** is shifted from 1.284 μm for pure silica to 1.383 μm for germania–silica glass (13.5 mol% GeO_2).

fiber multiplexer: A **fiber**-optic and electronic instrument that combines **laser beams** with different **wavelengths** or other properties in different ratios.

fiber near-infrared (NIR) transmission window: There are three **near-infrared wavelength** windows effective for biophotonic applications in the transmission of **light** with **fibers**. The 850-nm window, corresponding to the **wavelengths** of GaAs/AlGaAs **diode lasers**, and the 1300- and 1550-nm windows, corresponding to the **wavelengths** of InGaAsP/InP **diode lasers**. The lowest **attenuation** in the entire spectral range occurs at 1550 nm, while the **attenuation** at 1300 nm is slightly higher. The best silica **fibers** have **attenuation** as low as 0.15 dB/km at 1550 nm and 0.3 dB/km at 1300 nm, while **attenuation** at 850 nm is typically 2 dB/km. Plastic **fibers** in the **visible** range provide minimal **attenuation** on the level of 0.1–0.2 dB/m.

157

fiber nonlinear optics: The unique feature of **optical fibers** is that both a high **intensity** of light and a long interaction length, which are required efficient nonlinear-optical interactions, can be simultaneously fulfilled when operating at a modest **power** level. This is possible because of the small core diameter of a **single-mode fiber** and its high optical **transmittance**. Many nonlinear optical processes in **fibers** have direct bulk counterparts (see **nonlinear optics**). The use of a **fiber** may offer the advantages of improved efficiency, phase matching, or miniaturization of the nonlinear optical device. Examples are **fiber lasers**, **fiber** pulse compressors, and optical-**frequency** converters. Some nonlinear optical devices, such as all-optical switches and modulators that use **fiber interferometers** or **fiber couplers**, rely on the **waveguide** geometry for their functions and thus have no bulk counterparts. For isotropic core material, the first component of a nonlinear portion of the **refractive index** $n_1 = n_{1l} + n_{1n}$, $n_{1n} = N_{1n}I$, where I is the **intensity** and is defined by a cubic nonlinearity, i.e., three optical fields interact, $P^{(3)} = \varepsilon_0 \chi^{(3)} \vec{E}\vec{E}\vec{E}$, where $P^{(3)}$ is the cubic **nonlinear polarization density** of the core material, ε_0 is the dielectric **permittivity** of vacuum, and $\chi^{(3)}$ is the cubic **nonlinear susceptibility** of the core material. For silica $N_{1n} \approx 5 \cdot 10^{-16}$ cm^2 /W, which is negligible, but due to small core diameter of **single-mode fibers** and their high transparency, it can provide the **power density** up to 10^{10} W·cm^{-2} for the long interaction lengths. There are a variety of nonlinear processes in **fibers**, including **stimulated Raman scattering (SRS)**, which takes place at **laser power** of a few hundred milliwatts and is the basis for **NIR stimulated Raman scattering fiber lasers (SRS-fiber lasers)**. As the core **refractive index** depends on **light intensity**, the transportation of a short (with a broadband **spectrum**) pulse induces the phase self-**modulation** and correspondingly additional spectral broadening. If the middle **wavelength** of a pulse is within anomalous **light dispersion** of the core material and $n_{1n} > 0$, the **light** pulse will be compressed at its propagation to the limit defined by the resultant spectral width of the **radiation**, $\tau \sim 1/\Delta\omega$. The drawback of nonlinear effects is the increasing of **fiber attenuation** caused by utilizing of some of the **light energy** to support nonlinear processes. For **lasers**

with narrow **bandwidth** (≤1 MHz), the major nonlinear process is **stimulated Brillouin–Mandelshtam scattering (SBMS)**, which defines limits for the maximal **power** that can be transmitted through the long **fibers** (a few kilometers).

fiber numerical aperture: The **numerical aperture** of a **fiber**, which characterizes its **light**-gathering **power**, is $NA \equiv n \sin \theta_a = \sqrt{n_1^2 - n_2^2}$, where θ_a is the **fiber acceptance angle**, n, n_1, and n_2 are the refractive indices of surrounding medium contacting the **fiber tip**, **fiber** core, and cladding, respectively. For silica **multimode fibers**, $n_1 \approx 1.46$ and the relative refractive-index difference of the core and cladding $\Delta \cong (n_1 - n_2)/n_1 \leq 0.01$, thus, NA for a **fiber tip** in the air ($n \approx 1$), $NA \approx n_1 \sqrt{2\Delta}$ should be equal to or less than 0.2 (usually, 0.1–0.2), which corresponds to **acceptance angles** of $\theta_a \approx 5.7$–11.5 deg for medical **fibers**, which are typically high-aperture **fibers**, $\theta_a \geq 30$ deg($NA \geq 0.5$).

fiber optic destruction: Transportation of high-energetic **laser beams** through a **fiber** at levels above the **fiber radiation resistance** limit, can damage **fiber optics**. Characteristic **fiber** destruction occurs on the input and output faces, and on the core-cladding interface in the vicinity of the input **fiber** end, where high **energy** is applied because of nonoptimal **laser**-beam coupling, or for some transit areas, where optical defects or microbends exist. The distal end of a **fiber** is typically destroyed because of **absorption** by **tissue** debris. Because waves are summed at the **fiber**, output amplitudes of transmitted and backreflected waves are summed, and thus, in particular for **continuous wave radiation** of 4–5 kW/cm², the output **fiber tip** is destroyed. In addition, in **multimode fibers** the **speckle** structures of interfering waveguiding modes with high local intensities also may produce destruction of the distal **fiber** end. During **fiber tip** cooling, the destruction threshold could be increased up to ~40 kW/cm², and anti-**reflection** coatings of the input and output faces may increase **fiber transmittance** up to 25% and destruction threshold up to 50 kW/cm². The **power density** destruction limit for Ag-halide (0.25 AgCl/0.75 AgBr) cladding-free **fiber** with an antireflection face coating transporting **CW IR radiation** (λ = 10.6 μm) is 70 kW/cm^2. For highly energetic (up to 6.5 J/cm^2) short pulses (τ_p~0.1 μs) from **CO$_2$ lasers** and **Er:YAG lasers**, such **fibers** are not damaged up to **power density** of 8 MW/cm^2. For longer pulses (τ_p > 100 μs) the damage limit is of 36 J/cm^2. Sapphire **fibers** are effective for transport of the **erbium laser radiation** due to their high damage limit of 1.2 kJ/cm^2 for τ_p = 110 μs.

fiber optic catheter: A flexible single **fiber** or a **fiber bundle** used to move **light** into body cavities and back.

fiber optic device: Any type of device that uses **fiber** optic components.

fiber optic interferometer: Light **interference** of **light** underlies many high-precision measuring systems and displacement sensors. The use of **optical fibers** allows one to make such devices extremely compact and economic. Examples of **fiber optic interferometers** include **Michelson, Mach–Zehnder**, and **Fabry–Pérot interferometers**. For **fiber interferometers, lasers** and low-coherence optical sources with a high **spatial coherence**, such as **superluminescent light diodes**, are used. They may be easily configured for applications in many branches of medicine. **Single-mode fiber optic Michelson interferometers** are widely used in biomedical systems based on **optical coherence tomography (OCT)**. The **fiber** optic **Mach–Zehnder interferometer** is part of **swept-laser source OCT** systems as a generator of k-clock signal to monitor output **power** and **wavelength** of a **swept-laser source**. In a fiber optic **Fabry–Pérot interferometer**, the **interference** occurs at the partially reflecting end face surface of the **fiber** and an external mirror. The size of the sensitive element based on this principle can be as small as the diameter of the **fiber**, i.e., about 0.1 mm, and the sensitivity can achieve sub-**angstrom** level. **Fiber optic interferometers** are not sensitive to external electromagnetic interference and can be used in corrosive environments.

fiber optic probe: Fiber optic end (distal) instrument for irradiating **tissue** and/or **biological cells** or for collecting optical signals from **tissue** and/or **biological cells**, in the form of **light scattering**, back **reflectance**, **fluorescence**, **Raman scattering**, and so on.

fiber optic refractometer: Fiber optic device used to measure the **refractive index** of a medium (**tissue** or biological liquid). Such a device is usually used to explore the effect of disruption of the **total internal reflection** and is a robust instrument well fitted for biomedical applications.

fiber optic sensor: Sensor that uses **optical fiber** either as the sensing element (these are the so-called intrinsic sensors) or as a means of relaying signals from a remote sensor to the electronics that process the signals (extrinsic sensors). Combined **fiber** techniques are also widely used. Depending on the biomedical application, **fiber** may be used because of its small size, or because no electrical power interference is allowed at the **point-of-care testing** location, or because many sensors can be multiplexed along the length of a **fiber** by using different **wavelengths** of **light** for each sensor or by sensing the time delay as **light** passes along the **fiber** through each sensor.

fiber optic single-mode X-coupler: Fiber **coupler** that is made from a **single-mode fiber** and that provides connections between four optical components. It is usually used as a key part of the integrated **Michelson interferometer** when it connects a **light** source, reference mirror, the reflecting surface under study, and a **photodetector**. It is the basis for **fiber** optic **optical coherence tomography**.

fiber optics: Well-developed industrial field, where various **fiber** instrumentation is available, such as **fiber bundles**, **fiber connectors**, **fiber couplers**, **GRIN-** or **selfoc lenses**, tapered fibers, **fiber multiplexers** (dividers), **fiber lasers**, **fiber optic catheters**, **fiber optic interferometers**, **fiber optic probes**, **fiber optic refractometers**, **fiber optic sensors**, and so on.

fiber radiation resistance: Defined as a maximal value of **fiber** input **laser**-pulse **energy** E_{1max} or pulse-**energy density** W_{1max} for pulse **radiation, power,** or **power density** for **continuous wave radiation,** for which **fiber** material is not yet damaged (see **fiber optical destruction**). For example, W_{1max} depends on **laser**-pulse duration τ_p transporting **excimer-laser radiation** with $\lambda = 308$ nm through a commercial silica **fiber** of 400-μm core diameter, $W_{1max} \approx 12 \sqrt{\tau_p}$ (J · cm^{-2}) for $\tau_p \approx 10$–300 ns.

fiber stationary length: Independent of **light beam** and **multimode fiber** coupling conditions and **fiber** quality, not all desired modes can be excited. In the so-called **fiber stationary length** L_{st}, all **fiber** modes are excited. For the low-quality **fibers** with defects, L_{st} is small, a few centimeters only, but for high-quality **fibers**, it could be up to a few kilometers. To provide effective excitation of all propagating modes on a small length and to eliminate dependence of the output **light** distribution on the input coupling conditions, various mode mixtures are used (based on **fiber** bending, multiple microbendings, twisting, and so on). At excitation of a **step-index fiber** by a diffuse **light** source (see **Lambertian scatterer**), $L_{st} \approx [an_1/(2n \sin \theta_a)] \exp[V/2]$, and for **graded-index fiber,** $L_{st} \approx [\pi an_1/(n \sin \theta_a)] \cdot \exp[V/2]$, where $2a$ is the core diameter, n_1 and n are the refractive indices of the **fiber** core and surrounding medium contacting the **fiber tip**, θ_a is the **fiber acceptance angle,** and V is the **fiber waveguide** parameter. For the typical **multimode fiber,** $2a = 50$ μm, $(n/n_1) \sin \theta_a = 0.14, V = 30, L_{st} = 300$ m, and for $V < 10$, the stationary length is only a few centimeters.

fiber tip: Distal part of an **optical fiber.** Could be flat or have a more complex configuration to focus or defocus **light**, or it might not emit **light** in the open air, only at contact with a target **tissue**.

fiber waveguide parameter: For a **step-index fiber,** the **waveguide** parameter V, also called the V-number of the **fiber**, is defined as $V = (2\pi a NA)/\lambda$, where a is the core radius, NA is the **numerical aperture** of the **fiber**, n is the **refractive index** of a surrounding medium contacting the **fiber tip** (in particular, the end face of a **fiber core**), θ_a is the **fiber acceptance angle**, and λ is the **wavelength**. A **fiber** that has a **waveguide** parameter $V < 2.405$ supports only the fundamental HE_{11} mode and is called a **single-mode fiber**. A **fiber** with $V > 2.405$ can support more than just the HE_{11} mode and is called a **multimode fiber**.

fiber-cutoff wavelength: In addition to refractive-index step and core radius, the optical **wavelength** of guided **radiation** defines a **single-mode** or a **multimode fiber** regime. For a given **fiber**, $V = 2.405$ determines its cutoff **wavelength** λ_c for the single-mode guiding. The single-mode regime exits for $\lambda > \lambda_c$, but the same **fiber** turns to multimode for $\lambda < \lambda_c$ or for $2a < 0.76\lambda/NA$, where λ is the **wavelength** in free space (or air) and NA is the **fiber numerical aperture**.

fibril: Fine **fiber** or filament. In **muscles**, for example, their diameters are in the range of 5–15 nm, with a length of about 1–1.5 µm, and in the **eye cornea**, their diameters are in the range of 26–30 nm, with a mean length up to a few millimeters.

fibril D-periodicity: For example, corneal **fibrils** are D-periodic (axial periodicity of **collagen fibrils**, where $D \approx 67$ nm), uniformly narrow ($\approx$30–35 nm in diameter), and indeterminate in length, particularly in older animals. The D-periodicity of the **fibril** arises from side-to-side associations of triple-helical **collagen** molecules that are $\approx$ 300 nm in length (i.e., the molecular length $= 4.4 \times D$) and are staggered by D. The D-stagger of **collagen** molecules produces alternating regions of **protein** density in the **fibril**, which explains the characteristic gap and overlap appearance of **fibrils** negatively contrasted for transmission **electronic microscopy**.

fibroadenoma: **Benign tumor** originating in a **glandular epithelium**, having a conspicuous **stroma** consisting of the proliferating **fibroblasts** and other elements of **connective tissue**.

fibroblast: **Cell** that contributes to the formation of **connective tissue**.

fibrocystic: Pertaining to, of the nature of, or having a **fibrous cyst** or **cysts**.

fibroglandular tissue: **Glandular tissue** having a large number of **fibers**, such as the **tissue** of the female **breast**.

fibroid: (1) Resembling a **fiber** or **fibrous tissue**. (2) Composed of **fibers**, as a **tumor**. (3) A **tumor** largely composed of smooth **muscle**.

fibrous: Containing, consisting of, or resembling **fibers**.

fibrous cyst: Any **cyst** that is surrounded by or situated among a large amount of **fibrous connective tissue**.

fibrous plaque: Small, flat formation or area of **fibrous tissue**.

fibrous tissue: **Tissue** mainly consisting of conjunctive **collagen** (or **elastin**) **fibers**, often packed in lamellar bundles. In **fibrous tissues** or **tissues** containing **fiber** layers [**cornea**, **sclera**, *dura mater*, **muscle**, **myocardium**, **tendon**, **cartilage**, **vessel** wall, **retinal nerve fiber layer (RNFL)**, and so on] and composed mostly of **microfibrils** and/or **microtubules**, typical diameters of the cylindrical structural elements are 10–400 nm. Their length is in a range from 10–25 μm to a few millimeters.

field of view (FOV): Angular subtense (expressed in angular degrees or **radians** per side if rectangular and angular degrees or **radians** if circular) over which an instrument will integrate all incoming radiant **energy**. In **optical imaging**, the extent of an object that can be imaged or seen through an optical system. In thermography, for an **infrared radiation thermometer**, this defines the target spot size, and for an **IR** scanner or **infrared imager**, this defines the scan angle or picture size or total **field of view** (TFOV).

finite element method: Numerical method for finding approximate solutions of partial differential equations (PDEs) as well as of integral equations such as the **bioheat** or **radiation-transfer equations**. This approach is based on either eliminating the differential equation completely (steady state problems) or rendering the PDE into an equivalent ordinary differential equation, which is then solved using standard techniques such as the **finite-difference method**.

finite-difference method: In numerical analysis, finite differences play an important role—they are one of the simplest ways of approximating a differential operator and are extensively used in solving differential equations.

finite-difference time-domain (FDTD): Numerical solution applied to a finite in space and time numerical equivalent of the physical reality under investigation; for example, the solution of Maxwell's equations describing **light scattering** by a **cell**. The **FDTD** is widely used for simulation and modeling of the light interaction with single and multiple, normal and **pathological biological cells** and subcellular structures. This approach was first adopted as a better alternative of Mie theory allowing for the modeling of irregular cell shapes and inhomogeneous distributions of complex **refractive index** values. The emerging relevance of nanobiophotonics imaging research has established the **FDTD** method as one of the powerful tools for studying the nature of **light–cell** interactions. One could identify a number of research directions based on the **FDTD** approach: (1) studying the lateral **light scattering** patterns for the early detection of **pathological** changes in **cancerous cells**, such as increased nuclear size and degrees of nuclear **pleomorphism** and nuclear-to-cytoplasmic ratios; (2) exploring the application of **FDTD**-based approaches for time-resolved **diffused optical tomography (DOT)** studies; (3) modeling of advanced **cell** imaging techniques within the context of a specific biodiagnostics device scenario. For example, an emerging research direction consists of the extension of the **FDTD** approach to account for optical nanotherapeutic effects.

fissure: Groove, natural division, deep furrow, or cleft found in the **brain**, **spinal cord**, or **liver**; also, a tear in the anus (anal fissure). In dentistry, a **fissure** is a break in the **tooth enamel**.

fitting: Process of constructing a mathematical function that has the best fit to a series of data points, possibly subject to constraints. It can involve either interpolation, where an exact fit to the data is required, or smoothing, in which a "smooth" function is constructed that approximately fits the data. A related topic is regression analysis (see **linear regression** and **nonlinear regression technique**), which focuses more on questions of statistical inference, such as how much uncertainty is present in a curve that is fit to data observed with random errors. Fitted curves can be used as an aid for data visualization, to infer values of a function where no data are available, and to summarize the relationships among two or more variables. Extrapolation refers to the use of a fitted curve beyond the range of the observed data and is subject to a greater degree of uncertainty, because it may reflect the method used to construct the curve as much as it reflects the observed data. In **biomedical optics**, spectral and/or spatial data points are typically fitted.

fixation: In the fields of **histology**, pathology, and **cell** biology, **fixation** is a chemical process by which biological **tissues** are preserved from decay. **Fixation** terminates any ongoing biochemical reactions and may also increase the mechanical strength or stability of the treated **tissues**.

flagellum: Long, fine, thread-like process on a noncellular or unicellular organism, such as **bacteria** and spermatozoa. Usually, the organism possesses only one flagellum or possibly two flagella. Flagella are used for locomotion. Their movement is in 3D and undulates in a **wave**-like or helical fashion.

flame filter: Filter of a specific waveband used to minimize the effects of flame, enabling the **infrared camera** to "see" through the flame. The specific waveband is a region where the

transmittance of flame approaches unity. Center **wavelengths** are typically 3.9 μm for shortwave instruments and 10.6 μm for longwave.

flashlamp: An **arc lamp** designed to produce extremely intense, incoherent, full-spectrum white light with a short pulse duration. **Flashlamps** are widely used in biomedical research and applications.

flavin: Complex heterocyclic ketone that is common to the nonprotein part of several important yellow **enzymes**, the flavoproteins.

flavin adenine dinucleotide (FAD): Formed as the **flavin** moiety attached with an adenosine diphosphate. It is a **coenzyme** for many **proteins**, including monoamine **oxidase**, D-**amino acid oxidase**, **glucose oxidase**, xanthine **oxidase**, and Acyl-CoA dehydrogenase.

flavin mononucleotide (FMN): Prosthetic group found in, among other **proteins**, **NADH** dehydrogenase and old yellow **enzyme**. A phosphorylated form of **riboflavin**.

flicker noise: See **pink noise**.

flow cytometry: Technique for counting, examining and sorting microscopic particles (**cells**) suspended in a stream of fluid. It allows simultaneous multiparametric analysis of the physical and/or chemical characteristics of single **cells** flowing through an optical and/or electronic detection apparatus. **Flow cytometry** was invented in the late 1960s, and since then it has become an indispensable tool of research and clinical laboratories. The main recent technological improvements include high-speed sorting, on-chip **microfluidics**, phase-sensitive optical **flow cytometry**, multi-color optical **flow cytometry**, high-throughput multiplex bead assays, optical spectral detection—all of which provide the basis for extensive data collection. **Cells** may be stained with one

167

or more fluorescent dyes specific to cell components of interest, e.g., **DNA**, and **fluorescence** of each **cell** is measured as **cells** one by one rapidly transverse the excitation **light beam** (**laser** or **mercury arc lamp**). **Fluorescence** provides a quantitative measure of various biochemical and biophysical properties of the **cell**. Other measurable optical parameters, which are applicable to the measurement of **cell** size, shape, density, granularity, and stain uptake, include **light absorption**, **light scattering**, and **polarization degree**. Conventional **flow cytometry** is currently the method of choice for rapid quantification of **cells**, but it requires invasive extraction of cells from a living organism and associated procedures (e.g., **fluorescence** labeling and sorting), which may lead to unpredictable **artifacts** and prevents long-term **cell** monitoring in the native biological environment. Therefore methods of *in vivo* **flow cytometry** are rapidly developing.

flowmeter: Device for measurement of parameters of a flow, such as flow velocity (for example, **blood flow** velocity).

fluence: See **energy density**.

fluence rate (*Synonym*: total radiant energy fluence rate): Sum of the **radiance** over all angles at a point $\bar{r}$. The quantity that is typically measured in irradiated **tissues** in units of **watts** per square meter or centimeter (W/m^2 or W/cm^2).

fluorescein: **Fluorophore** commonly used in biological **microscopy** that has an **absorption** maximum at 494 nm and an emission maximum of 521 nm (in **water**). Fluorescein has an isoabsorptive point (equal **absorption** for all **pH** values) at 460 nm.

fluorescence: The **luminescence** that is the property of emitting **light** of a longer **wavelength** on **absorption** of **light energy** by a molecule. The **luminescence** that essentially occurs simultaneously with the excitation of a sample. Measured in units characteristic for any other **electromagnetic radiation**, such as **fluence rate** or **intensity**. Most commonly an object exposed to **UV light** will fluoresce in the **visible**. In **tissue** diagnostics (**spectroscopy, microscopy**, and **tomography**), more sophisticated **fluorescence** techniques allowing for in-depth **tissue** probing by a **visible** or even an **IR light** are now available. [See **4Pi-microscope, confocal microscopy, confocal microscopy time-lapse fluorescence imaging, fluorescence diffuse optical tomography (fDOT), fluorescence molecular tomography (FMT), fluorescence imaging, fluorescence-lifetime imaging microscopy (FLIM), fluorescence microscopy, fluorescence spectroscopy, fluorescence recovery after photobleaching (FRAP), multidimensional fluorescence imaging (MDFI), multiphoton laser scanning microscopy (LSM), stimulated emission depletion microscopy (STED)**, and **two-photon fluorescence microscopy**].

fluorescence anisotropy: Transition **dipole moments** have defined orientations within a molecule. On excitation with linear **polarized light**, one preferentially excites those molecules whose transition dipoles are parallel to the electric field vector of incident **light**. This selective excitation of an oriented population of molecules results in partially polarized **fluorescence**, which is described by **fluorescence anisotropy**.

fluorescence correlation spectroscopy (FCS): Fluctuation **spectroscopy** technique that makes use of temporal fluctuations in the detected **fluorescence** signal under equilibrium conditions in order to obtain information about processes that give rise to these fluctuations. Statistical analysis of measured **intensity** fluctuations is performed using an **autocorrelation function**, which provides information about the characteristic times and the relative weights of different processes that give rise to fluctuations, such as molecular translational **diffusion**, rotational motion, and singlet–triplet transition dynamics. **FCS** is close to **dynamic light scattering spectroscopy** methods, such as **quasi-elastic light scattering (QELS)**. Confocal **FCS** has considerable advantages caused by reduced background and larger relative fluctuations due to a smaller number of molecules inside the detection volume. In addition to its confocal implementation, **FCS** has been combined with many other modes of **fluorescence** excitation, such as **laser scanning microscopy (LSM)**, **two-photon fluorescence (TPF) microscopy**, and **STED microscopy**.

fluorescence diffuse optical tomography (fDOT) [*Synonym*: fluorescence molecular tomography (FMT)]: An *in vivo*, **noninvasive** technique that produces quantitative, 3D distributions of **fluorescence** and has so far been used in small-**animal models**. **fDOT** combines the use of fluorescent probes as a source of **contrast** with the principles of optical tomography. The sample bearing fluorescent probes is illuminated with a defined **wavelength** from different positions, and the emitted **light** is collected at detectors arranged in a specific order (**CCD**). The mathematical processing of the data obtained in this way results in the reconstruction of a tomographic image. **fDOT** incorporates the principles of **diffuse optical tomography (DOT)**, which models **light** propagation theoretically as being within the **diffusion approximation**, using **fluorescence** as a source of **contrast**. Advances in theoretical approaches that enable 3D measurements allow for the optimization of full-angle **fDOT** imaging, which results in an increase in the accuracy of the tomographic reconstructions.

fluorescence emission spectrum: Fluorescence spectrum measured at a certain excitation **wavelength**.

fluorescence excitation spectrum: Intensity of **fluorescence** measured at a certain emission **wavelength** as a function of the excitation **wavelength**.

fluorescence excitation–emission map: Map presenting combined data of **fluorescence** emission and excitation spectra, where excitation and emission **wavelengths** are presented on x–y axes and corresponding **fluorescence intensity** values as the isometric lines on the map.

fluorescence imaging: Powerful **optical imaging** method that uses excitation and detection of **fluorescence** of **endogenous** (**autofluorescence**) or **exogenous fluorophores** for imaging of **cell** and **tissue metabolism** and pathologies. This holds for intrinsic **fluorophores** (**proteins** or **coenzymes**) as well as for a number of **fluorescence** markers, including **green fluorescent protein (GFP)** and **quantum dots**, staining various organelles (**cell** nuclei, **mitochondria, lysosomes, cytoskeleton**, or **membranes**). For example, by fusion of **genes** coding for a specific cellular **protein** and a **GFP** variant, fluorescent **protein** chimera were thus created, which permitted a site-specific tracking in living **cells** or even whole organisms. The application of most fluorescent probes is restricted to *in vitro* systems, and only a few dyes are presently used *in vivo*, e.g., **fluorescein** or **indocyanine green** for **fluorescent angiography**, or **porphyrin** derivatives for **photodynamic diagnosis (PDD)** and **photodynamic therapy (PDT)** of **cancer** and inflammatory diseases. The development of highly sensitive detection systems significantly improved **fluorescence imaging** techniques. **CCD** cameras with a sensitivity around 10^{-7} W/cm^2 to highly sensitive **electron multiplying (EMCCD)** or **image intensifying (ICCD) cameras** with a sensitivity between 10^{-11} and 10^{-14} W/cm^2 are available, and even single-molecule detection could be provided. Axial resolution in the submicrometer range has been introduced into wide-field **microscopy** by **structured illumination microscopy (SIM)** or **selective plane illumination microscopy (SPIM)** techniques. Due to the availability of highly sensitive camera systems, wide-field techniques often require lower doses of exciting **light** than **laser** scanning techniques.

fluorescence-lifetime imaging microscopy (FLIM): **Fluorescence** lifetime is the average time the molecule spends in an upper **energy level** before returning to the ground state. For a large ensemble of identical molecules (or a large number of excitations of the same molecule), the time-resolved **fluorescence intensity** profile (detected **photon histogram**) following instantaneous excitation will exhibit a monoexponential decay. The presence of multiple **fluorophore** species (or multiple states of a **fluo-**

171

rophore species arising from interactions with the local environment) often results in more complex **fluorescence** decay profiles. Such complex **fluorescence** decays are commonly modeled by an N-component multiexponential decay model. **Frequency-domain fluorescence** lifetime measurements concern the **demodulation** of a **fluorescence** signal excited with modulated **light**. The **fluorescence** lifetime can be determined from measurements of the relative **modulation** m and the phase delay ϕ using appropriate electronic circuits for synchronous detection, such as a **lock-in amplifier**. If the **fluorescence** does not manifest a single exponential decay, it is necessary to repeat the measurement at multiple harmonics of the excitation **modulation frequency** to build up a more complete (multiexponential) description of the complex **fluorescence** profile. This is usually calculated by **fitting** the results to a set of **dispersion** relationships. Single-point time-domain measurement of **fluorescence** decay profiles has been implemented using a wide range of instrumentation. Ultrashort pulsed excitation is typically provided by **mode-locked solid-state lasers** or by **gain**-switched **diode lasers**. For detection, fast (GHz **bandwidth**) sampling oscilloscopes and **streak cameras** have been used for decades, but these have been increasingly supplanted by **photon** counting techniques that build up histograms of the decay profiles. The current most widely used **FLIM** detection technique is **time-correlated single-photon counting (TCSPC) technique.** Laser scanning microscopes are essentially single-channel detection systems and are widely used for **FLIM biological imaging** because their implementation as confocal or multiphoton microscopes provides improved **contrast** and optical sectioning compared to wide-field microscopes. The parallel nature of wide-field imaging techniques can support **FLIM** imaging rates of tens to hundreds of Hz, although the maximum acquisition speed is still of course limited by the number of **photons/pixel** available from the (biological) sample. Wide-field **FLIM** is most commonly implemented using modulated image intensifiers with **frequency**- or time-domain approaches. It is possible to implement wide-field **FLIM** at a single **modulation frequency** using only three phase measurements to calculate the **fluorescence** lifetime map, although it is common to use eight or more phase-resolved images to improve the accuracy.

fluorescence microscopy: Ordinary **fluorescence microscopy** using ordinary fluorescent microscopes has fairly good sensitivity for routine clinical studies and is often used in laboratory medical diagnostics. Enormous improvements in resolution have been achieved by using confocal and **multiphoton laser scanning microscopy (LSM)**, including **4-Pi microscopy** and **stimulated emission depletion microscopy (STED)** with a lateral and axial resolution of less than 60 nm. **Fluorescence microscopy** is extremely powerful due to its ability to show specifically labeled structures within a complex environment and also because of its inherent ability to provide 3D information about biological structures. For further improvement of the image **contrast**, the **deconvolution microscopy** could be used.

fluorescence quenching: Refers to any process that decreases the emitted **fluorescence** of a given molecule. A variety of processes can result in quenching, including **excited state** reactions, **energy** transfer, molecular complex formation, and collisions with other molecules. In general, quenching is considered an undesirable process, because it reduces the **fluorescence** signal. However, it is a valuable source of information about the interaction of a fluorescent molecule with a quenching one, and it is used for many biological applications, including studies of structure and dynamics of **proteins** and interactions with **nucleotides** [see also **Förster resonance energy transfer (FRET)**]. At high concentrations of **fluorophores**, there can be **fluorescence quenching** due to **aggregation** (dimerization), which is most pronounced in solutions where solvent consists of small, highly polar molecules, notably **water**. Excited state reaction also may contribute to quenching due to collisions of the **excited state** molecules with those in the ground state or with the sample **cell** wall.

fluorescence recovery after photobleaching (FRAP): Denotes an optical technique capable of quantifying the 2D lateral **diffusion** within a **cell** containing fluorescently labeled probes. The basic apparatus comprises an optical microscope, a **light** source, and some fluorescent probe. The technique begins by saving a background image of the sample before **photobleaching**. Next, the **light** source is focused onto a small patch of the viewable area either by switching to a higher magnification microscope **objective** or with **laser light** of the appropriate **wavelength**. The **fluorophores** in this region receive high-**intensity** illumination, which causes their **fluorescence** lifetime to quickly elapse (limited to roughly 10^5 **photons** before extinction). The image in the microscope is that of a uniformly fluorescent field with a noticeable dark spot. As **Brownian motion** proceeds, the still-fluorescing probes will diffuse throughout the sample and replace the nonfluorescent probes in the bleached region. This **diffusion** proceeds in an orderly fashion, analytically determinable from the **diffusion** equation. This technique is very useful in biological studies of **cell membrane diffusion** and **protein** binding, for characterization of **hydrophilic** (or **hydrophobic**) surfaces in terms of surface structure and free **energy**. Similar techniques have been developed to investigate the 3D **diffusion** and binding of molecules inside the **cell**.

fluorescence resonance energy transfer: See **Förster resonance energy transfer (FRET)**.

fluorescence spectroscopy: Type of **electromagnetic wave spectroscopy** that analyzes **fluorescence** from a sample. It involves using a beam of **light** that excites the electrons in molecules of certain compounds and causes them to emit **light** of a lower **energy**; typically, **visible** and **NIR light**. A complementary technique is **absorption spectroscopy**. Molecules have various states referred to as **energy** levels. **Fluorescence spectroscopy** is primarily concerned with electronic and vibrational states. Emission and/or excitation spectra are typically measured. By analyzing these spectra, the structure of the different vibrational levels can be determined.

fluorescence tomography: Optical tomography that is based on the detection of **fluorescence** signal. See **fluorescence diffuse optical tomography (fDOT)**.

fluorescent angiography: Technique for examining the **blood** circulation of the **retina** and other normal and **pathological tissues** using a dye tracing method that involves injection of sodium **fluorescein** or **indocyanine green (ICG)** into the systemic circulation. An angiogram is then obtained by imaging the **fluorescence** emitted after illumination of the **tissue** with blue (**fluorescein**) or **NIR (ICG) light**.

fluorometer (fluorimeter): Device that measures **fluorescence**.

fluorometry: Science that describes and quantifies **fluorescence**.

fluorophore: **Chromophore** that emits **light** with a characteristic spectral pattern at its excitation by a proper **wavelength**.

fluorophore-assisted light inactivation (FALI): Technique that is related to **chromophore-assisted light inactivation (CALI)**. In particular, it takes advantage of the great efficiency of the commonly used **fluorophore fluorescein** in the loss of a **protein** activity, which permits the use of nonlaser **light** sources (such as a slide projector) to simultaneously irradiate many samples in multiwell plates. The use of **green fluorescent protein (GFP)** would have advantages because it could be expressed in **cells** as a genetically encoded **photosensitizer**. The diarsenyl derivatives of **fluorescein** (FlAsH) have high efficiency in **CALI**-mediated damage and the **power** of molecular **genetics** by expressing the encoded binding domain, a tetracysteine domain that can bind tightly to FlAsH. FlAsH does not fluoresce in solution but does so when bound to a **protein** fusion containing the tetracysteine domain. Novel means of targeting the damage have been developed, including the use of environmentally sensitive **fluorophores**.

_f_-number (_f_/#): Refers to the **lens** optical system. It is the effective **focal length** F divided by the effective aperture diameter D, the diameter of its entrance **pupil**, $F/\# = F/D \equiv 1/(2\mathrm{NA})$.

f-number (*f*/#) coupling: When using **optical fiber** in an optical system, the acceptance cones (**numerical apertures**, or **NAs**) should match at each interface. In order to match **numerical apertures** between the **optical fiber** and the **lens** system with *f*-number, $F/\# = F/D \equiv 1/(2NA)$, where F is the effective **focal length** of the **lens** and D is the diameter of its entrance **pupil**, one needs **fiber numerical aperture** $NA_{fiber} = D/2 - F$, i.e., for $D = 4$ mm and $F = 10$ mm, $NA_{fiber} = 0.2$ to get an ideal match. This does not include any losses due to **Fresnel reflections** and **lens** focal-spot size versus core size mismatches.

focal depth: Every **lens** has a range of object positions that give an apparently focused image on a fixed screen. This range is called the depth of focus of the **lens**.

focal length: Measure of how strongly the optical system converges (focuses) or diverges (defocuses) **light**. In air, it is the distance over which initially **collimated** rays are brought to a focus. A system with a shorter **focal length** has greater optical power than one with a long **focal length**; that is, it bends the rays more strongly, bringing them to a focus in a shorter distance. In telescopy and most photography, longer **focal length** or lower optical power is associated with larger magnification of distant objects and a narrower **field of view** (**FOV**), and shorter **focal length** or higher optical power is associated with a wider **FOV**. In **microscopy**, on the other **hand**, a short **objective lens focal length** leads to higher magnification. For a thin **lens** in air, the **focal length** is the distance from the center of the **lens** to the principal foci (or **focal points**) of the **lens**.

focal plane: Focusing plane that is perpendicular to the principal axis and also passes through the principal focus. Rays parallel to each other, but at angle to the principal axis, are brought to a focus in the **focal plane**.

focal plane array (FPA): Linear or 2D matrix of detector elements, typically used at the **focal plane** of an instrument (**CCD**,

CMOS, infrared cameras). In thermography, rectangular **FPAs** are used in "staring" (nonscanning) **infrared imagers**. These are called **infrared focal plane array (IRFPA) imagers**.

focal point: Point where the spot size provided by an optical system is the smallest. In optical imagers, the point at which the instrument optics image the object onto a **photodetector**. In a scanning imager, this is where the **instantaneous field of view (IFOV)** is smallest.

focal spot: Spot obtained at the focus of a **lens**. The size of the spot depends on the **lens** and the **wavelength**, but its diameter is never smaller than the **wavelength** of **light**.

Food and Drug Administration (FDA): Government agency of the United States Department of Health and Human Services responsible for regulating and supervising food safety, tobacco products, dietary supplements, medication drugs, vaccines, biopharmaceuticals, **blood** transfusions, medical devices, **electromagnetic radiation** emitting devices, veterinary products, and **cosmetics**.

foot sole: Contains the thickest layers of **skin** on the human body due to the weight that is continually placed on them. Contains significantly less **pigment** than the **skin** of the rest of the body. One of the two areas of the human body that grow no vellus **hair**. Houses a denser population of **sweat glands** than most other regions of **skin**.

forearm: Lower part of the human **arm**, between the elbow and the **wrist**. An **arm** consists of the upper **arm** and the **forearm**.

foreground temperature: Temperature of the scene behind and surrounding the instrument as viewed from the target. See **instrument background temperature**.

177

formalin: Trade name of 37% aqueous solution of formaldehyde. In **water**, formaldehyde converts to the hydrate $CH_2(OH)_2$. Preserves or fixes **tissue** or **cells** by irreversibly cross-linking primary amine groups in **proteins** with other nearby nitrogen atoms in **protein** or **DNA** through a $-CH_2-$ linkage. Can be used as a disinfectant, because it kills most **bacteria** and **fungi cells** (including their spores).

form birefringence: **Birefringence** that is caused by the structure of a medium. For example, a system of long dielectric cylinders made from an isotropic substance and arranged in a parallel fashion shows **birefringence** of form.

Förster resonance energy transfer (FRET) (*Synonyms*: fluorescence resonance energy transfer, resonance energy transfer (RET), and electronic energy transfer (EET)): A mechanism describing **energy** transfer between two **chromophores**. A donor **chromophore**, initially in its electronic **excited state**, may transfer **energy** to an acceptor **chromophore** (in proximity, typically less than 10 nm) through nonradiative dipole–dipole coupling. **FRET** is analogous to near-field communication, in that the radius of interaction is much smaller than the **wavelength** of **light** emitted. In the near-field region, the excited **chromophore** emits a virtual **photon** that is instantly absorbed by a receiving **chromophore**. From quantum electrodynamical calculations, it is determined that radiationless (**FRET**) and radiative **energy** transfer are the short- and long-range asymptotes of a single unified mechanism. It is a technique in **fluorescence microscopy** for identifying where and when molecules with two different **fluorophores** are interacting with each other.

forward-scattering problem: Modeling of **light** propagation in a **scattering** medium by taking into account the experimental geometry, source, and detector characteristics and the known **optical properties** of a sample and predicting the measurements and associated accuracies that result. Such modeling is often needed for developing a strategy of **light** treatment or diagnosis.

Foscan®: PDT photosensitizer, which contains temoporfin. It requires **laser light** of a specific **wavelength** of 652 nm for activation.

Fourier optical microscope: Based on the principle that spatial variations in **optical density** in the object plane of the microscope are converted by a **Fourier transform** to spatial **frequency** variations in the **Fourier transform** plane in the rear **focal plane** of the **lens**. If the **optical density** changes slowly across the object, the **Fourier transform** places most of the scattered **light** near zero angles (low spatial **frequency**) in the **Fourier transform** plane (a good model of a **cell** with clear **cytoplasm**). If the **optical density** changes rapidly across the object, the **Fourier transform** moves more of the **energy** to larger **scattering** angles (higher spatial **frequency**) in the **Fourier transform** plane (a good model of a **cell** with highly granular **cytoplasm**).

Fourier transform (FT): Algorithm for the expression of any periodic function as a sum of sine and cosine functions.

Fourier transform infrared spectroscopy (FTIR): Spectroscopy based on **light dispersion** by using a **Michelson interferometer** with a tuned path length difference. In the **IR**, may provide $10^2–10^3$ higher **signal-to-noise ratio** than a grating **spectrometer**.

Fourier-domain OCT: See **frequency-domain OCT**.

fractal dimension: As the complexity of the object structure increases, its **fractal dimension** increases, being always higher than the topological dimension of the structure. For example, any structure described as a curve (**tissue fiber**) has a topological dimension $D = 1$; however, if we make this curve more complex by its bending infinite times, its **fractal dimension** will be equal to 2 when this curve densely covers a finite area, or even 3 when this curve "packs" a cube.

fractal object: An object with a self-similar geometry, i.e., each arbitrarily selected part of the object is similar to the whole object. The **fractal dimension** of the object (structure) is always higher than its topological dimension.

frame repetition rate: Time it takes an optical imager to scan (update) every image picture element (**pixel**), in frames per second.

frame-grabber: An electronic device that provides video data acquisition and converts it to digital form.

frame-transfer charge-coupled device (CCD): This device has a parallel shift register that is divided into two separate and almost identical areas, termed the image and storage arrays. The image array consists of a **light**-sensitive **photodiode** register, which acts as the image plane and collects incoming **photons** projected onto the **charge-coupled device (CCD)** surface by the camera or microscope **lenses**. After image data has been collected and converted to electrical potential by the image array, the data is then quickly, in 500 μs or less, shifted in a parallel transfer to the storage array for readout by the serial shift register. Typically, the storage array is not **light** sensitive. With the use of a mechanical shutter, a **frame-transfer CCD** can be used to quickly capture two sequential images, which is a useful feature in **fluorescence microscopy** and other applications that require simultaneous acquisition of images generated at different emission and/or excitation **wavelengths**.

Franck–Condon principle: States that an **electronic transition** is so fast that during this transition, a vibrating molecule could not noticeably change its internuclear distance.

Fraunhofer diffraction: Type of **diffraction** in which the **light** source and the receiving screen are effectively at an infinite distance from the **diffraction** object, i.e., parallel beams of **wave** trains are used.

Fraunhofer diffraction approximation: Description of forward-direction **scattering** caused by large particles (on the order of 10 μm).

Fraunhofer zone: Zone where **Fraunhofer diffraction** takes place.

freckle: Small tan spots of **melanin** on the **skin** of people with fair complexions.

free diffusion: **Diffusion** process in which molecules diffuse in the space free of any **membranes** and other barriers hindering **diffusion**.

free radical: Atom, molecule, or ion with unpaired electrons in an open shell configuration. **Radicals** may have positive, negative, or zero charge. The unpaired electrons cause **radicals** to be highly chemically reactive. These chemically reactive **radicals** are known to cause degenerative diseases such as **Alzheimer's disease**, Parkinson's disease, and **cancers**. Radicals play an important role in human physiology. For example, **superoxide** and **nitric oxide (NO)** regulate many biological processes, such as controlling **vascular** tone.

frequency: Number of occurrences of a repeated event per unit of time or the rate of change of phase of a sinusoidal waveform. **Frequency** ν has an inverse relationship to the **wavelength** λ of the **wave** and is equal to the speed v of the **wave** divided by the **wavelength** $\nu = v/\lambda$. In the special case of **electromagnetic waves (EMWs)** moving through a free space, then $v = c$, where c is the **speed of light** in a free space ($c = 3 \times 10^8$ m/s), and $\nu = c/\lambda$. When waves travel from one medium to another, their **frequency** remains exactly the same. Only their **wavelength** and speed change. Apart from being modified by the **Doppler effect** or any other nonlinear process, **frequency** is an invariant quantity; thus, it cannot be changed by any linearly physical process, unlike velocity of propagation or **wavelength**. **Frequency** ν is expressed

181

in **hertz (Hz)**, where 1 Hz is s^{-1}. Because of the high **frequency** of **light**, its **frequency** is typically expressed in **terahertz (THz)**: 1 THz is 10^{12} Hz. For example, **IR radiation** with a **wavelength** of 10 μm in free space is oscillating with a **frequency** of 30 THz.

frequency-domain optical coherence tomography (FD OCT): Also called **Fourier-domain OCT**, spectral **OCT**, or **spectral radar**. It is based on **backscattering** spectral interferometry with a parallel spectrograph as a detector. One of the main advantages of this technique is that it does not require scanning in the depth of a sample. This technique has great potential, in terms of speed and sensitivity. It demonstrates sensitivities that are two to three orders of magnitude greater than time-domain **optical coherence tomography (OCT)**. Since **FD OCT** measures the amplitude of **scattering** $E(z)$ along the axis from the surface toward the inside of an object during a single exposition of a detector without longitudinal scanning of the beam, the time of tomogram recording may be very small. For the superposition of the object and reference fields on the detector, the **intensity** of **light** $I(k) = |S(k)|^2 \int_0^\infty E(z)\cos(2kz)\,dz + \cdots$, where k is the **wave** vector, and $S(k)$ is the spectral distribution of the amplitude of the **light** source. Performing an inverse **Fourier transform** gives the dependence $a(z)$ of the **scattering** amplitude on the depth. Higher frequencies in the detected signal correspond to larger depths. The maximum depth of probing is defined by the spectral resolution of the **spectrometer**. Specifically, for a **spectrometer** with a resolution $\Delta\lambda = 0.05$ nm, $z_{max} = (1/4n)(\lambda^2/\Delta\lambda) \cong 2.4$ mm ($n = 1.5, \lambda = 853$ nm). To ensure a **signal-to-noise ratio (SNR)** at the level of 10^4, one should employ a highly sensitive **CCD** or **CMOS** camera at the output of the **spectrometer**. **Fourier-domain OCT** can be also realized using a **swept-laser source**, a rapidly **tunable laser** over a broad optical **bandwidth**. In **swept-laser source OCT**, instead of a **CCD** or **photodiode** arrays, a single **photodiode** in the detection path of the **interferometer** is employed, which allows for the spectral interferometric signal to be encoded with a characteristic heterodyne beat **frequency**. It was shown that heterodyne detection in **swept-laser source OCT** allows for resolution of complex conjugate ambiguity and the removal of spectral and **autocorrelation artifacts**, characteristic for spectral **OCT**.

frequency-domain (FD) spectrometer: **Spectrometer** that uses the **frequency-domain (FD)** method (**photon density wave**) for measuring the spectra of **absorption coefficient** and **scattering coefficient** of a **tissue**. **FD** technology is used also to detect time-resolved **fluorescence**, **photoacoustic**, and **photothermal** signals from **tissues** and **cells**.

frequency-domain (FD) technique (method): Spectroscopic or imaging technique (method) that exploits an **intensity**-modulated **light** and narrow-band heterodyne detection. Both temporal and spatial **modulation** versions are available.

Fresnel diffraction: Type of **diffraction** in which the **light** source and the receiving screen are both at a finite distance from the **diffraction** object, i.e., divergent and convergent beams of **wave** trains are used.

Fresnel equations: Equations that describe the behavior of **light** when it is moving from a plane-parallel medium of a given **refractive index** n_1 into a second plane-parallel medium with **refractive index** n_2. Both **reflection** and **refraction** of the **light** may occur. The **reflection** of **light** that the equations predict is known as **Fresnel reflection**. The angles that the incident, reflected and refracted rays make to the normal of the interface are given as θ_i, θ_r, and θ_t, respectively. The relationship between these angles is given by the law of **reflection** ($\theta_i = \theta_r$) and **Snell's law**. The fraction of the incident **power** that is reflected from the interface is given by the **reflectance** R, and the fraction that is refracted is given by the **transmittance** T. The calculations of R and T depend on **polarization** of the incident ray, its angle of incidence θ_i, and the relative **index of refraction** $m = n_1/n_2$.

Fresnel reflection: Reflection of a beam of **radiation**, such as **light**, that takes place at the interface between two media of different **refractive indexes**. Not all the **radiation** is reflected—some may be refracted.

Fresnel zone: Zone where **Fresnel diffraction** takes place.

frontal lobe: See **lobe**.

front chamber (segment) of the human eye: Includes the **cornea**, an anterior chamber of the **eyeball** filled by the **aqueous humor**, and the **iris** and **crystalline lens** in it.

fuchsine (*Synonym*: rosaniline hydrochloride): A magenta dye with chemical formula $C_{20}H_{19}N_3 \cdot HCl$. It becomes magenta when dissolved in **water**; as a solid, it forms dark green crystals. It is used to stain **bacteria** and sometimes as a disinfectant.

full scale: Span between the minimum value and the maximum value that any instrument is capable of measuring. In a thermometer, this would be the span between the highest and lowest temperature that can be measured.

full width at half maximum (FWHM): See **bandwidth**.

fullerene: Any molecule composed entirely of carbon, in the form of a hollow sphere, ellipsoid, or tube. Spherical **fullerenes** are also called buckyballs, and cylindrical ones are called **carbon nanotubes**. **Fullerenes** are similar in structure to graphite, which is composed of stacked graphene sheets of linked hexagonal rings. But they may also contain pentagonal (or sometimes heptagonal) rings. The discovery of **fullerenes** has greatly expanded the number of known carbon allotropes, which until recently were limited to graphite, diamond, and amorphous carbon. **Fullerenes** have been the subject of intense research, both for their unique chemistry and for their technological applications, especially in materials science, electronics, and nanotechnology, including biomedicine.

full-field optical coherence tomography (OCT): Conventional time-domain **optical coherence tomography** is a single-point detection technique. It can be used to generate 2D OCT images up to video rate; however, such systems have a limited sensitivity or a limited space-**bandwidth** product (resolved **pixels** per dimension). Full-field or parallel **OCT** uses linear or 2D detector arrays of, respectively, N and N^2 single detectors. The advantage of parallel **OCT** is that **signal-to-noise ratio (SNR)** when using linear or 2D detector arrays can be roughly, respectively, $\sqrt{N}$ and N times larger, compared to the single-detector signal. The disadvantages of using standard **CCD** sensors are connected with their time-integrating operation mode; therefore, no **alternating current (ac)** technique and no mixing and mode-lock detection are possible. To overcome these problems, synchronous illumination instead of the usual synchronous detection to obtain lock-in detection on every **pixel** of a **CCD** array-detector or **CMOS** detector arrays can be used. In the **CMOS** camera, each "smart **pixel**" consisting of a **photodetector** and analog signal processing performs heterodyne detection in parallel, thus dramatically increasing the dynamic range compared to a **CCD** array. A typical 2D smart **pixel** detector array makes it possible to record a data set of 58×58 **pixels** and 33 slices with an **acquisition rate** of 6 Hz. To improve depth resolution, a thermal **light** source can be used, with a 100-W tungsten halogen thermal lamp in a modified Linnik microscope allowed to obtained depth resolution of 1.2 μm. **Water** immersion can be used to compensate **dispersion**. The immersion **objective lenses** with an NA of 0.3 provide a transverse resolution of about 1.3 μm.

full-field technique: High-speed optical detection system based on irradiation of the whole object under study by a divergent **light beam** using an integrating digital camera (**CCD** or **CMOS**). For example, a **laser Doppler perfusion imaging (LDPI)** full-field system uses a **laser** source that is diverged to illuminate the area of the sample, and the **tissue** surface is imaged through the **objective lens** onto a **CMOS** camera sensor. The imaging time is 3–4 times faster than the current commercial raster scan **LDPI** systems. The refresh rate of the perfusion images is approximately 3.2 s for a

256 × 256 **pixel** perfusion image. This time includes acquisition, signal processing, and data transfer to the display.

functional imaging: An imaging technique for the visualization of the spatial distribution of **blood oxygenation**, **blood volume**, **blood** velocity, or any other functional parameter of a living **tissue**.

functionalized nanoparticle: In nanobiotechnology, metal **nanoparticles** are used in combination with recognizing biomacromolecules attached to their surface by means of physical adsorption or binding with molecular probes such as oligonucleotides, **proteins**, immunoglobulins, avidin, **antibodies**, peptides, **carbohydrates**, and so on. Such nanostructures are called bioconjugates, while the attachment of biomacromolecules to the **nanoparticle** surface is often called functionalization. A probe-conjugate molecule is used for unique coupling with a biological target, while a metal core serves as an optical label. For example, the carbon–gold nanotubes conjugated with folate are highly expressed in selected human **breast tumors** and are not expressed in normal endothelial **cells** in **lymphatics**.

function generator (FG): Piece of electronic test equipment or software used to generate electrical waveforms. These waveforms can be either repetitive or single-shot, in which case, some kind of triggering source is required (internal or external). Another type of function generator is a subsystem that provides an output proportional to some mathematical function of its input. For example, the output may be proportional to the square root of the input. Such devices are used in feedback control systems and in analog computers.

fundus: Base of an organ, or the part opposite to or remote from an aperture; for example, the **fundus** (bottom) of the **eye**.

fungi cell: Division of the subkingdom Thallophyta. Its members include the **yeasts**, mushrooms, molds, and rusts, i.e., fungal organisms. The characteristics of this division are that its members have **eucaryote cells**, they lack chlorophyll, there are unicellular or coenocytic tubular filaments for the main body of the organism, they are saprophytic or parasitic on plants and animals, and they reproduce by forming spores in very large numbers.

fusogenicity: Relates to the ability of **cell membrane** fusion by physical or chemical action.

FVB/N mouse strain: Inbred mouse strain that was established at the National Institutes of Health in 1970 from an outbred colony of Swiss mice. It is preferable for transgenic analyses.

GaAs laser: Laser based on the **semiconductor** material GaAs. The emission is in the **near-infrared (NIR)**, at about 830 nm.

gain: Measure of the ability of a circuit or a medium to increase the amplitude or **power** of a signal from the input to the output. It is usually defined as the mean ratio of the signal output of a system to the signal input of the same system. In electronics, most often this is the ratio of output to input voltages for audio and low-**frequency amplifiers**, especially operational **amplifiers**, but the ratio of **powers** for **radio frequency (RF) amplifiers**. It may also be defined on a logarithmic scale, in terms of the decimal logarithm of the same ratio, in **decibels (dB)**. The term **gain** is also applied to sensors, where the input and output have different units. In such cases, the **gain** units must be specified, as generated microvolts per **photon** for a **photodiode**, electrons per **photon** for a **photomultiplier tube (PMT)**, or electron-hole pairs per **photon** for an **APD**. In **lasers**, **gain** refers to the increment of **power** along the beam propagation in a **gain** medium, and its dimension is m^{-1}.

gall bladder: Small **bladder** situated between the lobes of the **liver**. It is connected to the **liver** through the cystic **duct** and the hepatic **duct**. Its function is to store **bile**, and its capacity in a human is 30–50 cm^3. The **liver** secretes **bile** continuously, but the **bile** enters the **duodenum** only during periods of digestion; otherwise, the liquid is stored in the **gall bladder**. The walls are contractile and empty the **gall bladder** when food, especially **fat**, passes through the **duodenum**. The contractions are probably activated by a **hormone** secreted by the intestinal walls.

gallstone (biliary calculus): Calculus, or hard stone, formed in the **gall bladder** or a **bile duct**. It contains **cholesterol** crystals combined with other substances (e.g., calcium salts). The different types of stones are called porcinement, **cholesterol**, and so on.

ganglion: Clusters of **neurons**.

gas-microphone method: Relates to **optoacoustic spectroscopy**, when an object under study is surrounded by a gas (or combination of gases) that serves as an acoustic **coupler** between the object and an acoustic receiver such as a **microphone**. The **spectroscopy** of the surrounding gas when an object's optical and acoustical properties are known or fixed can also be determined.

gastric juice: Secretion from **glands** in the **stomach** wall that contains hydrochloric acid (0.2–0.5%), digestive **enzymes** (e.g., pepsin), and, in young mammals only, rennin.

gastrointestinal tract: Also called the **digestive tract**, alimentary canal, or **gut**. It is a system of organs that takes in food, digests it to extract **energy** and nutrients, and expels the remaining waste.

gating: See **motion tracking**.

Gaussian correlation function: Correlation function described by a bell-shaped (Gaussian) curve.

Gaussian distribution: Normal distribution. In **probability** theory and statistics, this is an absolutely continuous **probability** distribution with zero cumulants of all orders higher than two. The graph of the associated **probability density function** is bell-shaped, with a peak at the mean, and is known as the Gaussian function or bell curve, where μ and σ^2 are the mean and the **variance** of the distribution. The **Gaussian distribution** with μ = 0 and σ^2 = 1 is called the standard normal distribution.

$$f(x) = \frac{1}{\sqrt{2\pi\sigma^2}} \cdot e^{-\frac{(x-\mu)^2}{2\sigma^2}}$$

Gaussian light beam: **Light beam** with a Gaussian shape for the transverse **intensity** profile. If the **intensity** at the center of the beam is I_0, then the formula for a **Gaussian light beam** is $I = I_0 \exp(-2r^2/w^2)$, where r is the radial distance from the axis and w is the beam "waist." The **intensity** profile of such a beam is said to be bell shaped. A **laser beam** is a **Gaussian light beam**. A **single-mode fiber** also creates a **Gaussian light beam** at its output.

Gaussian size distribution: Distribution size function of a Gaussian shape.

Gaussian statistics (*Synonym*: normal statistics): Statistics when a bell-shaped (Gaussian) curve showing a distribution of **probability** associated with different values of a variate is valid.

Gegenbauer kernel phase function (GKPF): One of the approximations of the actual **phase function** for **tissue**. The **Henyey–Greenstein phase function** is a special case of the **GKPF**. GKPF is a good function for simulating **light** transport in a **tissue** characterized by a high **scattering anisotropy**, such as **blood**.

gel: An intermediate stage in the **coagulation** of a solid. A mass of intertwining filaments enclose the whole of the **dispersion** medium to produce a pseudo-solid. A **gel** is jellylike in appearance and forms a distortable mass.

gelatin: Many substances that form lyophilic sols can be obtained in a jellylike condition. The process is called gelation. For example, **gelatin** mixed with **water** forms a colloidal solution. When cooled, this solution becomes a semisolid.

gene: Unit of heredity in a living organism. It is normally a stretch of **DNA** that codes for a type of **protein** or for an **RNA** chain that has a function in the organism. **Genes** correspond to regions within **DNA**, a molecule composed of a chain of four different types of **nucleotides**. The sequence of these **nucleotides** is the genetic information that organisms inherit. **DNA** occurs naturally in a double-stranded form, with **nucleotides** on each strand complementary to each other. Each strand can act as a template for creating a new partner strand. This is the physical method for making copies of **genes** that can be inherited. All **proteins** and functional **RNA** chains are specified by **genes**. **Genes** hold the information to build and maintain an organism's **cells** and pass genetic traits to offspring. **Genes** that encode **proteins** are composed of a series of three-**nucleotide** sequences called codons. The genetic code specifies the correspondence during **protein** translation between codons and **amino acids**. The genetic code is nearly the same for all known organisms.

gene expression: Process by which information from a **gene** is used in the synthesis of a functional **gene** product. These products are often **proteins**, but in nonprotein coding **genes** such as **rRNA genes** or **tRNA genes**, the product is a functional **RNA**. The process of **gene expression** is used by all known life (**eukaryotes**, **prokaryotes**, and **viruses**) to generate the macromolecular machinery for life. Several steps in the **gene expression** process may be modulated, including the transcription, **RNA** splicing, translation, and post-translational modification of a **protein**. **Gene** regulation gives the **cell** control over structure and function, and is the basis for cellular differentiation, morphogenesis, and the versatility and adaptability of any organism. **Gene** regulation may also serve as a substrate for evolutionary change, since control of the timing, location, and amount of **gene expression** can have a profound effect on the functions (actions) of the **gene** in a **cell** or in a multicellular organism.

gene knockout (KO): Genetic technique in which an organism is engineered to carry **genes** that have been made inoperative (have been "knocked out" of the organism). Such organisms are used in learning about a **gene** that has been sequenced but that has an unknown or incompletely known function. Researchers draw inferences from the difference between the knockout organism and normal individuals. The technique is essentially the opposite of a **gene** "knock in." Knocking out two or more **genes** simultaneously in an organism is also possible and is known as a double knockout (DKO), triple knockout (TKO), or quadruple knockout (QKO).

genetic inverse algorithm: Genetic **algorithms** (GAs) are now widely applied in science and engineering as adaptive **algorithms** for solving practical problems. Certain classes of problems are particularly suited to a GA-based approach. It is generally accepted that GAs are particularly suited to multidimensional global search problems where the search space potentially contains multiple local minima. Unlike other search methods, this approach does not generally have problems with **correlation** between the search variables; the basic GA does not require extensive knowledge of the search space, such as likely solution bounds or functional derivatives.

genetics: Science of heredity and variation in living organisms. In **genetics**, **gene expression** is the most fundamental level at which **genotype** gives rise to the **phenotype**. The genetic code is "interpreted" by **gene expression**, and the properties of the expression products give rise to the organism's **phenotype**.

genome: In molecular biology, the entirety of an organism's hereditary information. It is encoded either in **DNA** or, for many types of **virus**, in **RNA**. The **genome** includes both the **genes** and the noncoding sequences of the **DNA**.

genomics: Study of sets of **genes**, **gene** products, and their interactions. The term is derived from **genome** and used to refer to an organism's complete set of genetic information. It was originally applied to describe the mapping, sequencing, and analyzing of **genomes**, and is frequently termed structural **genomics**, which encompasses the construction of high-resolution genetic, physical, and transcript maps of an organism, including its complete **DNA** sequence. Functional **genomics** deals with the study of **gene** functions.

genotype: Inherited instructions that an organism carries within its genetic code. Not all organisms with the same **genotype** look or act the same way, because appearance and behavior are modified by environmental and developmental conditions. Similarly, not all organisms that look alike necessarily have the same **genotype**.

giant pulse: **Laser** pulses produced by the **Q-switching** technique and having extremely high (gigawatt) **peak power**. It is much higher than would be produced by the same **laser** if it were operating in a **continuous-wave (CW)** mode.

Giemsa stain: Mixture of **methylene blue** and **eosin**. The stain procedure includes **fixation** in pure methanol for 30 seconds of a thin film of the specimen on a microscope slide; slide immersion in a freshly prepared 5% **Giemsa stain** solution for 20–30 minutes; and then flushing with tap **water** and drying. It is used in cytogenetics and for the histopathological diagnosis of malaria and other parasites. It is specific for the phosphate groups of **DNA** and attaches itself to regions of **DNA** where there are high amounts of adenine-thymine bonding. It is used in G-banding to stain **chromosomes** to identify chromosomal **aberrations**. It is also a differential stain and can be used to study the adherence of pathogenic **bacteria** to human **cells** by staining human and bacterial **cells** purple and pink, respectively. **Giemsa stain** is a classical **blood** film stain for peripheral **blood smears** and **bone marrow** specimens. **Erythrocytes** stain pink, **platelets** show a **light** pale pink, **lymphocyte cytoplasm** stains sky blue, **monocyte cytoplasm** stains pale blue, and **leukocyte** nuclear **chromatin** stains magenta. The stain can also be used to identify **mast cells**.

gigabits per second (Gb/s): A unit of data transfer rate equal to 10^9 b/s (see **bit**).

Gimenez stain: Technique using biological stains to detect and identify bacterial infections in **tissue** samples. Although largely superseded by techniques like **Giemsa stain**, it may be valuable for detecting certain slow-growing or fastidious **bacteria**. Basic **fuchsin** stain in aqueous solution with phenol and **ethanol** colors many **bacteria** (both **gram-positive bacteria** and **gram-negative bacteria**) red, magenta, or pink. A **malachite green** counterstain gives a blue–green background cast to the surrounding **tissue**.

gingiva (*Synonym*: gums): The mucosal **tissue** that lays over the jawbone. The **gingiva** are naturally transparent, they are rendered red in **color** because of the **blood** flowing through **tissue**. The **gingiva** are connected to the teeth and **bone** by way of the **periodontal fibers**. They are divided in three portions: (1) free **gingiva**, which forms a cuff around a **tooth** and is not attached to **bone**; (2) attached **gingiva**, which is connected to **bone**; and (3) interdental papilla, which is the pointed portion of **gingiva** between teeth. Healthy **gingiva** is characterized by pale to coral pink **color**; there may be pigmentation in darker skinned individuals. Size, tone, and texture are firm, flat, and fit tightly around the **tooth**. Orange peel–like stippling is seen on the surface of attached **gingiva**. The shape is parabolic, with a knife-edged interdental papilla. The **gum** margin should be approximately at junction of **tooth** crown and root.

gingival: Pertaining to **gingiva** or **gums**.

gingival crevicular fluid (GCF): Fluid from **gum tissues** found in **gingival sulcus (crevice)**. It contains shed **epithelial cells**, **immune cells**, antimicrobial **proteins**, and **bacteria**. The fluid helps protect the **tooth** attachment area from bacterial invasion.

gingival sulcus (crevice): Thin **epithelial cell** layer of free **gingiva** that is not attached to the **tooth**. Under the **epithelial**

cell layer is **connective tissue** with **fibroblasts, collagen, nerves, blood vessels,** and **immune cells.**

gingivitis: Oral disease specified as an **inflammation** of the **gingiva.** In most cases, it is due to the presence of **dental plaque** and rarely viral infection (e.g., herpes); certain oral conditions can also cause **gingival inflammation.** Clinical signs include redness, swelling, bleeding, and changes in **gingival tissue** contour. The origin of the disease is **tissue immune response** to presence of **dental plaque**; bacterial products pass through the **epithelium** into **connective tissue** and stimulate **immune cells** such as neutrophils and **monocytes,** and in turn, **immune cells** release chemical mediators that further enhance **immune response** and result in **inflammation** and **tissue** loss, e.g., **collagen** breakdown, and further multiple bacterial species implication. Generally, **gingivitis** starts to develop after plaque is allowed to accumulate for 4–7 days; fully developed **gingivitis** is seen after 2–3 weeks, and if left untreated, can lead to further **tissue** destruction and may in many cases lead to **periodontitis.** Accumulation of **dental plaque** in sufficient quantity will cause **gingivitis** with severity that can vary among individuals; it can be reversed by plaque removal. Types of **gingivitis** include localized or generalized, further categorized as mild, moderate, or severe. The many subtypes include acute necrotizing ulcerative **gingivitis** (ANUG), with interdental **gum tissue** affected, associated with conditions of impaired host defense and **pain**; and **gingivitis** associated with systemic conditions (in the absence of plaque, some diseases mimic **tissue** changes seen in plaque-induced **gingivitis,** e.g., **leukemia**). Other conditions may be associated with a defective **immune response,** e.g., **diabetes** and **HIV. Hormone**-related **gingivitis** may see an exaggerated **immune response** to plaque, e.g., pregnancy.

gland: An organ that manufactures substances for secretion. It may be large (e.g., the **liver** or mammary **gland**), or it may be small (e.g., a **sweat gland**). It functions by taking chemical substances and **water** from the **blood** and synthesizing from these materials the compounds for secretion. **Glands** are either exocrine or endocrine, and their methods of secretion are either holocrine, merocrine, or apocrine. They are also described by their shape (e.g., tubular, racemose, flask-shaped).

glandular: Related to **gland** structure or function.

glandular tissue: Tissue-bearing **gland.**

Glan–Taylor polarization prism: Type of **prism** used as a **polarizer** or polarizing **beamsplitter**. The **prism** is made of two right-angled **prisms** of calcite (or other **birefringent** materials) that are separated on their long faces by an air gap. The optical axes of the calcite crystals are aligned parallel to the plane of **reflection**. **Total internal reflection** of *s*-**polarized light** at the air gap ensures that only *p*-**polarized light** is transmitted by the device. Because the angle of incidence at the gap can be reasonably close to **Brewster's angle**, unwanted **reflection** of *p*-**polarized light** is reduced.

glaucoma: Disease of the eye characterized by increased **pressure** within the **eyeball** and progressive loss of vision.

glioma: Tumor of the **brain** arising from and consisting of **neuroglia**.

globulin: One of the two types of **serum proteins**, the other being **albumin**. This generic term encompasses a heterogeneous series of families of **proteins**, with larger molecules that are less soluble in pure **water** than **albumin** and that migrate less than **albumin** during **serum electrophoresis**.

glucose: Sugar ($C_6H_{12}O_6$), having several optically different forms. The common or dextrorotatory form (dextroglucose or D-**glucose**) occurs in many fruits, animal **tissues**, and fluids, and so on, and has a sweetness about one-half that of ordinary sugar. The levorotatory form (levoglucose or L-**glucose**) is rare and not naturally occurring. Also called "starch syrup," a syrup containing dextrose, maltose, and dextrine, obtained by the incomplete hydrolysis of starch. It is used as an **optical clearing agent** for **blood**, **tissues**, and **cells**.

glucose clamp experiment: Monitoring **blood** sugar at basal (euglycemic) or elevated (hyperglycemic) levels during variable **insulin infusion**. It measures **tissue**-specific **insulin** action and **glucose metabolism**.

glucose tolerance test: In medical practice, the **administration** of **glucose** to determine how quickly it is cleared from the **blood**. The test is usually used to test for **diabetes, insulin** resistance, and sometimes reactive hypoglycemia. **Glucose** is given orally most often, so the common test is technically an **oral glucose tolerance test (OGTT)**.

glycated hemoglobin (GHb): Hemoglobin A1c, Hb_{1c}, Hb_{A1c}, or A1C. This form of **hemoglobin** is used primarily to identify the average **plasma glucose** concentration over prolonged periods of time. It is formed in a nonenzymatic pathway by hemoglobin's normal exposure to high **plasma** levels of **glucose. Glycation** of **hemoglobin** has been implicated in nephropathy and retinopathy in **diabetes mellitus**. Monitoring the Hb_{A1c} in type-1 diabetic patients may improve treatment. **Glucose** interacts with **plasma proteins** and **hemoglobin** in **erythrocytes**. In fact, **glycation** of **hemoglobin** occurs over the entire 120-day life span of the **red blood cell**, but within this timeframe, recent glycemia has the largest influence on the Hb_{A1c} value. Theoretical models and clinical studies suggest that a patient in stable control will form 50% of his or her Hb_{A1c} in the month before sampling, 25% in the month before that, and the remaining 25% in month two to four. More recent clinical studies suggest that in practice, a fall from an elevated Hb_{A1c} can be demonstrated within a few days of a change in therapy and certainly within 2 weeks or 4–8 weeks. **Glycated hemoglobin** is a useful marker for long-term **glucose** control in diabetics.

glycation: Result of a sugar molecule, such as **glucose**, bonding to a **protein** or **lipid** molecule without the controlling action of an **enzyme**. **Glycation** may occur either inside the body (**endogenous glycation**) or outside the body (**exogenous glycation**). **Enzyme**-controlled addition of sugars to **protein** or **lipid** molecules is termed glycosylation. **Glycation** is a haphazard process that impairs the functioning of biomolecules, while glycosylation occurs at defined sites on the target molecule and is required in order for the molecule to function. **Hemoglobin glycation** is the result of an irreversible nonenzymatic **fixation** of **glucose** on **hemoglobin** of the beta chain of **hemoglobin** A. **Glucose** combines with the α-amino group of the valine residue at the N-terminus of 18 globin chains to form an aldimine compound (**Schiff base**). This reaction is reversible, and **dissociation** to native **hemoglobin** and **glucose** occurs readily. Internal rearrangement of the aldimine intermediate by the Amadori reaction yields a stable ketoamine derivative. 60% of the **glucose** is bound to the N-terminal valines of the β chains. A small amount of **glucose** binding occurs at the α-chain N-terminal valines.

glycerin: See **glycerol**.

glycerine: See **glycerol**.

glycerol (*Synonyms*: glycerin, glycerine): Colorless, odorless, syrupy, sweet liquid (see **alcohol**) usually obtained by the saponification of natural **fats** and **oils**. It is used in the manufacture of **cosmetics**, perfumes, inks, and certain glues and cements; also used as a solvent and in medicine in suppositories and **skin** emollients. It is one of the most effective **optical clearing agents** of **tissues** due to its high **osmolarity** and **index of refraction**.

glycogen: Polysaccharide that is the principal storage form of **glucose** in animal **cells**. It is found in the form of granules in the **cytosol** in many **cell** types and plays an important role in the **glucose** cycle. It forms an **energy** reserve that can be quickly mobilized to meet a sudden need for **glucose**, but one that is less compact than the **energy** reserves of triglycerides.

glyco-lipid: Any of the class of **lipids** comprising the cerebrosides and gangliosides that on hydrolysis yield galactose or a similar sugar, a **fatty acid**, and sphingosine or dihydrosphingosine.

glycosaminoglycan: Long, unbranched **polysaccharide** consisting of a repeating disaccharide unit. They are synthesized in **endoplasmic reticulum** and **Golgi apparatus**. Glycosaminoglycans form an important component of **connective tissues**. Their chains may be covalently linked to a **protein** to form **proteoglycans**.

gold nanoparticles: Particles made of gold with dimensions typically of 10–160 nm. Relatively monodisperse and spherical particles with the controlled average equivolume diameter from 10–60 nm could be produced by citrate method. They have different chemical and **optical properties** than occur in bulk samples. Due to their **plasmon-resonant** property, high surface reactivity, and biocompatibility, **gold nanoparticles** can be used for *in vivo* molecular imaging and therapeutic applications, including **cancer** optical detection and **phototherapy**. **Surface-plasmon resonance** of gold nanorods (NRs) and silica (core)/gold (shell) particles can be easily tuned over 600–1500 nm by simple variation in NRs length or aspect ratio, or by variation of the ratio shell thickness/core radius. Other shapes of **gold nanoparticles** are also available, including nanocubes, nanocages, nanostars, and octahedrals. Fabrication of nanoparticle clusters by assembling them into 1D, 2D, and 3D structures allows one to explore the collective physical properties of the assemblies, which are different from those of isolated NPs.

gold vapor laser: An atomic metal-vapor **laser** with only pulse mode of generation. It generates a red **laser** line of 627.8 nm. It is similar to a copper vapor **laser**, but with fourfold to eightfold less mean **power** and pulse **energy**. This laser is widely used in **photodynamic therapy**.

Golgi apparatus (complex): Netlike mass of material in the **cytoplasm** of animal **cells**, believed to function in cellular secretion.

goniophotometric technique: See **goniophotometry**.

goniophotometry (*Synonym*: goniophotometric technique): Technique that allows for measurement of the angle-dependent **light intensity** distribution.

graded-index (GRIN) fiber: Fiber with a graded transverse profile of core **refractive index**. The index profile $n(r)$ in the core of the **fiber** is a function of the radial distance r from the center of the **fiber**. It starts at a value of $n(0) = n_1$ at the center of the **fiber** and gradually decreases to a value of $n(a) = n_2$ at the boundary between the core and the cladding. The properties of a **graded-index fiber** are determined by the specific functional dependence of $n(r)$ on r. The **numerical aperture**, for example, is a function of radial position: $NA(r) = \sqrt{n^2(r) - n_2^2}$, which decreases from $NA(r) = \sqrt{n_1^2 - n_2^2}$ at the core center to $NA(a) = 0$ at the core–cladding boundary. These **fibers** are primarily used as low-**dispersion multimode fibers** (see **fiber dispersion**). For the power-law index profile: $n(r) = n_1 \sqrt{1 - 2\Delta \left(\frac{r}{a}\right)^\alpha}, 0 \leq r \leq a$, and $n(r) = n_2, r > a$, where the relative **refractive index** difference of the core and cladding $\Delta \cong (n_1 - n_2)/n_1$. With $\Delta \ll 1$, the **fiber** core has a linear index profile for $\alpha = 1$. It becomes a **step-index fiber** for $\alpha = \infty$. Fiber **waveguide** parameter $V = (2\pi a NA/\lambda) \cong (2\pi a n_1/\lambda) \sqrt{2\Delta}$, and the total number of modes $M = [\alpha/(\alpha + 2)](V^2/2)$.

Gram-negative bacteria: **Bacteria** having a relatively thin layer (10% or less of **cell** wall) of peptidoglycan-made **cell** wall portion. **Gram-negative bacteria** also have an additional outer **membrane** that contains **lipids** and is separated from the **cell** wall by the periplasmic space. **Gram's stain** makes these **bacteria** red or pink in **color**.

Gram-positive bacteria: **Bacteria** having a thick, mesh-like **cell** wall made of peptidoglycan (50–90% of **cell** wall). **Gram's stain** makes these **bacteria** purple (dark blue or violet) in **color**.

Gram's stain: Empirical method of differentiating **bacteria** into two large groups (**Gram-positive bacteria** and **Gram-negative bacteria**) based on the chemical and physical properties of their **cell** walls. **Gram's stain** is almost always the first step in the identification of a bacterial organism. However, not all **bacteria** can be definitively classified by this technique. There are four basic steps of the **Gram's stain**, which include applying a primary stain (**crystal violet**) to a heat-fixed smear of a **bacterial** culture, followed by the addition of iodine as a trapping agent, rapid decolorization with **alcohol** or acetone, and counterstaining with positively charged **safranin** or basic **fuchsine**. After decolorization, the **Gram-positive bacteria** remain purple (dark blue or violet), and the **Gram-negative bacteria** lose their purple **color**. Counterstain gives decolorized **Gram-negative bacteria** a pink or red **color**.

grandular: Pertaining to **tissue** structures that contain granular inclusions. For example, **grandular**-cystic **hyperplasia**, **grandular tumor**, **grandular-squamous-cell carcinoma**.

grating spectrograph: Spectrograph that uses a **diffraction** grating to produce optical spectra. A **diffraction** grating is a band of equidistant, parallel lines, usually more than 5000 to the inch, ruled on a glass or polished metal surface for diffracting **light** to produce optical spectra with a high resolution.

graybody: Radiating object whose **emissivity** is a constant value less than unity (1.0) over a specific spectral range.

gray matter: **Nervous tissue** found in the **central nervous system**. It contains numerous **cell** bodies (cytons), **dendrites**, synapses, terminal processes of **axons**, **blood vessels**, and **neuroglia**. It is internal to **white matter** in the **spinal cord** and some other parts of the **brain**. It is external to **white matter** in the cerebral hemisphere and in the **cerebellum**. Coordination in the **central nervous system** is affected in **gray matter**. **Brain** nuclei and **nerve** centers are composed of **gray matter**.

green fluorescent protein (GFP): A protein comprised of 238 **amino acids** (27 kDa), coming from the jellyfish *Aequorea victoria* that fluoresces green when exposed to blue **light**. GFP has a unique can-like shape consisting of an 11-strand β-barrel with a single alpha helical strand containing the **chromophore** running through the center. This barrel permits **chromophore** formation and protects it from quenching by the surrounding microenvironment. In **cell** and molecular biology, the **GFP gene** is frequently used as a reporter of expression of the fluorescent compound. In modified forms, it has been used to make biosensors. After cloning of the **GFP gene**, variants emitting **light** in the blue, yellow, or red spectral region could be generated.

green photonics: Photonics solutions that generate or conserve **energy**, cut greenhouse gas emissions, reduce pollution, produce environmentally sustainable output, or improve public health.

ground substance: Homogeneous matrix in which the **fibers** and **cells** of **connective tissue** or other particles are embedded.

group refractive index: Refractive index associated with the group velocity of a train of waves traveling in a dispersive medium. The group velocity, and correspondingly the **group refractive index**, depends on the mean **wavelength** of a train of waves and the rate of change in velocity with **wavelength**. At propagation of very short pulses in **tissues** when a group of different **wavelengths** propagates in a media, the material **dispersion** ($dn/d\lambda$) should be accounted for by introducing the **group refractive index** $n_g = n - \lambda(dn/d\lambda)$. This is also an important phenomenon to be accounted for in low-coherence (broadband) optical systems, such as **OCT**, and low-coherence and **PCF**-based interferometry. For *in vivo* measured by **OCT refractive indices** of the human palm of **hand**

skin layers for central **wavelength** 1300 nm, $(nn_g)^{1/2} = 1.47 \pm 0.01$ for *stratum corneum* (**SC**); 1.43 ± 0.02 for epidermal granular layer; 1.34 ± 0.02 for epidermal basal layer; and 1.41 ± 0.03 for upper **dermis**. For central **wavelength** 980 nm, $(nn_g)^{1/2} = 1.50 \pm 0.02$ for SC of **dorsal** surface of a thumb, 1.56 for air-**skin** interface, and 1.34 for SC/**epidermis** interface of **volar** side of a thumb. For central **wavelength** 850 nm, $n_g = 1.51$ for human nail. For *in vitro* measured by **OCT** for central **wavelength** 855 nm, $n_g = 1.3817 \pm 0.0021$, and for 1270 nm, $n_g = 1.389 \pm 0.004$ for human **cornea**; for central **wavelength** 850 nm, $n_g = 1.59 \pm 0.08$ for black, 1.58 ± 0.06 for brown, 1.56 ± 0.01 for red, 1.57 ± 0.01 for blond, and 1.58 ± 0.01 for gray and white human **hair shafts**; $n_g = 1.53 \pm 0.02$ for dry and 1.43 ± 0.02 for fully **hydrated collagen** of type I; for central **wavelength** 856 nm $n_g = 1.62 \pm 0.02$ for **enamel** and 1.50 ± 0.02 for **dentin** of human **tooth**. See **tissue refractive index measurement**.

group-velocity dispersion: Defined as $D(\omega) = (2\pi c^2/\lambda)$ $(d^2k/d\omega^2)$ or $D(\lambda) = \lambda^2(d^2n/d\lambda^2)$, where $k = (\omega/c)n(\omega)$ is the **propagation constant of the electromagnetic wave (EMW)**. D is an important consideration in the propagation of optical pulses. It can cause broadening of an individual pulse, as well as changes in the time delay between pulses of different frequencies. The sign of D can be either positive or negative. In the case of $D > 0$, a long-**wavelength**, or low-**frequency**, pulse travels faster than a short-**wavelength**, or high-**frequency**, pulse. In contrast, a short-**wavelength** pulse travels faster than a long-**wavelength** pulse in the case of $D < 0$. In a given material, the sign of D generally depends on the spectral region of concern. **Group-velocity dispersion** and phase-velocity **dispersion** have different meanings; they should not be confused with each other.

Grüneisen parameter: Dimensionless, temperature-dependent factor proportional to the fraction of thermal **energy** converted into **mechanical stress**.

gums: See **gingiva**.

gut: See **gastrointenstinal tract**.

gynecological smear: Internal examination during which the doctor takes some cervical wall **cells** for testing. A small brush or swab collects a few **cells** from the surface of the **cervix**. The **cells** are placed on a glass slide and sent for staining and **microscopy** [see **Papanicolaou stain (Pap stain)**, **Pap smear**]. A **Pap smear** checks for the early warning signs of **cervical cancer**.

hair: Threadlike outgrowth from the **skin**. Each **hair** is a slender rod composed of dead **cells** strengthened by **keratin** but remaining soft and supple. It grows from a **hair follicle**, and its length varies according to species and the part of the body on which it is growing. A follicle surrounds the **hair** root and **hair shaft**. It penetrates deep into the **dermis**.

hair follicle: Part of the **skin** that grows **hair** by packing old **cells** together. It is attached to the follicle by a **sebaceous gland**.

hairless lab rat: Provides researchers with valuable data regarding compromised immune systems and genetic **kidney** diseases. There are over twenty-five **genes** that cause recessive hairlessness in laboratory rats. The more common ones are denoted as rnu (Rowett nude), fz (fuzzy), and shn (shorn). Rnu, first identified in 1953, have no **thymus**. Fuzzy rats were identified in 1976. The leading cause of death among these rats is ultimately a progressive **kidney** failure that begins around the age of one. Shorn rats were bred from **Sprague Dawley rats** in 1998. They also suffer from severe **kidney** problems.

hair shaft: Mature **hair shaft** is nonliving biological **fiber**. It is composed of a central pith (or medulla), surrounded by a more solid **cortex**, and is enclosed in a thin, hard, cuticle. Inside the **hair follicle**, it is surrounded by the inner and outer root **sheaths**.

half-width at half-maximum (HWHM): See **bandwidth**.

halitosis: Oral malodor. The components of breath that cause malodor are still being investigated. Currently, the principal compounds responsible for malodor are considered to be volatile sulfur compounds (VSCs), which are produced by **bacteria** as they break down certain **proteins**. **Bacteria** responsible for this are mainly **Gram-negative bacteria**; key are **anaerobic Gram-negative bacteria**, e.g., *Fusobacterium nucleatum*. Other identified compounds in malodor include indole, skatole, butyric acid, and cadavarine. The **oral cavity** is the main contributor of bad breath in most otherwise healthy **halitosis** patients, including the **tongue** surface, especially the back of the **tongue**, **gingiva** and **periodontium**, and oral **mucosa**; dental **caries** (although **tooth** decay itself does not cause malodor, food can get trapped in the irregular decay surface and contribute to **halitosis**); and oral **lesions**, oral **cancers**, and herpes, which lead to **tissue** breakdown and infection. Dry **mouth** symptoms include oral malodor as well as oral candidiasis, respiratory tract abnormalities, e.g., chronic **maxillary sinusitis**. Bad breath can be associated with food or **tissue** debris, and saliva that accumulate in tonsillar crypts; in the pharynx and the **lungs**, it may be associated with infections, **cancers**, and foreign bodies. **Lungs** are also a source of malodor due to normal **metabolism** of food (e.g., garlic, **alcohol**) and certain drugs; these compounds are carried in **blood** and released into the **lungs**. Gastrointestinal conditions that weaken closure of the **esophagus** and thus allow some stagnation of food in the **esophagus** can cause malodor, as can systemic conditions, e.g., **diabetes**, renal failure, and malodor due to buildup and subsequent release of certain compounds from the bloodstream into the **lungs**.

halogen lamp: Iodine-cycle tungsten incandescent lamp that is the **visible/NIR** (360 nm to > 1 μm) **light** source for **spectrophotometry** and **phototherapy**. As it is gas-filled, the tungsten electrode can be heated up to 4000 K. At this temperature, the maximum spectra of emission is about $\lambda_{max} = 750$ nm. About 30% of the total **power** is emitted at **wavelengths** shorter than λ_{max}, and the remaining 70% is emitted at **wavelengths** longer than λ_{max}.

hand: One of the two intricate, prehensile, multifingered body parts normally located at the end of each **arm** (medically: "terminating each anterior limb/appendage") of a human or other primate.

hard sphere approximation: Model of mutually impenetrable (hard) spheres. The interparticle forces are zero, except for the fact that two neighbor particles cannot interpenetrate each other.

hard tissue: Bone, **tooth enamel**, **dentin**, and **cementum**, as well as **tendon** and **cartilage**.

head: Part of the body that comprises the **brain**, eyes, **ears**, nose, and **mouth** (all of which aid in various sensory functions, such as sight, hearing, smell, and taste).

heart: Hollow, muscular organ that by rhythmic contractions and relaxations keeps the **blood** in circulation throughout the body.

heart attack: Common name of **myocardial infarction (MI)** or acute myocardial infarction (AMI).

heartbeat (*Synonym*: **cardiovibration**): Contraction of the **heart**. Usually, **heart** rate describing the **frequency** of the cardiac cycle is calculated as the number of **heartbeats** in one minute and expressed as "beats per minute" (bpm). The **heart** beats up to 120 times per minute in childhood. When resting, the adult human **heart** beats at about 70 bpm (males) and 75 bpm (females).

heart valve leaflet: Valves in the **heart** maintain the unidirectional flow of **blood** by opening and closing depending on the difference in **pressure** on each side. The mitral **valve** is the **heart valve** that prevents the backflow of **blood** from the left **ventricle** into the left **atrium**. It is composed of two leaflets (one anterior, one posterior) that close when the left **ventricle** contracts. Each leaflet is composed of three layers of **tissue**: atrialis, fibrosa, and spongiosa.

heat capacity: Measurable physical quantity that characterizes the ability of a material or structure to store heat as it changes in temperature. It is defined as the rate of change of temperature as heat is added to a body at the given conditions and state of the body (foremost, its temperature). It is the product of the volumetric **specific heat capacity** (c_p) and the density (ρ) of the material. This means that denser materials generally will have higher heat capacities than porous materials. Capacity is expressed in units of **joules** per kelvin.

heat conductance: Process of transfer of heat through a body without **visible** motion of any part of the body. The process takes place where there is a temperature gradient. The heat energy diffuses through the body by the action of particles of high kinetic energy on particles of lower kinetic energy. For solids with covalent bonding, they will be molecules whose motion is restricted to vibrations about fixed positions; the energy is transferred by high-frequency waves. Conductance measures the ability of a material of defined thickness and cross-sectional area to conduct heat. It is related to the material property, **heat conductivity**, and it is the inverse of thermal resistance.

heat conduction: The only mode of **heat flow** in solids, which can also take place in liquids and gases. It occurs as the result of atomic vibrations (in solids) and molecular collisions (in liquids and gases), whereby energy is transferred from locations of higher temperature to locations of lower temperature.

heat conductivity: Material property defining the relative capability to carry heat by conduction in a static temperature gradient. Conductivity varies slightly with temperature in solids and liquids and with temperature and pressure in gases. It is high for metals and low for porous materials and gases. It is measured in $W \cdot m^{-1} \cdot K^{-1}$.

heat convection: Form of **heat transfer** that takes place in a moving medium and is almost always associated with transfer between a solid (surface) and a moving fluid (such as air), whereby energy is transferred from higher temperature sites to lower temperature sites.

heat flow: Describes heat propagation due to various mechanisms such as **heat conduction**, **heat convection**, and **thermal radiation**. See **heat transfer**.

heat light source: All bodies emit **electromagnetic radiation** in the **IR wavelength** spectral range and with intensities that correspond to their temperature. This is called heat radiation or **blackbody radiation** (see **Planck curve**). **Spontaneous** and **stimulated emission** by atoms are the basis for the **Planck curve**, which gives the **intensity** radiated by a **blackbody** as a function of **wavelength** for a definite body temperature. The normalized spectral irradiancy of heat sources versus **wavelength** shows that the emitting **spectrum** is very broad and is shifted to the **IR** range by decreasing temperature. The peak in the emitted **energy** moves to the shorter **wavelengths** as the temperature is increased in accordance with **Wien's displacement law**, for which the maximum of the heat **radiation spectrum** is the function of body temperature to the **power** of four. Thus, strongly heated metals are used in **light** sources with broadband **visible** and **IR radiation**. For example, a filament lamp with a temperature of 2000 K emits **light** with peak **wavelength** at approximately 1400 nm.

heat transfer: Variety of processes that provide transfer of heat through a body and surroundings, such as **heat conduction**, **heat convection**, **thermal radiation** and **absorption**, **latent heat** of fusion, and **vaporization**.

heat-absorbing filter: See **infrared filter**.

helium–cadmium (He–Cd) laser: One of the ionic metal-vapor **lasers**. The output **power** of **He–Cd lasers** is typically higher and **wavelengths** are shorter than those of **He–Ne lasers**; they are applicable in many biomedical diagnostic and therapeutic optical technologies. **He–Cd lasers** with two main lines, blue (λ = 441.6 nm) and **UVA** (λ = 325.0 nm), are widely used. Hollow **cathode** discharge systems allow for generation of a much richer **spectrum** of **laser** lines from **UV** to **IR**, including 325.0, 441.6, 533.7, 537.8, 635.5, 636.0, 723.7, 728.4, 806.7, 853.1, 865.2, and 887.8 nm.

helium–neon (He–Ne) laser: Gas-discharge **laser** whose medium is a mixture of He and Ne. **Lasers** with the red emission (632.8 nm) are widely used. **Lasers** with other **wavelengths** are also available: green (543.3 nm), yellow (594 nm), orange (604, 612.0 nm), far red (730.5 nm), and **IR** (1152.3, 1523, 3391.2, 4218.3, and 5404.8 nm). They can be multimode, single-mode, and single-**frequency** with extremely narrow **bandwidth** (a few **hertz**) and linear or circularly polarized. Their **power** is from a few milliwatts to a few hundred milliwatts. These **lasers** are typically used for **tissue** imaging and **spectroscopy**, **blood flow** and perfusion monitoring, **tissue fluorescence** excitation, and so on. These are also common **lasers** for **low-level laser therapy (LLLT)** (or **laser** biostimulation) and **photodynamic therapy**.

helium–selenium (He–Se) laser: Belongs to the ionic metal-vapor **lasers**. The output **power** of **He–Se lasers** is typically higher than that of **He–Ne lasers**. **He–Se lasers** generate more than 20 lines in the range 460.4–653.5 nm.

helium–zinc (He–Zn) laser: Belongs to the ionic metal-vapor **lasers**. The output **power** of **He–Zn lasers** is typically higher than that of **He–Ne lasers**. **He–Zn lasers** generate around 10 lines in the range 491.2–775.8 nm, with two more intensive lines at 747.9 and 758.8 nm.

helix: Connected series of concentric rings of the same radius, joined together to form a cylindrical shape.

hemangioma: Native abnormality caused by **proliferation** of endothelial **cells**. It is formed by aggregates consisting chiefly of dilated or newly formed **blood vessels** that look like **tumors**. Types of **hemangioma** include **capillary hemangioma, cavernous hemangioma** (see **port wine stain**), senile **hemangioma**, and verrucous **hemangioma**.

hematocrit: Relative volume of the **red blood cells** in **blood** expressed in percentages. The abbreviations are Ht or Hct. It also can be presented as packed **cell** volume (PCV) or **erythrocyte** volume fraction (EVF). It is normally about 48% for men and 38% for women. It is independent of body size and considered as an integral part of a person's complete **blood** count results, along with **hemoglobin** concentration, **white blood cell** count, and **platelet** count.

hematoporphyrin: Complex mixture of monomeric and aggregated **porphyrins** used in the **photodynamic therapy** of **tumors**. A purified component of this mixture is known as dihematoporphyrin **ether**.

hematoporphyrin derivative (HpD): **Photosensitizer** with an excitation band around 620–630 nm. It is used in **cancer** diagnostics and **photodynamic therapy. Photofrin II (Photofrin®)**, Photosan®, and Photogem® are the commercialized products. At **PDT**, a typical **laser** dose is of 150 J/cm^2.

hematoxylin: Other names are Natural Black 1 or C.I. 75290. It is extracted from the wood of the logwood tree. When oxidized, it forms hematein, a compound that forms strongly colored complexes with certain metal ions, notably Fe(III) and Al(III) salts. Metal–hematein complexes are used to stain **cell** nuclei in **microscopy** and **histology**. Structures that stain with iron– or aluminum–hematein are often called basophilic, even though the mechanism of the staining is different from that of staining with basic dyes.

Hematoxylin and Eosin (H&E) stain: A staining method in **histology** widely used in medical diagnosis including **cancer**. In **histology**, it is termed an H&E, H + E, or HE section. It

209

involves application of hemalum, which is a complex formed from aluminium ions and oxidized **hematoxylin**. This stain colors the nuclei of **cells** (and a few other objects, such as **keratohyalin granules**) blue. The staining of nuclei by hemalum does not require the presence of **DNA** and is probably due to binding of the dye-metal complex to **arginine**-rich basic nucleoproteins such as histones. The nuclear staining is followed by counterstaining with an aqueous or alcoholic solution of **eosin** Y, which colors other structures in various shades of red, pink, and orange. The mechanism is different from that of nuclear staining by basic (**cationic**) dyes such as thionine or **toluidine blue O**. Staining by basic dyes is prevented by chemical or enzymatic extraction of **nucleic acids**. Such extractions do not prevent staining of nuclei by hemalum. **Red blood cells** are stained intensely red. Other colors, e.g., yellow and brown, can be caused by intrinsic **pigments**, such as **melanin**. Some structures do not stain well: **basal laminae** need to be stained by **periodic acid-Schiff (PAS)** stain or **silver stain**. Hydrophobic structures also tend to remain clear, such as those rich in **fats, adipocytes, myelin** around **neuron axons**, and **Golgi apparatus membranes**.

heme: An iron-containing substance, it is the basic unit of the **hemoglobin** molecule. Mammals have four heme units in their **hemoglobin**.

hemodynamics: Physiology branch dealing with the forces involved in the circulation of the **blood**.

hemoglobin: Red iron-containing respiratory **pigment** found in the **blood**. It conveys **oxygen** to the **tissues** and occurs in reduced form (**deoxyhemoglobin**) in venous **blood** and in combination with **oxygen** (**oxyhemoglobin**) in arterial **blood**. It consists of **heme** combined with globin, a **blood protein**. It is chemically related to chlorophyll, **cytochrome**, hemocyanin, and **myoglobin**.

hemoglobin spectra: Main bands include the following: Soret band, 400–440-nm segment; Q bands, 540–580-nm segment.

It has the **isobestic point** for two forms of **hemoglobin**: **oxyhemoglobin** and **deoxyhemoglobin** at the **wavelength** 805 nm. At the shorter than **isobestic point wavelength**, λ = 700 nm, **deoxyhemoglobin** is 6.7-fold more absorptive than **oxyhemoglobin**, but for the longer **wavelength**, λ = 1000 nm, **oxyhemoglobin** is 5-fold more absorptive than **deoxyhemoglobin**. This property is very important for a quantitative evaluation of **hemoglobin** concentration in these two forms in **tissues**, which is the basis for many disease diagnostics and monitoring. **Methemoglobin** has a four-banded **absorption spectrum** with a strong band in the orange–red at 630 nm.

hemolysis: Breaking open of **red blood cells** and the release of **hemoglobin** into the surrounding fluid (**plasma**, *in vivo*).

hemolytic disease: **Hemolytic disease** of the newborn is an alloimmune condition that develops in a fetus, when the IgG **antibodies** that have been produced by the mother and have passed through the placenta include ones that attack the **red blood cells** in the fetal circulation. The **red blood cells** are broken down, and the fetus can develop reticulocytosis and anemia. Hemolysis leads to elevated **bilirubin** levels. After delivery, **bilirubin** is no longer cleared (via the placenta) from the neonate's **blood**, and the symptoms of yellowish **skin** and yellow discolouration of the whites of the eyes increase within 24 hours after birth.

hemorheological status: Status determined on the basis of study of **blood** rheology parameters, such as **whole blood** and **plasma** viscosity, **cell** transit time, **cell** deformability, clogging rate, and clogging particle changes.

hemorrhage: Discharge of **blood**, as from ruptured **blood vessels**.

Henyey–Greenstein phase function (HGPF): One of the practical semiempirical approximations of the **scattering phase function**.

hertz (Hz): Unit of **frequency** that is equal to 1 cycle per second. It is often used to indicate the pulse repetition rate of a **laser** (e.g., a 10-Hz **laser** emits 10 pulses per second): 1 kilohertz (kHz) is 10^3 Hz, 1 megahertz (MHz) is 10^6 Hz, 1 gigahertz (GHz) is 10^9 Hz, and 1 **terahertz** (THz) is 10^{12} Hz.

heterodyne microscopy: **Microscopy** technique that uses optical heterodyning to enhance the registered signal and image **contrast**.

heterodyne phase system: See **cross-correlation measurement device**.

heterodyne spectrum: Spectrum of the **intensity** fluctuations registered by a **photodetector** at the intermediate (beat) **frequency** as a central **frequency** of the measured **spectrum**. The intermediate **frequency** is chosen for technical reasons: it has the best **signal-to-noise ratio**.

heterodyne system with zero cross-phase detectors: Phase measuring system that uses amplitude **modulation** at two close **radio frequencies** f_1 and f_2.

heteropolymer: See **copolymer**.

heterostructure: **Semiconductor** junction that is composed of layers of dissimilar **semiconductor** materials with nonequal **bandgaps**. A quantum **heterostructure** has a size restricting the movements of the charge carriers and forcing them into a quantum confinement that leads to formation of a set of discrete **energy** levels with sharper density than for structures of more conventional sizes. It is important for fabrication of the short-**wavelength light-emitting diode (LED)**, **superluminescent diode (SLD)** and **diode lasers (DLs)**, and **IR photodiodes**.

Hexvix®: **PDT photosensitizer**, which contains hexaminole-vulinate [hexyl ester of **ALA (delta (δ)-aminolevulenic acid)**, hexyl **ALA**, or HAL]. It is approved in Europe for **photodynamic**

diagnoses (PDDs) of early **bladder cancer** and visualization of flat **lesions**. Because of this prodrug's superior pharmacokinetics and selectivity, it also has potential for **PDT**.

high-pass filter (HPF): Filter that rejects the low-**frequency** components in electronic devices.

Hispanic skin: Darker than northern European **skin (Caucasian skin)** because of the increased amount of **melanin** in the **skin**. The **melanin pigment** protects the **skin** from sunlight and slows down the **skin** aging process. See **skin type**.

histogram: One of the forms of representation of distribution of experimental data as a bar diagram.

histology: Study of **tissue** sectioned as a thin slice, using a microtome. It can be described as microscopic anatomy.

hollow waveguide: The air core of these special optical **waveguides** gives them an inherent advantage over solid-core **IR fibers** because **IR** materials used in these **fibers** have **laser** damage thresholds that are frequently very low. The air-core **waveguides** are capable of delivering close to 30 kW of **CW carbon dioxide (CO_2) laser power**, far in excess of any **IR** solid-core **fiber**. The major losses for **hollow waveguides** are due to **interference** effects resulting from the thin-film coatings used to make the guides. They are an ideal instrument for **laser-power** delivery at all **IR laser wavelengths**. They are good for gas sensing, as the core of these **fibers** can be filled with gas so that **light** propagating through the **waveguide** is partially absorbed by the gas. Temperature measurements are also possible over a large temperature range using these **waveguides**. Due to their unique mechanical and **radiation** strength, suitable flexibility, and relatively low losses (0.25–2.0 dB/m), these **waveguides** are widely used in **IR laser** surgery. **Transmittance** of the 1-m **waveguide** with cross section of 0.5 × 8.0 mm for 30-W CO_2 **laser radiation** is 70%. The typical output **power density** of the laser scalpel built on the basis of the **hollow waveguide** is of $10 \ kW/cm^2$ (two-**lens** focusing using cylindrical and spherical **lenses**, focused beam spot of 500 μm). Plastic **hollow waveguides** on the basis of Teflon® [polytetrafluoroethylene (PTFE)] or tubes with a **micrometer** thickness thin-film metal-dielectric internal coating are also designed to guide **radiation** from a CO_2 **laser**. These **light guides** are flexible, easily sterilized, and appropriate for multiple use in **laser** surgery and therapy for internal organs. The polymer Arton-coated silver hollow **fiber** is 0.7 mm in diameter and 1 m in length and has **transmittance** of 94% (losses of 0.25 dB/m) for **radiation** of CO_2 **lasers** and **Er:YAG lasers**.

holmium:yttrium aluminium garnet (Ho:YAG) laser: Solid-state **laser** whose lasing medium is the crystal Ho:YAG with emission in **NIR** at 2.09–2.15 μm. This **laser** could be optimal for many applications in **laser** medicine, such as **tissue laser welding** and **coagulation** within not small volumes and in some depth, because its **radiation** penetrates **tissue** more effectively than **radiation** of an **erbium laser**, but **absorption** is still high to provide **tissue** damage. A **holmium laser** (a crystal 4 mm in diameter and 76 mm long) operating on $\lambda = 2.088$ μm in a free-run regime provides 8 J of optical **energy**, whereas in the single-mode **Q-switching** regime for a **laser** with a crystal (3 mm in diameter and 54 mm long), it is possible to obtain a **giant pulse energy** of 50 mJ ($\tau_p = 50$ ns, $f_p = 1$ Hz).

hologram: Negative produced by exposing a high-resolution photographic plate to two interfering waves: A subject **wave**, which is formed by illumination of a subject by monochromatic, **coherent radiation**, as from a **laser**, and a reference **wave**, which goes directly from the same **light** source (**laser**). When a **hologram** is placed in a beam of **coherent light**, a true 3D image of the subject is formed.

holographic interferometry: In **holography** under identical environmental conditions, the superposition of two scattered fields from an object are identical. However, with small **deformation**

214

applied to the object, the relative phases of these two **light** fields will alter, and it is possible to observe **interference**. This technique is known as live **holographic interferometry**. It enables static and dynamic displacements of objects with optically rough surfaces to be measured to optical interferometric precision. These measurements can be applied to stress, strain, and vibration analysis. It can also be used to detect optical path length variations in low **scattering** transparent **media**, for example, to visualize fluid flows. It can also be used to generate contours representing the form of the body organ surface.

holographic microscopy: **Microscopy** that uses holographic principles, i.e., mode of **light microscopy** in which a highly **coherent laser beam** is split into a reference and main beam, with the reference beam (usually traveling outside the microscope) being made to interfere with the main beam that has passed through the specimen. The **interference** of the two mutually **coherent** beams forms a **hologram**. The **depth of field** gained by viewing the **hologram** is essentially infinitely great, and the **contrast** mode or observation can be switched to dark field, phase **contrast**, **interference contrast**, and so on, after the **hologram** has been formed by the microscope in the bright field.

holography: Process or technique of making **holograms**. It enables the **light** field scattered from an object to be recorded and replayed.

homodyne phase system: System that does not down-convert the **radio frequency** prior to phase measurements.

homodyne spectrum: Self-beat **spectrum** of the **intensity** fluctuations registered by a **photodetector**. It is like the **heterodyne spectrum**, but with a central **frequency** equal to zero and with overlapping negative and positive **spectrum** wings.

homogeneous medium: Medium that has common physical properties, including **optical properties**, throughout.

homologous series: In chemistry, this is a series of organic compounds with a similar general formula, possessing similar chemical properties due to the presence of the same functional group, and showing a gradation in physical properties as a result of increase in molecular size and mass.

hormone: Chemical released by one or more **cells** that affects **cells** in other parts of the organism. Only a small amount of **hormone** is required to alter **cell metabolism**. It is essentially a chemical messenger that transports a signal from one **cell** to another. All multicellular organisms produce **hormones**. **Hormones** in animals are often transported in the **blood**. **Cells** respond to a **hormone** when they express a specific receptor for that **hormone**. The **hormone** binds to the receptor **protein**, resulting in the activation of a signal transduction mechanism that ultimately leads to **cell**-type-specific responses. Endocrine **hormone** molecules are secreted (released) directly into the bloodstream, while exocrine **hormones** (or ectohormones) are secreted directly into a **duct**, and from the **duct** they flow either into the bloodstream or from **cell** to **cell** by **diffusion** in a process known as paracrine signaling.

horny skin layer: See *stratum corneum*.

hue: One of the main properties of a **color**, defined technically as the degree to which a stimulus can be described as similar to or different from stimuli that are described as red, green, blue, and yellow (the unique **hues**). The other main correlates of **color** appearance are **colorfulness**, **chroma**, **saturation (color):**, **lightness**, and **brightness**. Usually, **colors** with the same **hue** are distinguished with adjectives referring to their **lightness** and/or **chroma**, such as **light** blue, pastel blue, and vivid blue. Exceptions include brown, which is a dark orange, and pink, a **light** red with reduced **chroma**.

human epidermal membrane (HEM):   Skin flap containing **epidermis** and used to perform *in vitro* permeability experiments under varied experimental conditions for different deliverable agents and drugs. Two-chamber **diffusion cells** are typically used.

human papilloma virus (HPV): Belongs to a diverse group of **DNA**-based **viruses** that infect the **skin** and **mucous membranes** of humans and a variety of animals. More than 100 different **HPV** types have been characterized. Some **HPV** types cause benign **skin** warts, or papillomas, for which the **virus** family is named. **HPVs** associated with the development of such "common warts" are transmitted environmentally or by casual **skin**-to-**skin** contact.

humidity: Measure of the extent to which the atmosphere contains moisture (**water** vapor). Absolute **humidity** (AH) is the mass of **water** vapor, m_w, in the air volume, V_a. AH $= m_w/V_a$, measured typically in $g \cdot m^{-1}$. AH ranges from zero in dry air to $30 \ g \cdot m^{-1}$ when the vapor is saturated at 30 °C. It changes as air **pressure** changes. More rigorous for heat and mass balance calculations is the so-called **humidity** (mixing) ratio MRi, which is also absolute **humidity** expressed as a ratio of mass of **water** vapor, m_w, per unit mass of dry air, m_d, at a given **pressure** and usually measured in $g \cdot kg^{-1}$: MRi $= m_w/m_d = \delta \cdot p_w/(p_a - p_w)$, where $\delta = 0.62197$ is the ratio of molecular weights of **water** vapor and dry air, p_w is the partial **pressure** of **water** vapor in moist air, and p_a is the atmospheric **pressure** of moist air. Relative **humidity** (RH) is defined as the ratio of the partial **pressure** of **water** vapor (in a gaseous mixture of air and **water** vapor) to the saturated vapor **pressure** of **water** at a given temperature. RH is expressed as a percentage and is calculated as RH $= [p(H_2O)/p^*(H_2O)] \times 100\%$, where $p(H_2O)$ is the partial **pressure** of **water** vapor, and $p^*(H_2O)$ is the saturation vapor **pressure** of **water** at the temperature of the gas mixture. The relative **humidity** should be kept between 30% and 60% because at high **humidity**, sweating is less effective, and at low **humidity**, the dry **skin** syndrome is characteristic. Control of environmental **humidity** is important for measurements of **optical properties** of **skin** *in vitro* and *in vivo*.

hyaluronic acid: Natural moisturizing component in **tissues**. The quantity of **hyaluronic acid** in an organism decreases with aging.

hydrated: Being associated with **water** molecules. The degree of **hydration** of **tissues** ranges from 4% (**tooth enamel**) to 75% (**soft tissue**).

hydration: **Absorption** of **water** by **tissues** and **cells**. Organic **hydration** is a reaction in which **water** is added across a double bond. Mineral (component of **tooth** or **bone tissue**) **hydration** is a reaction in which **water** is combined into the **crystalline** structure of a mineral. **Hydration** H is usually defined as $H = \left(Weight_{wet} - Weight_{dry}\right)/Weight_{dry}$.

hydraulic conductivity: Property of material that describes the ease with which **water** can move through pore spaces or fractures. It depends on the intrinsic permeability of the material and on the degree of saturation. Saturated **hydraulic conductivity** describes **water** movement through saturated media.

hydrocephalus: An abnormal increase in the amount of **cerebospinal fluid (CSF)**.

hydrocortisone: Corticosteroid that is similar to a natural **hormone** produced by adrenal **glands**.

hydrodynamic radius of a particle: Radius that is determined from the measurements of the translation **diffusion coefficient** for an ensemble of identical particles in the medium. It is larger than the initial one due to interactions with molecules of the medium.

hydrogen peroxide (H_2O_2): Very pale blue liquid that appears colorless in a dilute solution, slightly more viscous than **water**. It is a weak acid that has strong oxidizing properties and is therefore a powerful bleaching agent that has found use as a disinfectant.

hydrophilic: Having affinity for **water**.

hydrophobic: Having little or no affinity for **water**.

hydrostatic pressure: **Pressure** at a point in a liquid is the force per unit area on a very small area around the point. If the point is at a depth h in the liquid of density ρ, then **pressure** $p = \rho g h$. The **pressure** at a point in a liquid at rest acts equally in all directions. The force exerted on a surface in contact with a liquid at rest is perpendicular to the surface at all points. **Hydrostatic pressure** is measured in N/m^2 or Pa (Pascal).

hydroxyapatite (HAP): See **apatite**.

hydroxyethyl cellulose: Nonionic, **water**-soluble polymer that can thicken, suspend, bind, emulsify, and form films.

hygroscopic: Ability of a substance to attract **water** molecules from the surrounding environment through either **absorption** or adsorption. **Hygroscopic** substances include **glycerol**, **ethanol**, methanol, concentrated sulfuric acid, and concentrated sodium hydroxide. Calcium chloride is so **hygroscopic** that it eventually dissolves in the **water** it absorbs.

Hypaque: Commonly used **x-ray contrast** medium. As diatrizoate meglumine and as diatrizoate sodium, it is used for gastrointestinal studies, angiography, and urography. Very good agent for **optical clearing** of **fibrous tissue** owing to its high **osmolarity** and high **index of refraction**. An analog of **trazograph**.

hyperchromaticity: Defined as the increase in **optical density** of **DNA** molecules in solution that increase on nuclease digestion due to the release of **nucleotides** that absorb more **UV light**. Such chromic shift is also seen during the process of **denaturation** due to temperature of **DNA** separation.

hyperdermal: Refers exclusively to the **skin**, when, for instance, intradermal injection is provided. See **cutaneous**.

hyperglycemia: Condition in which an excessive amount of **glucose** circulates in the **blood plasma**. It is primarily a symptom of **diabetes** in which there are elevated levels of **blood** sugar, or **glucose**, in the bloodstream. In type I **diabetes**, **hyperglycemia** results from malfunctioning in the supply of **insulin**, the chemical that enables **cells** to receive energy from **glucose**. Type II **diabetes** is due to a combination of defective **insulin** secretion and defective responsiveness to **insulin**, often termed reduced **insulin** sensitivity.

hypericin: Naphtodianthrone, a red-colored anthraquinone derivative, which, together with hyperforin, is one of the principal active constituents of *Hypericum* (Saint John's wort). **Hypericin** is believed to act as an **antibiotic** and nonspecific kinase inhibitor. The large **chromophore** system in the molecule means that it can cause photosensitivity of **tissues**. Because **hypericin** accumulates preferentially in **cancerous tissues**, it is used as an indicator of **cancerous cells**. It is under research as an agent in **photodynamic therapy (PDT)**, for example, for treatment of transitional **cell carcinoma**.

hyperinsulinemic-hypoglycemic clamp: Procedure that suppresses **endogenous insulin** secretion by hyperinsulinemia- and hypoglycemia-mediated feedback inhibition of beta **cells**.

hyperosmotic: Term describing a liquid with a lower concentration of **water** and higher solute concentration than fluids in a **tissue** or **cell** have. This term also means that if a **cell** is **hyperosmotic**, it absorbs **water** from the surroundings to dilute the higher solute concentration, thus making the **cell isotonic** to the environment.

hyperplasia: Enlargement of a part due to an abnormal increase in the number of its **cells**.

hyperpolarizability: Nonlinear **polarizability** β characterizes the nonlinear part of the induced **dipole moment** of the molecule, which is proportional to the squared external electric field with the coefficient of proportionality equal to $(1/2)\beta$.

hyperspectral imaging: Image technology that collects and processes information from across the **UV** to **IR spectrum** (typically from 0.3–25 µm). Sensors (imaging **spectrometers**) collect information as a set of "images," where each image represents a **wavelength** range, i.e., spectral band. These images are then combined and form a 3D hyperspectral cube for processing and analysis. Spectral and **spatial resolution**, as well as **signal-to-noise ratio**, are important to provide reliability of object-measured features. The acquisition and processing of hyperspectral images is also referred to as imaging **spectroscopy** or spectral imaging. In contrast to **multispectral imaging**, hyperspectral data is a contiguous set of dozens to hundreds of bands. Typically, hardware is based on spectral **reflectance** measurements, such as hemispherical, directional (when the fraction of the **light** incident on a sample at a given angle is reflected back into the hemisphere), bidirectional (when the distribution of **light**, described as a function of two angles, is reflected back into the hemisphere from **light** incident at a given angle on a sample), diffuse, and **specular**. Enhanced backscatter measurements using a **laser** interferometric reflectometer are also exploited. **Hyperspectral imaging** systems provide the real-time processing requirements of **microscopy**, biological screening, and analysis. The typical imager acquires up to a 1024×1024 **pixel** image that is more than 100 bands deep in as little as a few seconds. This technique allows for accurate, rapid, and **noninvasive** measurement of **blood** oxygenation and its mapping.

hyperthermia: An acute condition that occurs when the body produces or absorbs more heat than it can dissipate. It is usually due to excessive exposure to heat. It can be created artificially by drugs or medical devices (based on acoustics, microwaves, **light**, and so on); in these instances, it may be used to treat **cancer** and other conditions. When the **tissue** temperature approaches and exceeds 40 °C, there is an increased **blood flow** in both **tumor** and normal **tissues**. As **tumor** temperature reaches 41.5 °C, cellular

221

cytotoxicity occurs. Temperatures above 42.5 °C can result in **vascular** destruction within **tumor tissue**. The thermal impact on **tissue** changes drastically when temperature exceeds 43 °C. The rate of "**cell** kill" doubles for every 1 °C increase beyond 43 °C and decreases by a factor of 4 to 6 for every 1 °C drop below 43 °C. It has been observed that **tumor tissue** is more sensitive to temperature increase than normal **tissue**.

hypertonic: A solution that has a higher concentration of solutes than that in a **cell** is said to be **hypertonic**. This solution has more solute particles and, therefore, relatively less **water** than the **cell** contents.

hypodermic: Situated or lying under the **skin**, as a **tissue**. Performed or introduced under the **skin**, as an injection by a syringe, and so on.

hypo-osmotic: Describes a **cell** or other **membrane**-bound object that has a lower concentration of solutes than its surroundings. For example, a **cell** in a high-salt-concentration medium is **hypo-osmotic**. **Water** is more likely to move out of the **cell** by osmosis as a result. This is the opposite of **hyperosmotic**.

hypothesis of Roy and Sherrington: Widely accepted to account for the phenomenon whereby increased neuronal metabolic activity will give rise to the accumulation of vasoactive catabolites, which decrease **vascular** resistance and thereby increase **blood flow** until normal homeostasis is reestablished.

hypotonic: Conditions or bathing **media** owing to the osmotic flow of **water** into the **cell cytoplasm**.

hypoxia: Lack of **oxygen** in air, **blood**, or **tissue**.

hysterectomy: Excision of the **uterus**.

IC-GREEN^{TM}: Sterile, **lyophilized** green powder containing 25 mg of **indocyanine green (ICG)** with no more than 5% sodium iodide. It is packaged with aqueous solvent consisting of sterile **water** for injection used to dissolve the **ICG** and is to be administered intravenously.

ileum: Final section of the **small intestine**. It follows the **duodenum** and **jejunum** and is separated from the **cecum** by the ileocecal **valve** (ICV), or Bauhin's **valve**. In humans, the **ileum** is about 2–4 m long, and its **pH** is usually between 7 and 8 (neutral or slightly alkaline).

image cytometry: Numerous clinical and research applications especially in anatomic pathology for detection and study of **malignant lesions** have a so-called **image cytometry**. This technique uses morphometry and densitometry, as measuring techniques, and neural networks and expert systems to process collected data. Improvements in image cytometric techniques applying more and more sensitive detectors and introducing **nonlinear optics** (two-photon excitation), lifetime measurements **(FLIM)**. The latest developments were able to break the diffraction limit, such as **scanning near-field optical microscopy (SNOM)**, the **total internal reflection (TIRF) microscopy**, **fluorescence resonance energy transfer (FRET)**, **stimulated emission depletion (STED)** and **4Pi** and multi-objective microscopy.

image display tone: Gray shade or **color hue** on an image.

image reconstruction: See **time-resolved optical absorption and scattering tomography (TOAST)** and **tomographic reconstruction**.

image segmentation: The process of partitioning a digital image into multiple segments (sets of **pixels**). The goal of segmentation is to simplify and/or change the representation of an image into something that is more meaningful and easier to analyze. It is typically used to locate objects and boundaries in images. The result of **image segmentation** is a set of segments that collectively cover the entire image, or a set of contours extracted from the image. All of the **pixels** in a region are similar with respect to some characteristic or computed property, such as **color**, **intensity**, or texture. Adjacent regions are significantly different with respect to the same characteristic(s).

image-carrying photons: Group of **photons** selected for producing an image of a certain macro-inhomogeneity within a **scattering** medium.

imaging (image) contrast: To point to differences between two or more objects or points on the object. A parameter that characterizes differentiation (visibility) of the visualized object (objects) hidden in the **scattering** surroundings. The following contrasting parameters may be used: **light intensity**, **reflectance**, **degree of polarization (DOP)**, **fluorescence intensity** and lifetime, **refractive index**, reconstructed **absorption** and **scattering coefficients**, and so on (see **contrast**).

imaging radiometer: **Infrared thermal imager** that provides quantitative **thermal images**.

imaging resolution: When two objects are close together, they may not form two distinguishable images on the **retina** of the eye or matrix detector. The measure of the ability to detect two such images of two objects close together is the resolving power of the instrument. For a microscope, two objects are resolved if the angular separation of the objects is not less than λ/D, where λ is the **wavelength** of the **light** used, and D is the diameter of the **objective**. The minimum separation of two objects if they are to be resolved is $0.61\lambda/NA$, where NA is the **numerical aperture**. The **spatial resolution** of imaging systems can be quantified by the **point spread function (PSF)** (the image of a point object).

immersion liquid: See **immersion medium**.

immersion medium (*Synonym*: immersion liquid): Liquid that provides optical matching between a **light microscope objective** and a biological specimen. It enhances the **numerical aperture** of the **objective** and the microscope resolution. In addition, optical matching reduces surface **reflection** and **scattering** and consequently allows for receiving higher **contrast** images. When immersion liquid penetrates into **tissue**, it may provide **optical clearing** due to reduction of **tissue** bulk **scattering**.

immersion technique: Technique used to reduce **light scattering** in an inhomogeneous medium by matching the **refractive index** of the **scatterers** and **ground substance** (**optical clearing**). Immersion liquids with an appropriate **refractive index**, rate of **diffusion**, and **osmotic pressure** are usually used.

immobilize: To deprive of mobility.

immune cell: See, for example, **macrophage** and **lymphocytes**.

immune response: How the body recognizes and defends itself against **bacteria**, **viruses**, and substances that appear foreign and harmful to the body. The immune system protects the body from potentially harmful substances by recognizing and responding to **antigens**. The immune system recognizes and destroys substances that contain these **antigens**. Even the body's own **cells** have **proteins** that are **antigens**. The immune system learns to recognize these **antigens** as normal and does not usually react against them.

impedance: Quantity that determines the current flowing in an inductive or capacitive component of a circuit when an alternating potential difference is applied. The magnitude of the **impedance** varies with the **frequency** of the **ac**.

implant: Material grafted (implanted) or introduced into a **tissue**.

incision: Surgical cut of a **tissue**; separating of **soft tissues** using a scalpel.

index of refraction: Number n indicating the **speed of light** in a given medium as either the ratio of the **speed of light** in a vacuum to that in the given medium (absolute **index of refraction**), or the ratio of the **speed of light** in a specified medium to that in the given medium (relative **index of refraction**, $m = n_1/n_2$). For different **tissues** and **tissue** components, **refractive index** n in the **visible/NIR wavelength** range varies from a value slightly higher than for **water** due to the influence of some organic components, ~1.35 for **interstitial fluid**, to 1.62 for **tooth enamel**. Average data for bulk **tissue** of human organs measured in the spectral range 456–1064 nm are as follows: **intima** (1.39), **media** normal (1.38) and calcified (1.52), and **adventitia** (1.36) of **aorta**; **bladder mucosa** (1.37) and wall (1.40); **brain** gray (1.36) and **white matter** (1.38); **colon muscle** (1.36); **submucosa** (1.36) and **mucosa** (1.38); esophageal **mucosa** (1.37); **subcutaneous** (1.44) and **abdominal** (1.46) **fat**; **heart** trabecula (1.40) and myocard (1.38); femoral **vein** (1.39); **lung** (1.38); **muscle** (1.37); **spleen** (1.37); and **stomach mucsa** (1.38) and **muscle** (1.39). In the spectral range 400–700 nm: **cell cytoplasm** (1.350–1.367), **cerebral spinal fluid** (1.335), eye **aqueous humor** (1.336), **cornea** (1.376) with **collagen fiber** (1.47) and extrafibrillar material (1.35), **lens** surface (1.386) and center (1.406), **vitreous humor** (1.336), **tooth enamel** (1.62), **dentin** matrix (1.553 ± 0.001), **hair** strands (1.45–1.50), and **skin** *stratum corneum* (SC) (1.55). And on separate **wavelengths**: 632.8 nm **kidney** (1.417±0.006) and **liver** (1.367±0.006); 800 nm normal (1.403) and **malignant** (1.431) female **breast tissue**; 1300 nm mesenteric **fat** (1.467±0.008) and left ventricular cardiac **muscle** (1.382 ± 0.007); **whole blood** 488 nm (1.395 ± 0.003), 632.8 nm (1.373 ± 0.004), 1079.5 nm (1.363 ± 0.004), 1341.4 nm (1.360 ± 0.005); human **blood plasma** 488 nm (1.350 ± 0.002), 632.8 nm (1.345 ± 0.002), 1079.5 nm (1.332 ± 0.003), 1341.4 nm (1.327 ± 0.004); and human **hemoglobin** (**oxygenated**, 287 g/l) 500 nm (1.413 ± 0.03), 700 nm (1.404 ± 0.03) and 900 nm (1.401 ± 0.03).

India ink: Used in preparation of **tissue phantoms** as an **absorbing medium** with a smooth **absorption spectrum** close to **melanin** in the **visible** and **NIR**.

indirect thermography: Thermal imaging and measurement of a surface that is indirectly affected by the target of concern; that is, the target of concern is thermally decoupled from the surface due to thermal insulation, such as an air gap or a radiant barrier.

indium antimonide (InSb): Material from which fast, sensitive **photodetectors** used in **infrared** scanners and imagers are made. Such detectors usually require cooling while in operation.

indocyanine green (ICG): **Water**-soluble tricarbocyanine dye with **infrared** absorbing and fluorescing properties developed in the Kodak Research Laboratories in 1955. **ICG** was approved by the **Food and Drug Administration (FDA)** in 1956, 1958, and 1975 for cardiocirculatory measurements, **liver** function tests, and ophthalmic **fluorescent angiography**, including retinal angiography. An intraoperative video angiography device for the viewing of **blood flow** in the cerebral **vascular** area using **ICG** as a fluorescent agent was also approved by the **FDA** (2006). The molecular formula for **ICG** is $C_{43}H_{47}N_2O_6S_2Na$, molecular weight 774.98, green powder. It has peak **absorption** at 775 nm in **water** and has little or no **absorption** in the **visible** below 700 nm. This dye is used as a diagnostic aid for **blood volume** determinations, eye **vessel** angiography (choroidal circulation), cardiac output, or hepatic function. For instance, the typical dye concentrations used for *in vivo* retinal and choroidal angiography are in the range of 20–25 mg/ml of ICG applied by injection into a peripheral **arm vein**. The dye is soluble in **water** and less soluble in **ethanol**. The principal advantages are the presence of an **absorption** maximum near the **isobestic point** of **oxyhemoglobin** and **deoxyhemoglobin** around 805 nm, the confinement to the **vascular** compartment by binding to **plasma proteins** (**albumin**), the very low toxicity, and the rapid excretion, almost exclusively, into the **bile**. **ICG** has been used extensively in **tissue laser welding** and **photothermal cancer** treatments because of its **absorption** properties at the **laser diode wavelength** of 805–810 nm. In **tissues** and **cells**, the **NIR absorption** peak due to binding with **cell proteins** is moved to longer **wavelengths** to 805 nm for **blood** and human **skin** *in vivo*, and to 810 nm for epidermal **cell cultures**. It has a photodynamic effect and is used for **bacteria** killing in **tissue** depth such as *Propionibacterium acnes* for **skin** acne treatment using **photodynamic therapy (PDT)** with a **NIR diode laser** (810 nm).

inelastic scattering: From quantum electrodynamics, it follows that an individual **light scattering** event is considered as an **absorption** by a particle of the scattering medium of the incident photon having **energy** $h\nu$, momentum $(h/2\pi)k$, and polarization p, and then emission of the photon having **energy** $h\nu'$, momentum $(h/2\pi)k'$, and polarization p'. When $\nu \neq \nu'$, **light scattering** is accompanied by redistribution of **energy** between the radiation, and the medium is called inelastic; for example, **Raman scattering**. When $\nu = \nu'$, no redistribution takes place, and **light scattering** is called elastic or **Rayleigh scattering**.

infiltrate: To perform infiltration, i.e., to penetrate a **cell** or **tissue** with a substance. It also refers to the substance infiltrated.

infiltrating: Refers to infiltration, the process of **percolation** and impregnation of a material, **cell**, or **tissue** by a gas, liquid, or solution. It is also related to **cell** migration. Examples include adipose infiltration appearance of **fat cells** in the places where they are normally absent, calcareous infiltration (see **calcification**), and fatty infiltration (a **pathological** storage of **fat** drops in **cell cytoplasm**).

inflammation: Traditionally, Western medicine has recognized the four signs of **inflammation** as *tumor*, *rubor*, *calor*, and *dolor* (swelling, redness, heat, and **pain**). In addition to these physical changes, there are also important psychological ones, including lethargy, apathy, loss of appetite, and increasing sensitivity to **pain**. In response to acute damage or entrance of foreign material, **monocytes** enlarge and synthesize increased amounts of **enzymes**, which help to break down the material. In doing so, they are transformed to more active phagocytes called **macrophages**.

Infracyanine® **25 (IC25):** **NIR** contrasting agent. It is the trade name of **indocyanine green (ICG)**.

infrared (IR): See **light wavelength range**.

infrared atmospheric window: Spectral intervals within the **IR spectrum** in which the atmosphere transmits radiant **energy** well (atmospheric **absorption** is at a minimum). These are roughly defined as 3–5 µm and 8–14 µm.

infrared calibration source: **Blackbody** or other target of known temperature and **effective emissivity** used as a **calibration** reference.

infrared camera: An **infrared thermal imager** that creates pictures of heat rather than **light**. It measures radiated **IR energy** and converts the data to corresponding maps of temperatures. It provides temperature data at each image **pixel**. **Indium antimonide (InSb)** and **mercury cadmium telluride (HgCdTe)** materials are often used as fast, sensitive **infrared** matrix detectors [see **focal plane array (FPA)**]. Images may be digitized, stored, manipulated, processed, and printed out.

infrared detector: Transducer element that converts incoming **IR** radiant **energy** impinging on its sensitive surface to a useful electrical signal. See **optical detector**, **photodetector**, and **infrared camera**.

infrared fiber: Can be made from glass, **crystalline** material, or **hollow waveguides** that may be further subdivided based on the **fiber** material or structure or both. The key property of **infrared**

fibers is their ability to transmit **wavelengths** longer than most oxide glass **fibers**, in particular from 2–20 μm. In some cases, the **transmittance** of the **fiber** can extend well beyond 20 μm, but there are few applications requiring the transmission of **IR radiation** longer than about 12 μm. The losses for most of the **infrared fibers** are a few **decibels** per meter (**dB**/m) rather than less than 1 dB/km, which is common for silica **fibers**. The losses are because of impurities and imperfections, which give rise to a large **absorption** and **scattering** (see **fiber losses**). An exception is fluoride glass **fiber**, which can have losses as low as a few **dB**/km. Typically, **IR fibers** are much weaker than silica **fiber** and, therefore, more fragile. **IR fibers** usually have higher loss, larger **refractive indices** and temperature gradient dn/dT, lower melting or softening points, and greater thermal expansion than silica **fibers**. For example, **chalcogenide glass** and polycrystalline Ag-halide **fibers** have **refractive indices** greater than 2. This means that the **reflection** or loss due to **Fresnel reflection** exceeds 20% for two **fiber** ends. The higher dn/dT and low melting or softening point leads to thermal lensing and, as a result, low **laser**-induced damage thresholds for the solid-core **IR fibers**. **Fibers** composed of ZrF_4, BaF_2, AlF_3, LiF_3 and other fluorides have a low loss in the **MIR** range of 2–8 μm, and despite their unsatisfactory mechanical and **hygroscopic** properties, their high **transmittance** for the shorter **IR radiation**, especially for **erbium lasers** ($\lambda =$ 2.94 μm), makes them useful for biomedicine. **Fibers** composed of **chalcogenide glasses** are transparent up to 12–20 μm have losses less than 1 dB/m (about 20% per meter) in the range of 2–6.5 μm. Their main disadvantages are toxicity and dissolving in **water**; however, they could be used in biomedical applications at distant measurements of temperature or **IR** imaging. Sapphire (Al_2O_3) mono-**crystalline fibers** are nontoxic and nonhygroscopic and have a high melting temperature. Using pulling technology, they could be made up to 10 meters in length with total losses about 0.9 dB/m ($\lambda =$ 2.94 μm). Their main disadvantage is lack of flexibility. The best **IR fibers** are polycrystalline Ag-halide **fibers** (for example, AgBrCl-**fiber**) transparent in a wide **wavelength** range, 2.5–20.0 μm. Solid-core **IR fibers** are ideal **evanescent-wave sensors** for monitoring chemical processes in the sensitive fingerprint region of the **IR spectrum**. In these applications, the **fiber** core is surrounded by the chemical or biological agent, and some portion of the **light** is coupled out of the core into the surrounding medium. This type of chemical sensor is potentially very sensitive and selective. **Blackbody radiation** from a source is well transmitted through the **IR fiber**, and the temperature can be determined by **calibration** to a **blackbody** of known temperature. Since **blackbody radiation** from room temperature objects and physiological temperature living objects peaks near 10 μm, **IR fibers** are excellent candidates for use in measuring these temperatures, below 50 °C.

infrared filter: Designed to block or reflect **mid-infrared wavelengths** but pass **visible light**. They are often used in microscopes with bright incandescent **light** bulbs to prevent unwanted heating of biological materials.

infrared focal plane array (IRFPA): Linear or 2D matrix of individual **infrared detector** elements, typically used as a detector in an **infrared imager**.

infrared focal plane array (IRFPA) imager: An **infrared thermal imager** that incorporates a 2D **IRFPA** and produces a thermogram without mechanical scanning. See **infrared camera**.

infrared imager: Infrared instrument that collects the **infrared** radiant **energy** from a target surface and produces an image in monochrome (black and white) or **color**, where the gray shades or **color hues** correspond respectively to target radiant exitance.

infrared molecular laser: Laser in which the lasing medium is molecular gas with an **IR** emission, such as **CO (carbon monoxide) lasers** (λ = 5–6.5 μm) and **CO_2 (carbon dioxide) lasers** (λ = 9.2–11.1 μm). There are many other **IR** molecular **lasers** whose energetic parameters are close to those of **CO lasers** and **CO_2 lasers**, such as N_2O **lasers** with two bands 10.5 and 11.0 μm, H_2O **lasers** (28.78 and 118 μm), D_2O **lasers** (171 μm),

SO_2 (141 and 193 μm), DCN **lasers** (311 and 337 μm), and DCN **lasers** (190–204 μm).

infrared photodetector: Type of a **photodetector** sensitive in the **infrared** spectral range that has fast response (on the order of **microseconds**), has limited spectral response, and usually requires cooled operation. **IR photodetectors** are used in **infrared radiation** thermometers, **infrared** scanners, and **infrared imagers**. **Indium antimonide (InSb)** and **mercury cadmium telluride (HgCdTe)** are materials from which fast, sensitive (at cooled operation) **IR photodetectors** are made. See **infrared detector**.

infrared radiation thermometer: Instrument that converts incoming **infrared** radiant **energy** from a spot on a target surface to a measurement value that can be related to the temperature of that spot.

infrared spectroscopy: Spectroscopy of **mid-** and **far-infrared wavelength** range that uses **light**-excited vibrational **energy** states in molecules to get information about the molecular composition, molecular structures, and molecular interactions.

infrared thermal imager: Instrument or system that converts incoming **infrared** radiant **energy** from a target surface to a thermal map, or thermogram, on which **color hues** or gray shades can be related to the temperature distribution on that surface.

infusion: Administration of drug parenterally by the intravenous route or by **subcutaneous** or intramuscle injection.

inhomogeneous medium: Medium with regular or irregular spatial distribution of physical properties, including **optical properties**.

injury: **Tissue** damage, **wound**, **trauma**.

in situ: In biology, to examine the phenomenon exactly in place where it occurs (i.e., without moving it to some special medium). When used in laboratory science, such as **cell** science, this term can mean something intermediate between *in vivo* and *in vitro*. For example, examining a **cell** within a whole organ **intact** and under perfusion may be *in situ* investigation. This would not be *in vivo*, but it would not be also the same as working with the **cell** alone (a common scenario for *in vitro* experiments), actually this would be more similar to *ex vivo*, as before experimentation animal or human organs are excised from the living body and kept in conditions very close to the natural ones,.

instantaneous field of view (IFOV): Angular subtense (expressed in angular degrees or **radians** per side if rectangular and angular degrees or **radians** if round) found by the ratio of the detector dimension divided by the instrument **focal length**. IFOV is the projection of the detector at the target plane. In a **radiation** thermometer, this defines the target spot size. In a line scanner or imager, it represents one resolution element in a scan line or thermogram and is a measure of **spatial resolution**.

instrument background temperature: The apparent temperature of the radiant **energy** impinging on an object that is reflected off the object and enters the temperature-measuring instrument. It originates from the scene behind and surrounding the instrument, as viewed from the target. The **reflection** of this background appears in the image and affects temperature measurements. Good-quality, quantitative thermal-sensing and thermal-imaging instruments provide a means for correcting measurements for this **reflection**.

insulin: Polypeptide **hormone** that regulates **carbohydrate metabolism**. It is produced in the islets of Langerhans in the **pancreas**. It has effects on **fat metabolism**, and it changes the liver's activity in storing or releasing **glucose** and in processing **blood lipids**, and in other **tissues** such as **fat** and **muscle**. **Insulin** is used medically to treat some forms of **diabetes mellitus**.

integrating sphere (IS): Photometric sphere with a highly reflecting white or metallic coating and **photodetector** inside. Used for precise measurements of **diffuse reflectance** or **total transmittance** of **scattering** materials (**tissues**). As coating materials having smooth and high **reflectance** in the **visible** and **NIR**, barium-sulfate, **MgO**, Spectralon®, and Zenith® are usually used. For **IR** applications, gold coatings are available.

integrating sphere spectrophotometry: Spectrophotometry of the **scattering** objects, including **blood** and **tissues**. It provides precise measurements of **diffuse reflectance** or **total transmittance** in a wide spectral range using single- or double-**integrating sphere spectrometers** (see **double-integrating sphere (DIS) technique**). To reconstruct reduced **scattering** and **absorption coefficients** from these measurements, simple the **Kubelka–Munk model (KKM)** or more sophisticated **algorithms** such as the **inverse adding-doubling (IAD) method (technique)** or **inverse Monte Carlo (IMC) method (technique)** are used.

integration time: Time interval over which measurements are taken. Longer **integration times** allow more averaging in order to filter out background noise and boost the **signal-to-noise ratio**.

intensified charge-coupled device (ICCD): A **CCD** that is optically connected to an image intensifier that is in turn mounted in front of the **CCD**. An image intensifier includes three functional elements: a **photocathode**, a **micro-channel plate (MCP)**, and a phosphor screen. These three elements are mounted closely behind each other in the sequence described. The **photons** that are coming from the **light** source fall onto the **photocathode**, thereby generating photoelectrons. The photoelectrons are accelerated toward the **MCP** by an electrical control voltage, applied between **photocathode** and **MCP**. The electrons are multiplied inside of the **MCP** and thereafter accelerated toward the phosphor screen. The phosphor screen finally converts the multiplied electrons back to **photons**, which are guided to the **CCD** by a **fiber**

optic or a **lens**. An image intensifier inherently includes shutter functionality by reversing the control voltage at the **photocathode**, in a process called gating, and therefore **ICCDs** are also called gateable **CCD** cameras. They have extremely high sensitivity, which enables single-**photon** detection; the gateability is one of the major advantages of the **ICCD** over **EMCCD** cameras. The highest performing **ICCD** cameras enable shutter times as short as 200 **picoseconds**.

intensity: Several measures of **light** are commonly known as **intensity**. Radiant **intensity** is a radiometric quantity. Luminous **intensity** is a photometric quantity, measured in **lumens** per steradian (lm/sr), or **candela** (cd). Radiance (**irradiance**) is commonly called "**intensity**," measured in **watts** per meter squared (W/m^2) or centimeter squared (W/cm^2).

intensity diffusion wave (*Synonym*: photon diffusion wave): See **photon-density wave**.

intensity matrix: See **light-scattering matrix (LSM)**.

intensity probability density distribution function: Function that describes the distribution of **probability** over the values of the **light intensity**.

intercellular: Between **cells**, as in an **intercellular** bridge.

interference: Process in which two or more **light**, sound, or **electromagnetic waves** of the same **frequency** combine to reinforce or cancel each other, the amplitude of the resulting **wave** being equal to the algebraic sum of the amplitude of the combining **waves**.

interference filter: See **dichroic (dichromatic) filter**.

interference fringe: Series of alternating dark and bright bands produced as a result of **light interference**. With a monochromatic source of **light**, the bands (fringes) are alternately bright and dark. With white **light**, the **interference** bands are colored.

interference microscopy: Uses two separate **light beams** with much greater lateral separation than that used in **phase-contrast microscopy** or in **differential interference contrast (DIC) microscopy**. In variants of the **interference** microscope where object and reference beam pass through the same **objective**, two images are produced of every object (one being the "ghost image"). The two images are separated either laterally within the visual field or at different **focal planes**, as determined by the optical principles employed. These two images can be a nuisance when they overlap, because they can severely affect the accuracy of mass or thickness measurements. Rotation of the preparation may thus be necessary, as in the case of **DIC**. The main advantage offered by **interference microscopy** measurements is the possibility of measuring the projected dry mass of living **cells**. The main original disadvantage (difficult interpretation of translated **interference** bands or complex colored images) can now be easily surmounted by means of digital camera image recording, followed by the application of computer **algorithms** that rapidly deliver the processed data as false-**color** images of projected dry mass.

interference of photon-density waves (intensity waves): Process in which two or more **photon-density waves** of the same **frequency** combine to reinforce or cancel each other, the amplitude (**light intensity**) of the resulting **wave** being equal to the algebraic sum of the amplitude (**light intensity**) of the combining **waves**.

interference of speckle fields (speckle-modulated fields): Interference of the fields in which amplitudes and phases are randomly modulated due to their interaction (**scattering**) with **inhomogeneous media**.

interference pattern: Pattern of **interference fringes**. **Light** from any source can be used to obtain **interference patterns**— for example, Newton's rings can be produced with a low coherent sunlight. However, in general, white **light** is less suited for producing clear **interference patterns**, as it is a mix of a full **spectrum** of **colors**, each of which has different spacing of **interference fringes**. The most suitable is **laser light** because it is almost perfectly monochromatic with a large **coherence length**.

interferometer: Instrument that splits a **light beam** into a number of coherent beams and then superimposes the beams to obtain **interference fringes**. The instrument is used in accurate determinations of **wavelengths** of **light**, for examination of the hyperfine structure of spectra, testing of optical elements for **refraction** purposes, and accurate measurement of distance, displacement, and vibrations.

interferometry: Science and technology that deals with the measurements using various types of **interferometers**.

interferon (IFN): Natural **proteins** produced by the **cells** of the immune system of most vertebrates in response to challenges by foreign agents such as **viruses**, **bacteria**, parasites, and **tumor cells**. They belong to the large class of glycoproteins known as cytokines and assist the **immune response** by inhibiting viral replication within other **cells** of the body.

interfibrillar spacing (IFS): Spacing between **fibrils**. For example, **x-ray diffraction** was used to measure **IFS** of **collagen** in bovine **cornea** and **sclera** as functions of **pH**, **ionic strength**, and **tissue hydration**. The packing of **fibrils**, defined as $(\text{IFS})^2$, is an important parameter that determines control of **tissue light scattering**. For **cornea** at physiological **pH** 7.4, the squared **IFS** decreased linearly from approximately 9.2×10^3 nm^2 for a highly **hydrated tissue** ($H = 9.7$) to approximately 2.1×10^3 nm^2 at 10-fold less **hydration** and was equal to 4.2×10^3 nm^2 at physiological **hydration** $H = 3.2$.

intermolecular spacing (IMS): Spacing between molecules. For example, **x-ray diffraction** was used to measure **IMS** of **collagen** in bovine **cornea** and **sclera** as functions of **pH, ionic strength,** and **tissue hydration**. The **IMS** in both **tissues** decreased as the **ionic strength** was increased; for scleral **hydration** $H \cong 2.5$ and **pH** 7.0, **IMS** changed from 1.71 to 1.61 nm at 33-fold increase of **ionic strength**. The **IMS** has virtually no change on **hydration**, when $H > 1, H = 3.2$ is physiological **hydration**. The corresponding mean value for the **cornea** was 1.75 ± 0.04 nm ($n = 12$) and for the **sclera** was 1.65 ± 0.02 nm ($n = 9$) at **pH** 7.4. For dehydrated **tissues** ($H = 0$), the mean spacing was 1.25 ± 0.02 nm ($n = 2$) for the **cornea** and 1.27 ± 0.01 nm for the **sclera**.

internal conversion: Defined as a transition between one set of atomic (or molecular) electronic excited levels to another set of the same spin multiplicity (for example, the second **singlet state** to the first **singlet state**). It is sometimes called "radiation less de-excitation," because no **photons** are emitted. It differs from inter-system crossing in that, while both are radiation less methods of de-excitation, the molecular spin state for **internal conversion** remains the same, whereas it changes for inter-system crossing.

internal reflectance: Ratio of the **intensity** of **light** reflected from a surface to the incident **intensity** at **internal reflection** conditions. It is a dimensionless quantity. See **optical reflectance**.

internal reflection: When **light** is incident on a medium of lesser **index of refraction**, the ray is bent away from the normal, so the exit angle is greater than the incident angle. See **total internal reflection**.

interstitial fluid: Solution that bathes and surrounds the **cells** of multicellular animals. It is the main component of the **extracellular** fluid, which also includes **plasma** and transcellular fluid. On average, a subject has about 11 liters of **interstitial fluid**, providing the **cells** of the body with nutrients and a means of waste removal.

interstitial space: Space where **interstitial fluid** is circulating.

intersystem crossing: A photophysical process. It is an isoenergetic nonradiative transition between two electronic states having different multiplicities. It often results in a vibrationally excited molecular entity in the lower electronic state, which then usually deactivates its lowest vibrational level.

intestine: Part of the alimentary canal, in the shape of a long tube, that is concerned with the digestion and **absorption** of nutrients and the reabsorption of **water** from feces. Most of the digestion and almost all the **absorption** takes place in the **intestine**. The internal surface area of the **intestine** is increased by folds in the lining and projections on the lining. The **intestine** is coiled in the **abdominal cavity**. Its length is greater than the length of the body. The anterior part of the **intestine** contains **glands** for secreting digestive **enzymes** and receives **ducts** from the large digestive **glands**.

intima: Innermost **membrane** or lining of some organ or part, especially that of an **artery**, **vein**, or **lymph vessel**.

intracellular fluid: See **cytoplasm**.

intracellular motility: Motility of **cytoplasm** components.

Intralipid: Nutralipid or Liposyn. It is travenously administered nutrients that are **fat** emulsions containing soybean **oil**, egg phospholipids, and **glycerol**. In **biophotonics**, it is often used as a **tissue phantom** due to its **scattering** properties being very close to **scattering** properties of **tissues**. Typically, mixtures of approximately close to 10%-**Intralipid** (**scatterers**) and ~0.01%-**India ink** (absorbers) are used to model **tissue optical properties** in the far-red/**NIR** range.

intravital microscopy (IVM): Currently a gold standard for microvascular imaging. With chamber window preparation, conventional **optical microscopy** can be adopted to quantify the **vessel** count, diameter, length, density, permeability, and **blood** and **lymph** flow within the targeted thin **tissues** (see **transillumination digital microscopy**). However, **IVM** generally involves invasiveness and lacks depth information—a crucial morphological parameter.

invariant embedding method: Applied to the study of the propagation of various types of **waves** (acoustic, gravity, and electromagnetic) in **inhomogeneous media**. This method is used to reduce the initial boundary value problems to problems with initial data, permitting the solution of both determinate and statistical problems. It is applicable to both stationary (linear and nonlinear) and nonstationary **wave** problems.

invasive: Characterized by invasion, denoting (1) a procedure requiring insertion of an instrument or device into the body through the **skin** or a body orifice for diagnosis or treatment, (2) a **diffusion** of **malignant tumor** by its growing into or destruction of the adjacent **tissue**, or (3) a spreading of infection.

inverse adding-doubling (IAD) method (technique): Method that provides a tool for the rapid and accurate solution of the **inverse scattering problem**. It is based on the general method for the solution of the **radiation-transfer equation (RTE)** for plane-parallel layers. An important advantage of the **IAD** method when applied to **tissue** optics is the possibility of rapidly obtaining iterative solutions with the aid of up-to-date microcomputers. It is flexible enough to take into account anisotropy of **scattering** and the **internal reflection** from the sample boundaries. The method includes the following steps: (1) choosing the **optical parameters** to be measured, (2) counting the **reflections** and transmissions, (3) comparing the calculated and measured **reflectance** and **transmittance**, and (4) repeating the procedure until the estimated and measured values coincide with the desired accuracy. The method allows any intended accuracy to be achieved for all the parameters being measured, provided the necessary computer time is available. An error of 3% or less is considered acceptable. Also, the method may be used to directly correct experimental findings obtained with the aid of **integrating spheres**. The term doubling means that the **reflection** and transmission estimates for a layer at certain ingoing and outgoing **light** angles may be used to calculate both the **reflectance** and **transmittance** for a layer twice as thick by means of superimposing one upon the other and summing the contributions of each layer to the total **reflectance** and **transmittance**. Reflection and transmission in a layer having an arbitrary thickness are calculated in consecutive order, first for the thin layer with the same optical characteristics (**single scattering**), and then by consecutive doubling of the thickness, for any selected layer. The term adding indicates that the doubling procedure may be extended to heterogeneous layers for modeling **multilayer tissues** or taking into account **internal reflections** related to abrupt change in **refractive index**. The **IAD** is a numerical method for solving the one-dimensional **RTE** in slab geometry. It can be used for media with an arbitrary **phase function** and arbitrary angular distribution of the spatially uniform incident **radiation**. The **IAD** method has been successfully applied to determine **optical parameters** of **blood**; human and animal **dermis**; ocular **tissues** such as **retina**, choroids, **sclera**, **conjunctiva**, and **ciliary body**; **aorta**; and other **soft tissues** in a wide range of **wavelengths**. It provides accurate results in cases when the side losses are not significant, but it is less flexible than the **IMC** technique.

inverse Monte Carlo (IMC) method (technique): Iterative method that is based on the statistical simulation of **photon** transport in the **scattering media** and that provides a tool for the most accurate solutions of **inverse scattering problems**. It takes into account the real geometry of the object, the measuring system, and **light beams**. The Monte Carlo technique is employed as a method to solve the forward problem in the inverse **algorithm** for the determination of the **optical properties** of **tissues**. A number of **algorithms** that use the **IMC** method are now available. The **standard deviation** of a quantity (**diffuse reflectance**, **transmittance**, and so on) approximated by the MC technique decreases proportionally to $1/\sqrt{N}$, where N is the total number of launched **photons**. It is worthwhile to note that stable operation of the **algorithm** was maintained by generation of $(1-5) \times 10^5$ **photons** per iteration. Two to five iterations were usually necessary to estimate the **optical parameters** with approximately 2% accuracy. The main disadvantage is the long computation time.

inverse problem: Task where the values of some model parameters must be obtained from the observed data. The transformation from data to model parameters is a result of the interaction of **radiation** with an object under study—for example, **light** with a **tissue** (**light scattering** or **fluorescence**)—this is the **inverse problem** that arises in medical optical **spectroscopy** and imaging. Limitations to a finite number of measurements and the practical need to reconstruct only a few unknown parameters may lead to the problems being considered in discrete form. The **inverse problems** are typically ill-conditioned. In these cases, regularization, such as **Tikhonov regularization**, is usually used to introduce mild assumptions on the solution and prevent over-**fitting**.

inverse scattering problem: Attempt to take a set of measurements and error estimates, and only a limited set of parameters describing the sample and experiment, and to derive the remaining parameters. Usually, the geometry is known, intensities or their parameters are measured, and the **optical properties** or sizes of **scatterers** need to be derived. If these properties are considered to be spatially varying, then the resultant solutions can be presented as a 2D or 3D function of space, i.e., as an image.

*in vitro***:** In medicine and biology, a procedure performed not in a living organism but in a controlled environment, such as in a test tube, cover glass, or Petri dish. Many experiments in cellular biology are conducted outside organisms or **cells**. Because the test conditions may not correspond to the conditions inside the organism, this may lead to results that do not correspond totally to the situation that arises in a living organism. In **tissue** optics, one of the approaches is to measure **optical properties** of freshly excised (not fixed) cadaver **tissue** at conditions kept close to the living **tissue** (temperature, **hydration**, **pH**, and so on).

in vivo: In medicine, pertaining to experiments on living animals and humans.

in vivo **flow cytometry:** Flow **cytometry** that is based on **cell** imaging by a high-resolution, high-speed **CCD** or **CMOS** cameras [see **transillumination digital microscopy (TDM)**] and detection of single-photon, or two-photon **fluorescence**, **optoacoustic/photoacoustic** or **photothermal** signals from **cells** [see **photothermal flow cytometry**, **photoacoustic (PA) method**, **optoacuostic flow cytometry**] within the **blood** or **lymph** stream in **vessels**. For example, **TDM** allows one to provide *in vivo*, label-free, high-speed (up to 40,000 frames per second), high-resolution (up to 300 nm), real-time continuous imaging with successive framing of circulating individual **erythrocytes**, **leukocytes**, and **platelets** in fast **blood flow**. It is applicable for fundamental study of cell–cell interactions in native flow, identification of rare abnormal **cells** (e.g., **cancerous** or sickle **cells**) on the basis of their different deformability in flow, imaging of **platelets** during thrombus formation, study of the influence of drugs or **x-ray radiation** on individual **blood cells**, estimation of **blood** viscosity and velocity profiles in fast flows, and study of the dynamics of intravascular **cell aggregation** and **adhesion** to endothelial **cells**.

ionic strength: Characterizes a solution, and is a function of the concentration of all ions present in a solution. Generally, multivalent ions contribute strongly to the **ionic strength**.

ionizing radiation: Either particle **radiation** or **electromagnetic radiation** in which an individual particle/**photon** carries enough **energy** to ionize an atom or a molecule by completely removing an electron from its orbit. These ionizations, if enough occur, can be very destructive to living **tissue** and can cause **DNA** damage and mutations. Examples of particle **radiation** that is ionizing may be energetic electrons, neutrons, atomic ions, or **photons**. **Electromagnetic radiation** can cause ionization if the **energy** per **photon**, or **frequency**, is high enough, and thus the **wavelength** is short enough. The amount of **energy** required varies between molecules being ionized. **X rays** and gamma rays will ionize almost any molecule or atom. Far **UV**, near **UV**, and **visible light** are ionizing to some molecules. Microwaves and radio waves are nonionizing **radiation**.

iontophoresis: **Noninvasive** method of propelling high concentrations of a charged substance, normally medication or bioactive agents, transdermally by repulsive electromotive force using a small electrical charge applied to an iontophoretic chamber containing a similarly charged active agent and its vehicle. One or two chambers are filled with a solution containing an active ingredient and its solvent, termed the vehicle. The positively charged chamber, termed the anode, will repel a positively charged chemical, while the negatively charged chamber, termed the **cathode**, will repel a negatively charged chemical into the **skin**.

in-phase quadrature (IQ) circuit: A device that allows one to measure the amplitude and phase of an **ac** signal using the 0-deg/90-deg phase-mixing technique of the receiving and reference signals. See **0-degree hybrid (or splitter)** and **90-degree hybrid (or splitter)**.

IRDye 800CW carboxylate: One of the forms of **indocyanine green (ICG)** dye. Unfortunately, the clinically approved form of **ICG** does not have a reactive functional group and cannot be used to label targeting agents. In contrast, **IRDye 800CW carboxylate** is a **NIR** dye that can be functionalized with either an NHS or maleimide reactive group, allowing it to be attached to a number of biomolecules. **UV/visible** and **fluorescence** ($1 \times$ **PBS**) measurements yielded an **absorption** maximum of 774 nm and an emission maximum of 789 nm. **IRDye 800CW carboxylate** is more than 50 times brighter than **ICG**, and it may be especially suited for molecular imaging of disease markers at picomolar to femtomolar **tissue** concentrations.

iris: Thin, circular, colored sheet of **muscular tissue** at the front of the **eyeball**, forming the colored part of the eye. The central opening, the **pupil**, allows **light** to enter the **eyeball**. The **iris** controls the amount of **light** that enters the **eyeball** and assists in accommodation for near objects.

irradiance: Radiometric quantity, measured in **watts** per meter squared (W/m^2). Used when **electromagnetic radiation** is incident on the surface. This quantity characterizes the total amount of **radiation** present at all frequencies. It is also common to consider each **frequency** in the **spectrum** separately. This is called spectral **irradiance** and is measured in $W/(m^2 \cdot nm)$.

irreversible thermodynamics: If the change from initial state to final state of the system is so slow that the process can be assumed to be proceeding through a series of closely spaced quasi-equilibrium states, then such a process is called a reversible process, and the entire time evolution of each of the state variables can be obtained from the conventional theory of thermodynamics. But almost all the processes in living systems are irreversible processes, and the system is not in an equilibrium state for most of the time the system is evolving. A general theory of nonequilibrium thermodynamics does not exist. The thermodynamics of steady state processes is relatively well established, at least when the system does not deviate from equilibrium substantially.

irritation: Enhanced inflammatory reaction (see **inflammation**) of **tissue** on its **injury**.

ischemia: Restriction in **blood** supply, generally due to factors in the **blood vessels**, with resultant damage or **dysfunction** of **tissue**.

isobestic point: Point (**wavelength**) in the spectra having an identical **absorption** for different forms of a molecule. For example, a **hemoglobin** molecule in the form of **oxyhemoglobin** and **deoxyhemoglobin** has the **isobestic point** of 805 nm.

245

isoosmotic: Pertaining to solutions that exert the same **osmotic pressure**.

isopropyl laurate: Synthetic compound derived from **fatty acids**. It is an emollient and a **moisturizer**.

isopropyl myristate: $C_{17}H_{34}O_2$. It has a refractive index n_D = 1.435–1.438 at 20 °C, and is used in cosmetic and **topical** medicinal preparations, where good **absorption** through the **skin** is desired. It is a binding agent, emollient, **moisturizer**, and solvent.

isopropyl palmitate: Ester of palmitic acid from coconut **oil** used to impart silkiness to the **skin** and **hair**. It is a synthetic antistatic agent, binding agent, emollient, **moisturizer**, and solvent.

isotherm: Pattern superimposed on a thermogram or on a line scan that includes or highlights all points that have the same apparent temperature.

isotonic: (1) Noting or pertaining to solutions characterized by equal **osmotic pressure**; (2) noting or pertaining to a solution containing just enough salt to prevent the destruction of the **erythrocytes** when added to the **blood**.

isotropic scattering: Equality of **scattering** properties along all axes. **Rayleigh scattering** is an example.

Jablonski diagram: Representation of molecular **energy** levels and transition rates using potential curves, which are plotted without regard to the variable nuclear distances.

Jacobian matrix: Matrix of all first-order partial derivatives of a vector-valued function. The **Jacobian matrix** of a function describes the orientation of a tangent plane to the function at a given point. For example, if (x_2, y_2) = $f(x_1, y_1)$ is used to transform an image, the **Jacobian matrix** of function f, $J(x_1, y_1)$, shows how much the image in the neighborhood of (x_1, y_1) is stretched in the x, y, and xy directions. The **Jacobian matrix** is the derivative of a multivariate function, its importance is due to fact that it represents the best linear approximation to a differentiable function near a given point. The **Jacobian matrix** is a generalization of the gradient, which is the first derivative of a scalar function of several variables, because it is the first derivative of a vector function of several variables. According to the inverse function theorem, the matrix inverse of the **Jacobian matrix** of a function is the **Jacobian matrix** of the inverse function. Similarly, the (scalar) inverse of the **Jacobian matrix** determinant (often simply called the Jacobian) of a transformation is the Jacobian determinant of the inverse transformation. The Jacobian determinant at a given point gives important information about the behavior of the functions near that point, including functions describing the behavior of dynamic systems.

jejunum: Middle section of the **small intestine** that lies between the **duodenum** and the **ileum**. In adult humans, the **small intestine** is usually between 5.5–6.0 m long, 2.5 m of which is the **jejunum**. The **pH** in the **jejunum** is usually between 7 and 9 (neutral or slightly alkaline). The **jejunum** and the **ileum** are suspended by the **mesentery**, which gives the bowel great mobility within the abdomen. It also is wrapped by smooth **muscle** that helps to move food along by a process known as peristalsis.

Johnson–Nyquist noise: See **thermal noise**.

Jones matrix: See **amplitude-scattering matrix**.

joule: Derived unit of **energy** in the **SI**. It is the **energy** exerted by a force of one newton acting to move an object through a distance of one meter. In terms of dimensions, $1 \text{ J} = 1 \text{ kg} \cdot \text{m}^2/\text{s}^2$.

kalium dihydrophosphate (KDP): Material widely used in nonlinear optics, for example, for **light modulation** and **optical frequency doubling**.

keloid: Kind of **fibrous tumor** forming hard, irregular, clawlike excrescences upon the **skin**, especially postburn.

keratectomy: Incision of part of the **cornea**.

keratin: Family of filamentous structural **proteins**. Tough and insoluble, they form the hard but nonmineralized structures found in humans, animals, and other living objects.

keratinization: See **cornification**.

keratinocyte: Mature **epithelial cell** producing keratins, which comprise its distinctive **cytoskeleton**. It can be found in areas of abrasion of **epithelial tissues**. **Keratinocyte** is the principal **cell** type of **skin epidermis**.

keratohyalin granules: Basophilic granules of 0.2 to 4.5 μm diameter found in **cells** of the *stratum granulosum* that are presumed to play a role in keratinization.

keratotomy: Incision of the **cornea**.

kidney: Either of a pair of bean-shaped **glandular** organs in the back part of the abdominal cavity that excrete urine. A **kidney** contains numerous nephrons and their associated **blood** supply. It consists of two zones, a **cortex** and **kidney medulla**, encased in a fatty protective capsule.

kidney medulla: Inner, paler-colored region of a **kidney**, surrounded by the **cortex**. In it are situated the collecting tubules leading from the uriniferous tubules to the pyramid.

KillerRed: Genetically encoded **photosensitizer** providing **light**-induced production of reactive **oxygen** species. Its advantages include direct expression in **cells**, easy targeting to various subcellular compartments, and no **exogenous** chemical compound requirements. It is not toxic before activation by green **light** irradiation with maximum at 585 nm. Maximum **fluorescence** is at 610 nm. It is recommended for selective **light**-induced **protein** inactivation and **cell** killing.

Kirchhoff approximation: Approximate method for solving **wave diffraction** problems that is applicable for finding the diffracted field at **wave diffraction** on inhomogeneities with sizes much larger than the **wavelength**.

Kirchhoff's law: In thermal equilibrium, the **absorptivity** of an opaque surface equals its **emissivity**.

knee: Lower extremity joint connecting the femur and the tibia. Since in humans the **knee** supports nearly the entire weight of the body, it is vulnerable both to acute **injury** and to the development of osteoarthritis.

Kramers–Kronig relations: Mathematical properties, connecting the real and imaginary parts of any complex function that is analytic in the upper half-plane. They are often used to relate the real and imaginary parts of response functions in physical systems. They allow one to calculate the **wavelength** dependence of both real and imaginary parts of a specimen's **light** optical **permittivity**, together with other **optical properties** such as the **absorption coefficient** and **index of refraction**.

krypton (Kr) arc lamp: Discharge **arc lamp** filled with krypton. It gives out very bright **UV** and **visible light** in the range from 200 nm to >1.0 μm.

krypton (Kr) laser: **Laser** with a lasing medium composed of ionized krypton gas. The emission is mostly in the **UV** and **visible wavelength range**: 337.5–356.4 nm, 350.7–356.4 nm, and 647.1–676.4 nm. Constructive and technical parameters are close to that of an Ar **laser**. Ar–Kr **lasers** working on mixtures of these two gases may have a number of lines—for example, 13 lines between 467 and 676 nm.

K-space spectral analysis: Near-field **wave** technique that relies on a series of 2D fast **Fourier transforms** and that is employed for fast image reconstruction.

Kubelka–Munk model (KKM): Two-flux model describing transportation of **radiation** in a **scattering** medium. It employs simple relations for evaluating **optical parameters** using the diffuse **transmittance** and **reflectance** measurements.

labeling: Specific marking of **cells** or **cell** compartments to provide tracking of probes and measurements of functional parameters from molecular- and cellular-based studies to *in vivo* systems to understand how marked components impact human physiology and disease. For instance, in cellular transplantation technology, **labeling** provides information about location, tracking, and quantifying of implanted **cells** in *in vivo* systems. A wide variety of **labeling** probes and systems are available. They are mostly based on fluorescing molecules and **nanoparticles** with a possibility of specific binding to **cell** and **tissue** compartments. **CW** and time-resolved **fluorescence** techniques are typically used to monitor these markers.

lab-on-a-chip (LOC): Device that integrates one or several laboratory functions on a single chip of only a few square millimeters/centimeters in size. The handling of extremely small fluid volumes down to less than picoliter is possible (see **microfluidics**). Lab-on-a-chip devices often use **MEMS** devices or related manufacturing technologies. Micro- and nanocapillary glass technology, such as used in **PCF**-based capillary biosensors fabrication, is also prospective. Lab-on-a-chip technology indicates generally the scaling of single or multiple lab processes down to chip format, whereas related **micro total analysis systems** (μTAS) technology is aimed to the integration of the total sequence of lab processes to perform biochemical analysis.

Laboratory Virtual Instrumentation Engineering Workbench (LabVIEW): A platform and development environment for a visual programming language from National Instruments. Commonly used for data acquisition, instrument control, and industrial automation.

lactic acid: Also known as milk acid, its chemical formula is $C_3H_6O_3$. Systematic name is 2-hydroxypropanoic acid. It is a chemical compound that plays a role in several biochemical processes. It has a hydroxyl group adjacent to the carboxyl group, making it an **alpha (α)-hydroxy acid (AHA)**. In solution, it can lose a proton from the acidic group, producing the lactate ion $CH_3CH(OH)COO^-$. It is miscible with **water** or **ethanol** and is **hygroscopic**. **Lactic acid** is chiral and has two optical isomers. One is known as L-(+)-**lactic acid** or (S)-**lactic acid**, and the other, its mirror image, is D-(−)-**lactic acid** or (R)-**lactic acid**. L-(+)-**lactic acid** is the biologically important isomer. In animals, L-lactate is constantly produced from pyruvate via the **enzyme** lactate dehydrogenase (LDH) in a process of fermentation during normal **metabolism** and exercise. The concentration of **blood** lactate is usually 1–2 mmol/L at rest but can rise to over 20 mmol/L during intense exertion. Industrially, **lactic acid** fermentation is performed by Lactobacillus **bacteria**, among others. These **bacteria** can operate in the **mouth**, and the acid they produce is responsible for the **tooth** decay known as **caries**.

lambda (λ)/4-phase plate (*Synonym*: quarter-wave plate):   A device that provides an optical **phase shift** of 90 deg ($\pi/2$ **radians**) or an optical path difference equal to a quarter of the **wavelength**. A thin plate of **birefringent** substance, such as calcite or quartz, is cut parallel to the optical axis of the crystal and of a specific thickness that is calculated to give a **phase difference** of 90 deg ($\pi/2$ **radians**) between the emergent ordinary ray and the emergent extraordinary ray for **light** of a specified **wavelength**. Quarter-**wave** plates are usually constructed for the **wavelengths** of sodium light (589 nm). If the angle between the plane of **polarization** of **light** incident on the plate and the optic axis of the plate is 45 deg, then circularly **polarized light** is produced and emerges from the plate. If the angle is other than 45 deg, elliptically **polarized light** is produced. See **optical retarder**.

Lambertian radiator: Radiator whose **radiance** is proportional to the cosine of the viewing angle. (See **Lambert's cosine law**). For example, in the **visible spectrum**, the sun is not a **Lambertian radiator**. Its **brightness** is a maximum at the center of the solar disk, an example of limb darkening. A **blackbody** is a perfect **Lambertian radiator**.

Lambertian scatterer: When an area element is radiating as a result of being illuminated by an external **light** source, the **irradiance** falling on that area element will be proportional to the cosine of the angle between the illuminating source and the normal. A **Lambertian scatterer** will then scatter this **light** according to the same **Lambert's cosine law** as a **Lambertian radiator**. This means that although the **radiance** of the surface depends on the angle from the normal to the illuminating source, it will not depend on the angle from the normal to the observer. This phenomenon is of great importance in diffuse **tissue** optics.

Lambert's cosine law: States that the **radiant intensity** observed from a "Lambertian" surface is directly proportional to the cosine of the angle θ between the observer's line of sight and the surface normal. The law is also known as the cosine emission law or Lambert's emission law. An important consequence of this law is that when such a surface is viewed from any angle, it has the same apparent **radiance**. This means, for example, that to the human eye, it has the same apparent **brightness** (or **luminance**). It has the same **radiance** because, although the emitted **power** from a given area element is reduced by the cosine of the emission angle, the size of the observed area is increased by a corresponding amount. Therefore, its **radiance** (**power** per unit solid angle per unit projected source area) is the same.

lamella: Term for a plate-like structure, appearing in multiples, that occurs in various situations, such as biology (**connective tissue** structures) or materials sciences.

lamina fusca: Layer of the eye **sclera**.

lamina propria: Thin **vascular** layer of areolar **connective tissue** beneath the **epithelium**; part of the **mucous membrane**. It is dense **tissue** containing **fibroblasts**, **collagen**, **nerves**, and **immune cells**.

laminar flow: Occurs when a fluid flows in parallel layers, with no disruption between the layers. In fluid dynamics, **laminar flow** is a flow regime characterized by high-momentum **diffusion**, low-momentum convection, and **pressure** and velocity independence from time. It is the opposite of **turbulent flow**.

Langer's skin tension lines: Local **skin**-tension-directed lines caused by bundles of fibroconnective **tissues** within the reticular **dermis**.

Laplace transform: Technique for analyzing linear time-invariant systems such as electrical circuits, harmonic oscillators, optical devices, and mechanical systems. It gives a simple mathematical or functional description of an input or output to a system.

large intestine: Second to last part of the digestive system—the final stage of the alimentary canal is the anus. Its function is to absorb **water** from the remaining indigestible food matter and then to pass useless waste material from the body. It consists of the **cecum** and **colon**. It starts in the right iliac region, where it is joined to the bottom end of the **small intestine**. It is about 1.5 meters long.

larynx: Muscular and cartilaginous structure lined with **mucous membrane** at the upper part of the **trachea**, in which the vocal cords are located.

laser: Acronym for **light** amplification by the **stimulated emission** of **radiation**. A device that generates a beam of **light** that is **collimated**, monochromatic, and coherent. **Laser radiation** is characterized by its **wavelength**, **power**, and pulse-

or **continuous-wave (CW)**—mode of generation. Normally, **laser power** (rate of **radiation** emission from a **laser**) is expressed in **watts** (W), milliwatts (mW), or microwatts (μW). To provide a high precision of **laser beam** focusing and to transport its **radiation** through **single-mode fibers, single-mode lasers** are used. A pulsed **laser** is a **laser** that generates a single pulse or a set of pulses. Two technologies are typically used to produce **laser** pulsing: **Q-switching** and **mode-locking**. Most **lasers** emit at a particular **wavelength**. In **tunable lasers**, the **wavelength** is varied over some limited spectral range. There are a huge variety of **lasers** and **laser** systems available on the market. **Lasers** can be classified in accordance with active **media** used, such as gas, solid-state, liquid, and **semiconductor (diode) lasers**. For example, a gas **laser** is a **laser** whose active medium is a gas or mixture of gases. **Fiber laser** is an example of a **laser** system that combines principles of **solid-state lasers** with lightwave guiding by a **fiber**. Any **CW laser** can work in pulse mode by a switch-on and switch-off pumping **power**, but many pulse **lasers** cannot work in **CW**. Normally, **lasers** are characterized by the output **wavelength** (nm or μm), spectral **bandwidth** (nm), **energy** characteristics such as **power** (mW, W, kW) for **CW laser**, and **energy** per pulse (J), pulse width (ns, μs, ms, s), repetition rate (Hz), **average power** (mW, W, kW), and **peak power** (W, kW, MW, and TW) for pulse **lasers**. An important practical characteristic of a **laser** is its efficiency, which is the ratio of the output **laser power** to the input electrical **power** of **laser** pumping and expressed in percentage. **Lasers** of higher efficiency normally have the smallest size and lower cost. Lasing **media** of **UV excimer lasers** are excited molecular complexes such as ArF (193 nm), KrF (248 nm), XeCl (308 nm), and XeF (351 nm). An N_2 **(nitrogen) laser** is a molecular gas-discharge pulse **laser** that works on electronic-**vibrational transitions** with generation in **UVA** with the main line at 337.1 nm. **He–Cd (helium cadmium) laser** is an ionic metal-vapor **laser** with two main lines: blue (441.6 nm) and **UVA** (325.0 nm). An **Ar (argon) laser** is an ion arc gas-discharge **laser** with a powerful emission mostly in the **UV** and **visible wavelength range**: 336.6–363.8 nm, 454.5 nm, 457.9 nm, 488 nm, 514 nm, and

528.7 nm. A **Kr (krypton) laser** is also an ion arc gas-discharge **laser** with a powerful emission at 337.5–356.4 nm, 350.7–356.4 nm, and 647.1–676.4. A **He–Ne (helium neon) laser** is a gas-discharge **laser** whose red emission (632.8 nm) is widely used; green, yellow, orange, far-red, and **IR lasers** are also available. **Dye lasers** use as a **gain media** liquid dyes, such as **Rhodamine 6G**, and emit in a broad spectral range of **UV–visible–NIR**; they are **wavelength**-tunable and can be highly energetic with a short pulse and high pulse repetition rate. **Solid-state lasers** use as active **media** crystal matrices doped by active ions—for example, a Cr^{3+} doping sapphire (**ruby laser**) provides lasing at 694 nm, the same ions doping alexandrite crystal (alexandrite **laser**) give **radiation** at 755 nm; a **titanium sapphire (Ti:sapphire) laser** provides **laser radiation** tunable in the **wavelength** range from 700 to 960 nm. An **Nd:YAP (perovskite) laser** emits at 1054 and 1341 nm, **Nd:YAG (neodymium) laser** at 1064 nm, **Ho:YAG (holmium) laser** at 2.09–2.15 µm, and **Er:YAG (erbium) laser** at 2.79–2.94 µm. **Diode lasers** are **semiconductor** injection **lasers** pumped by electrical current. The **GaAs laser** (830 nm) is one of the most widely used **diode lasers**. **CO lasers** and **CO_2 lasers** are **infrared** gas-discharge molecular **lasers** with **IR** emission from 5 to 6.5 µm and from 9.2 to 11.1 µm, respectively. Optically pumped gas **lasers** are submillimeter **lasers** covering a wide range of **wavelengths** from 70 to 1990 µm; for example, the CH_3I **laser** emits **radiation** at 1250.0 µm. See **Appendix: Laser Specifications** for more information.

laser analytical spectroscopy: Generally, analytical **spectroscopy** aims to identify substances by observing the **spectrum** emitted, scattered, or absorbed by them. The nature, structure, and density of various species existing in the probe volume can be screened and quantitatively detected at low concentration of excited species (on the order of parts per billion or even less for a single molecule level). Sometimes, the separation of materials is accomplished using chromatography, **electrophoresis**, or atomization in flame or **plasma**. **Lasers** are widely accepted tools in classical analytical **spectroscopy**. Many **laser** techniques based on **laser-induced fluorescence (LIF)**, **Raman scattering**, or **laser**

light absorption are applied to detect atoms or molecules in given energetic states. For example, **UV-LIF** is used for detection in capillary **electrophoresis**. Red **diode lasers** or **Ti:sapphire lasers** are used principally in **laser** techniques, such as **multiphoton fluorescence scanning microscopy**. All kinds of Raman spectroscopies, such as **resonance Raman scattering (RRS)**, **surface-enhanced Raman scattering (SERS)**, **stimulated Raman scattering**, **coherent anti-Stokes Raman scattering (CARS)**, as well as **laser microspectral analysis (LMA)** and **laser microprobe mass analysis (LAMMA)**, are **laser** analytical tools widely used in **biophotonics**.

laser-assisted subepithelial keratectomy (LASEK): Includes **laser epithelial** keratomileusis. It refers to **laser refractive surgery** that permanently changes the shape of the anterior central **cornea** using **excimer laser ablation** of a small amount of **tissue** from the corneal **stromal layer (stroma)** at the front of the eye, just under the corneal **epithelium**. Prior to **laser stromal ablation**, an **alcohol** solution is used to cause the **epithelial cells** to weaken. The surgeon will fold the **epithelial cell** layer out of the **laser** treatment field, and fold it back in its original place after the **cornea** has been reshaped by the **laser**, allowing the **cells** to regenerate after the surgery. A computer-aided tracking system automatically centers the **laser beam** on the patient's visual axis. The procedure is distinct from **LASIK**, a form of **laser** eye surgery where a permanent flap is created in the deeper layers of the **cornea**.

laser-assisted *in situ* keratomileusis (LASIK): Type of **laser refractive surgery** for correcting myopia, hyperopia, and astigmatism. **LASIK** is similar to other surgical corrective procedures such as **photorefractive keratectomy (PRK)**, although it provides benefits such as faster patient recovery. It is performed in three steps: The first step is to create a flap of corneal **tissue** with a mechanical microkeratome using a metal blade or a **femtosecond laser** microkeratome (IntraLASIK), the second step is to remodel the **cornea** underneath the flap (the middle section of the **cornea**) with **excimer ArF laser** (193 nm) **ablation**, and the third is to reposition the flap. **Lasers** use an eye-tracking system that follows the patient's eye position, redirecting **laser** pulses for precise placement within the treatment zone. Typical pulses are around 1 millijoule (mJ) of **pulse energy** in 10 to 20 **nanoseconds**.

laser beam: Group of nearly parallel rays generated by a **laser**. A **light beam** with a Gaussian shape for the transverse **intensity** profile (see **Gaussian light beam**).

laser calorimetry: Measuring technique based on detection of a temperature rise in a sample induced by **absorption** of a **laser beam**.

laser coagulation: **Coagulation** of **tissue** by **laser heating**.

laser cyclophotocoagulation: See **cyclophotocoagulation**.

laser diode: See **diode laser**.

laser Doppler anemometry (LDA):   Technique of measuring the velocity of flows by the Doppler method using a **laser** (see **Doppler effect**, **Doppler microscopy**, and **Doppler spectroscopy**).

laser Doppler flowmetry (LDF):   Refers to the general class of techniques using the optical **Doppler effect** to noninvasively measure changes in **blood flow** microscopically. This technique operates by using a coherent **laser light** source to irradiate the **tissue** surface. A fraction of this **light** propagates through the **tissue** in a random fashion and interacts with the different components within the **tissue**. The **light** scattered from the moving components such as **RBCs** will undergo a **frequency** shift that is due to the **Doppler effect**, while the **light** scattered from the static components will not undergo any shift in **frequency**. To measure this **frequency** shift, the backscattered **light** from the **tissue** is allowed to impinge on the surface of a **photodetector** where a **beat signal** is produced. Typical frequencies of these beat notes

257

detected, using a **wavelength** of 780 nm, range from 0–20 kHz. From these beat frequencies, it is possible to determine **blood perfusion** within the **scattering** volume.

laser Doppler imaging (LDI): Tissue functional imaging technique based on **laser** Doppler measurement of **blood flow** velocity as an image parameter. **Laser beam** scanning systems and full-field systems on the basis of **CCD** and **CMOS** cameras are available.

laser Doppler interferometry: Technique of measuring the velocity of the particles in a flow by the Doppler method using a **laser interferometer** when a particle's velocity is measured by its traversing of **interference fringes**.

laser Doppler line scanning (LDLS) imaging: New **LDPI** technique that does not utilize the standard point raster approach but works by scanning a **laser** line over the **skin** or other **tissue** surfaces while photodetection is performed in parallel by a **photodiode** array. This technique allows for numerous perfusion measurements to be performed in parallel. This arrangement greatly reduces **acquisition time** and is bringing **LDPI** one step closer to real-time imaging.

laser Doppler microscope (LDM): Laser Doppler imaging **(LDI)** system working at a microscopic scale.

laser Doppler perfusion imaging (LDPI): Developed for imaging of **skin blood perfusion**. The **laser beam** illuminates the **tissue** by way of a single scanning point (point raster scanning **LDPI**), a scanning line (**LDLS**), or static uniform illumination over the entire **skin** surface (**full-field technique**). The rationale for moving from point raster scanning to line scanning and **full-field technique** is to be able to update a complete image at increased speed. However, the main drawback with the **LDPI** technique is the limited update rate, which currently does not allow real-time video-rate imaging.

laser Doppler perfusion monitoring (LDPM): Developed for point-wise measurement of **tissue blood perfusion**.

laser flow cytometry: Flow cytometry (see **cytometry**) with **laser** excitation of **fluorescence**, **light scattering**, **polarization** transform, **photoacoustic**, or **photothermal** signals from **cells** under investigation (see **photoacoustic cytometry** and **photothermal flow cytometry**).

laser heating: Heating of an object by **laser radiation**. **Laser beam** interaction with a **tissue** finally leads to **light absorption** and heat generation. Generated heat induces several reversible and irreversible effects in **tissue**, which can be presented in the order of amount of heat deposition (see, for example, **ablation**).

laser interferential retinometer: Device for determining retinal **visual acuity** in the human eye by projecting the **interference fringes** produced by a **laser interferometer** at the **retina**.

laser microprobe mass analysis (LAMMA): Refers to a mass-spectrometry method that is based on the following steps: ionization of molecules of the matter under study, separation of ions, and their analysis in respect to the ratio of their mass to charge m/z. Laser **photoionization** provides enhanced selectivity of the analysis, high ion-emission yield (up to 100%), and the possibility to analyze short-lived products. **Laser**-induced **photoionization** occurs in a broad range of **laser** intensities, from 10 to 10^{11} W/cm^2; thus, many types of high-**intensity lasers**, including CO_2, **ruby**, **Nd:YAG**, N_2, **excimer**, **dye**, and **diode lasers**, are used. In **laser** mass spectrometry, time-of-flight ionic systems with ion selection in the sectioned electrical and magnetic fields and static systems with double-ion focusing and dynamic mass-**spectrometers**, such as 'mass-reflectrons', are found in a wide range of applications. This method is used for detection of atomic and molecular clusters, foreign molecules and **radicals** in gases, and molecules of different synthetic and natural materials important for biology, medicine, and pharmacology. For example, close to 100% efficiency of two-photon **photoionization** of organic molecules by **KrF excimer laser** (248 nm) allows one to detect single molecules within the irradiation volume at a single **laser** pulse. As a result, the sensitivity is equal to their partial **pressure** of 10^{-12} Pa or relative concentration in the air of 10^{-9}. Femtosecond **laser ablation** for microsampling can be regarded as a new tool for elemental mass spectrometry of biological materials.

laser microprobe mass analysis (LAMMA) tool: Specifically designed for biomedical use to determine any element of the periodic system in biological substances with a **micron** or submicron **spatial resolution**. It does not need etalons and allows for analysis of many elements simultaneously: drugs, dried **whole blood** and its components, and soft and **hard tissues**. The **spatial resolution** is 0.5–1.0 μm, the absolute detection limit for many elements is 10^{-19} g, and the concentration detection limit is 10^{-4}–$10^{-5}\%$. To complete analysis, only 1 pg of material is needed or even less, which is important in the pharmaceutical industry. In addition to analysis of elements, this method is used to study mass spectra of many classes of organic and bioorganic compounds such as **carbohydrates**, organic acids, **amino acids** and micro-peptides, organic salts, aromatic molecules, metalloorganic complexes, and many others. There are a few commercially available **LAMMA** systems, such as **LAMMA**-500, **LAMMA**-1000 (Germany), LIMA (UK), EMAL-2 (Russia). **LAMMA**-500 based on a Q-switched **Nd:YAG** ($\tau_p \approx$ 15 ns) **laser** with **frequency** conversion up to the fourth harmonic (λ = 264 nm) is often used in biology and medicine. Tight focusing provides a **laser beam** diameter of 0.5 μm on the sample surface. Its resolution of ion mass $m/\Delta m$ could be from 200 to 1000. Minimal mass of the analyzed material is of 10^{-13} g, absolute detection limit is 10^{-18}–10^{-20} g, and concentration detection limit is 10^{-2}–$10^{-3}\%$.

laser microspectral analysis (LMA): Usually refers to **emission spectroscopy** of **laser** microprobes conducted materials, including biological ones. It is related to methods of **laser analytical**

spectroscopy that use **laser** techniques for **photoexcitation** and photoionization of biological specimens pre-prepared by their local **evaporation** or atomization by **laser**, electron, or ion beams or by other means. These methods have a high sensitivity and allow for the extraction of quantitative information about the element content of the **tissue**. In general, **LMA** can use any suitable spectroscopic technique to analyze matter at its transition from liquid/solid to gas state during **laser**-focused beam **ablation**. More often, **emission spectroscopy** and **absorption spectroscopy** or mass spectrometry [see **laser microprobe mass analysis (LAMMA) tool**] are applied. Despite **laser**-induced **plasma** creation, which is a self-source of **radiation** for spectral analysis, sometimes additional excitation of ablated material by arc discharge is needed. A typical **LMA** instrument (**LMA**-10, Carl Zeiss, Jena) with a grating **spectrometer** allows for a probe area of $10 \times 10 \ \mu m^2$ and analytic sensitivity of 10^{-11}–10^{-13} g for a Q-switched **ruby laser** as a probe **light** source. **LMA** is applicable for specimen analysis placed in a vacuum camera ($p \leq 10^{-3}$ Pa), in a buffer gas ($p \approx 10^2$–10^4 Pa), and in the open air. Commercially available **LMA** instruments provide high absolute and relative sensitivity, selectivity of probing, high specificity regarding studied elements, and the possibility to determine a group of elements; they do not need preliminary preparation of the samples (*in situ* measurements are possible). Absolute sensitivity is of 0.1 pg. **Femtosecond laser radiation** is prospective for **LMA** studies of **tissues**. For example, for human **tooth** dentine, in **plasma** produced at **laser** intensities of $\sim 10^{13}$–10^{15} W/cm^2 C, O, Ca, Zn, Na, and Cu spectral lines were identified, and **x-ray radiation** with energies $E > 30$ keV has been observed with **laser beam** intensities of $\sim 5 \times 10^{15}$ W/cm^2.

laser mirror: See **Bragg mirror (reflector)**.

laser nanosurgery: Tool in biology for the dissection or deletion of specific structures that can work without using genetic methods or chemical agents (see **optical injection** and **optical transfection**). Different **laser** systems, such as **nanosecond** or **picosecond UV** or **visible** short-wavelength **lasers**, have been used for subcellular disruption. Because of low **penetration depth** for these **wavelengths**, the disruptions are limited to surfaces or thin samples, including a single **cell** in **cell culture**. In contrast, **multiphoton absorption** is a new tool for the selective disruption and dissection of cellular structures in living **cells** in *in vivo* **tissue** conditions because of the use of sharply focused **NIR femtosecond laser** irradiation (see **ablation by femtosecond NIR lasers**). By varying the **laser** repetition rate, pulse **energy**, number of pulses irradiated, and the focusing conditions, **femtosecond** nanosurgery can be performed with different interaction regimes. The combination of multiphoton nanosurgery and *in vivo* imaging in the framework of the same system (see **nonlinear optical imaging**) allows for probing and selective and direct disruption of intracellular structures in the investigation and treatment of many vital processes, including cellular division, locomotion, cytoskeletal plasticity, and neuronal network organization and functioning.

laser photoionization: At **laser** interaction with gaseous or condensed **media**, such as biological liquid or **tissue**, single-**photon**, step-wise, or multiphoton ionization processes could be expected. Direct single-photon ionization of organic materials could by provided by **UV lasers**. However, to provide a step-wise ionization from the excited atomic or molecular state, **lasers** with much longer **wavelength** could be used. An application of intense pulsed **lasers** makes it possible for several **photons** of **energy** below the ionization threshold to combine their energies and ionize an atom or molecule. In the perturbative regime (below about 10^{14} W/cm^2 at optical frequencies), the **probability** of absorbing N **photons** depends on the **laser-light intensity** I as I^N.

laser power: Rate of **radiation** emission from a **laser**, normally expressed in microwatts (μW), milliwatts (mW), **watts** (W), kilowatts (kW), megawatts (MW), or terawatts (TW).

laser pyrometer: Infrared radiation thermometer that projects a **laser beam** to the target, uses the reflected **laser energy** to compute target **effective emissivity**, and automatically computes target temperature (assuming that the target is a **diffuse reflector**).

laser radiation: Radiation emitted by a **laser**.

laser refractive surgery: A special **laser** (typically, a **UV excimer laser**) reshapes the **cornea** by precise and controllable removal of corneal **tissue** and therefore changes corneal focusing **power**. **Laser** technologies such as **LASIK** (**laser-assisted** *in situ* **keratomileusis**), **LASEK** (**laser-assisted subepithelial keratectomy** or **laser epithelial** keratomileusis), and **photorefractive keratectomy** (**PRK**) are currently on use. Wavefront-guided **LASIK** is a variation of **LASIK** surgery in which, rather than applying a simple correction of focusing **power** to the **cornea**, a spatially varying correction, guiding the computer-controlled **excimer laser** with measurements from a wavefront sensor, is used to provide more precise surgery. New **laser** technologies based on all-**femtosecond** correction by intrastromal **ablation** that avoid weakening the **cornea** with large **incisions** and deliver less **energy** to surrounding **tissues** are prospective.

laser scanning microscopy (LSM): **Microscopy** with a highly focused **laser beam** as a **light** source that is scanned to get 2D (*xy*-scan) or 3D (*xyz*-**scan**) images of a specimen. Different modes of **LSM** are available—**light transmittance** and **reflectance** for 2D imaging, and confocal **reflectance** and **fluorescence** for 3D imaging. For example, the confocal **LSM** Zeiss 510 Meta is equipped with four **lasers**: blue diode **laser**, 405 nm; **argon laser**, 458/477/488/514 nm; **diode-pumped solid-state** (**DPSS**) **laser**, 561 nm; and **He–Ne laser**, 633 nm. Nomarski optics allow superimposition of signals from the **fluorophores** overlaid with a **differential interference contrast** (**DIC**) **microscopy** of **cells**. Software is available for reconstruction of 3D images, presentation of image "galleries," *z*-sectioning, time series, and so on. The Zeiss Axiovert inverted microscope used by the system has $10\times, 20\times, 40\times, 63\times,$ and $100 \times$ **oil** as well as **water**

immersion **objectives** and z-axis and xy-stage motors. Controlled environment chambers are available for studies of live **cells**. Zeiss 410 confocal **LSM** is equipped with an argon-krypton **laser**, 488/568/647 nm.

laser scattering matrix meter (LSMM):   Instrument for the measurement of the **LSM elements** of transparent biological **tissues** and fluids. The principle of operation is based on the **modulation** of the **polarization** of the incident **laser beam** followed by the scattered **light demodulation** (transformation of **polarization modulation** to **intensity modulation**) and described by the following matrix equation: $\mathbf{S} = \mathbf{AF'MFPS_0}$, where $\mathbf{S}$ and $\mathbf{S_0}$ are the **Stokes vectors** of the recorded and source **radiation**, respectively. $\mathbf{P}$, $\mathbf{A}$, and $\mathbf{F'}$, $\mathbf{F}$ are the Mueller matrices for the linear **polarizers** and the **phase plates** (or electro-optic modulators) placed respectively ahead of and after the **scattering** medium. As the **phase plates** are rotated (or electrical signals modulate optical properties of the electrooptic modulators), the **intensity** recorded by a **photodetector** depends on time and can be represented as a Fourier series with coefficients defined by the values of the matrix $\mathbf{M}$ elements of the object under study, whose measurement ensures a system of linear equations to determine the matrix $\mathbf{M}$. The number of equations and the degree of stipulation for this system of equations are dependent on the choice of the ratio between the rotation rates of the **phase plates** (**retarders**) (or **modulation frequency** of electrooptic modulators). An optimal choice of the rotation rates relationship at $1:5$ allows for an optimally stipulated system of linear equations to be derived to find the full matrix $\mathbf{M}$ of the object under study. A scheme with rotating **retarders** [**lambda (λ)/4-phase plates**] has a comparatively simple software and allows one to avoid many of the experimental **artifacts** peculiar to **DC measurements** and to systems utilizing electrooptic modulators.

laser speckle contrast analysis (LASCA):   Fully digital, real-time **full-field technique** for the mapping of **skin capillary blood flow**. It uses only a **laser** with diverging optics, a **CCD** camera, a **frame-grabber**, and a personal computer that computes the local

speckle contrast and converts it to a false-**color** map of **contrast** (and hence of velocity). The basic principle is very simple: a time-integrated image of a moving object exhibits blurring, which in the case of a **laser speckle** pattern appears as a reduction in the **speckle contrast** $K = (\sigma/\langle I \rangle) \le 1$, where σ is the variation of the **intensity** fluctuations, and $\langle I \rangle$ is the mean **intensity**. The higher the velocity of the red **blood cells**, the faster are the fluctuations and the more blurring occurs in a given **integration time**. For the particular case of a Lorentzian velocity distribution of moving particles, the following equation is used for calculation of the **speckle contrast**: $K = \sqrt{\left\{\frac{\tau_C}{2T}\left[1 - \exp(-2T/\tau_C)\right]\right\}}$, where τ_C is the **speckle correlation** time, and T is the camera **integration time**. LASCA suffers the same problem as all of the temporal **frequency** measurement techniques, such as **photon-correlation spectroscopy**, **laser Doppler flowmetry**, and **laser speckle perfusion imaging**, which is the relation of the **correlation** time τ_C to the velocity distribution of the **scatterers**. This relation depends on many factors, including **multiple scattering**, the size and the shape of the **scattering** particles, non-Newtonian flow, and non-**Gaussian statistics** resulting from a low number of **scatterers** in the resolution **cell**. Because of the uncertainties caused by these factors, it is common in all these techniques to rely mainly on **calibration** rather than on absolute measurements.

laser speckle imaging (LSI): See **LASCA** and **LSPI**.

laser speckle perfusion imaging (LSPI): This technique is very fast and allows for real-time video-rate **blood perfusion** imaging. It is based on the same fundamental principle as **LDPI** but with a different and faster way of signal processing. **LSPI** is generally described as based on analysis of a time-varying **speckle** pattern appearing on a remote screen or a detector array being produced by diffusely backscattered **laser light** from an object with particles in internal motion (such as **RBCs**). See **LASCA** and **LSI**.

laser-induced-breakdown spectroscopy (LIBS): Technique for analyzing a sample by heating it with a **laser** to ionize a small amount of material and then observing the spectral emission lines as the gas cools. This is a type of atomic **emission spectroscopy** that uses a highly energetic **laser** pulse as the atomization and excitation source due to **laser plasma** formation. **LIBS** is applicable to solids, liquids, and gases; in principle, any element can be detected. The detection limit is defined by the **plasma** excitation temperature, the **light** collection optical window, and the line strength of the viewed transition. Laser **ablation** provides typically from nanograms to picograms of the sample material for investigation at material atomization [the ablated material dissociates (breaks down) into excited ionic and atomic species] at high initial temperatures exceeding 100,000 K. The data collection is provided by a time-gating after approximately 10 μs of cooling, when local thermodynamic equilibrium is established and **plasma** temperatures are of 5,000–20,000 K, and when the characteristic atomic emission lines of the elements can be observed. **LIBS** makes use of optical **emission spectroscopy** and is to this extent very similar to arc/spark emission spectrometry. It is also technically very similar to a number of other **laser**-based analytical techniques, sharing much of the same hardware, such as **Raman spectroscopy** and **laser-induced fluorescence (LIF) spectroscopy**, that **LIBS** allow for the atomic, molecular, and structural characterization of a biological specimen. Related techniques are **laser microspectral analysis (LMA)** and **laser microprobe mass analysis (LAMMA)**.

laser-induced coagulation (LIC): **Laser** treatment providing **tissue** temperatures above 60 °C when thermal damage with **coagulation** occurs (see **photocoagulation**). Nd:YAG **lasers** (1,064 nm) and **diode lasers** (805 nm) are the most popular **lasers** for **tissue coagulation**, in particular for **coagulation** of gastric **ulcers**.

laser-induced fluorescence (LIF): Related to **fluorescence spectroscopy** and used for studying the structure of molecules, detection of selective species, and flow visualization and measurements. The species to be examined is excited with a **laser**. The

signal-to-noise ratio of the **fluorescence** signal is very high, providing a good sensitivity to the process. It is also possible to distinguish between more species, since the lasing **wavelength** can be tuned to a particular excitation of a given species that is not shared by other species. **LIF** is useful in the study of the electronic structure of molecules and their interactions. It has also been successfully applied for **quantitative measurement** of molecular species concentrations in **cells** and **tissues** and of **blood flow** (*in vivo* **fluorescence cytometry**), in some cases visualizing concentrations down to nanomolar levels. See also related **fluorescence** techniques with **laser** excitation: **laser scanning microscopy (LSM)**, **confocal laser scanning microscope**, **multidimensional fluorescence imaging (MDFI)**, **multiphoton fluorescence scanning microscopy**, **two-photon fluorescence microscopy**, **three-photon fluorescence microscopy**, **fluorescence-lifetime imaging microscopy (FLIM)**, **fluorescence recovery after photobleaching (FRAP)**.

laser-induced hyperthermia (LIHT): Kind of **photothermal therapy** at **laser** irradiation using heating temperatures from the upper limit of physiological temperature 42 °C up to (not above) thermal damage temperature, typically less than 60 °C. There are multiple **hyperthermia** mechanisms behind treatment, from increased **blood flow** to cellular cytotoxicity associated with heat-induced **cell apoptosis**.

laser-induced interstitial thermotherapy (LIITT): A kind of **photothermal therapy** where an **optical fiber** guiding an intense **laser beam** is positioned directly into the **pathological** section. The distal **fiber** ends are designed to provide more diffuse **radiation** patterns to avoid carbonization and **vaporization** of the **tissue**. Due to **light absorption** and heat **diffusion**, coagulative as well as hyperthermic effects are reached, leading to immediate or delayed **tissue** destruction, respectively. Through physiological remodeling and decomposition, this leads to a regression of the treated area. This is a reliable procedure in various medical disciplines, including treatments of **liver**, **brain**, **prostate**, and gynecological disease.

laser-induced pressure transient (LIPT): See **pressure transient**.

Laserphyrin®: **PDT photosensitizer** that contains **mono-L-aspartyl chlorine e6** (NPe6, or LS11, or talaporfin sodium). It requires **laser light** of a specific **wavelength** of 664 nm for activation. It was approved in Japan in 2004 for **PDT** of **lung cancer**.

latent heat: Also called "hidden heat," as heat is added or removed without changing the temperature. The amount of heat required (or released) for a change of phase from solid to liquid and liquid to gas (or vice versa). The **latent heat** of **vaporization** is the amount of heat required to change one gram of liquid to vapor without change of temperature. The **latent heat** of fusion is the amount of heat to melt one gram of solid to liquid with no temperature change.

latex: Suspension of **micron**-sized polystyrene spheres.

Lauth's violet: See **thionine**.

L-curve method: A method for the selection of regularization parameters. It is a log–log plot of the regularized solution against the squared norm of the regularized residual for a range of values of regularization parameters. The name implies that the shape of the curve should resemble the letter L (see **Tikhonov regularization**).

least-squares: Standard approach to the approximate solution of overdetermined sets of equations in which there are more equations than unknowns. Term means that the overall solution minimizes the sum of the squares of the errors made in solving every single equation. The most important application is in data **fitting**, where the best fit minimizes the sum of squared residuals, a residual being the difference between an observed value and the value provided by a model. Depending on whether the residuals are linear in all unknowns, linear and nonlinear **least-squares** problems are recognized. The linear **least-squares** problem with a closed-form solution occurs in statistical regression analysis. The nonlinear **least-squares** problem has no closed solution and is usually solved by iterative method, where the system is approximated by a linear one with each iteration.

lecithin: A synthetic substance that contains 60% natural phospholipids (major phosphatidylcholine), 30–35% plant **oil**, **glycerol**, and so on. It is a basis for many nourishing (nutritive) creams due to its ability to penetrate deep into the **skin**.

length of thermal diffusivity: Length within a medium (**tissue**) characterizing the distance of heat **diffusion** at medium heating by a short localized **laser** or acoustic pulse. See also **thermal length**.

lens: Optical device with perfect or approximate axial symmetry that transmits and refracts **light**, converging or diverging the beam. A simple **lens** is a **lens** consisting of a single optical element. A compound **lens** (for example, **objective**) is an array of simple **lenses** (elements) with a common axis. The use of multiple elements allows more optical **aberrations** to be corrected than is possible with a single element. Manufactured **lenses** are typically made of glass or transparent plastic. See also **crystalline lens**.

lenslet: Set of spatially distributed **lens**-like (phase) irregular inhomogeneities.

lens syneresis: **Water** is released from the bound state in the **hydration** layers of **lens proteins** and becomes bulk **water**. This increases the difference in **refractive index** between the **lens proteins** and the surrounding fluid. See **crystalline lens**.

lesion: An **injury** or an alteration of an organ or **tissue**.

leukemia: **Cancer** of the **blood** or **bone marrow** characterized by an abnormal **proliferation** (production by multiplication) of

blood cells, usually **leukocytes (white blood cells)**. **Leukemia** is a broad term covering a **spectrum** of diseases. In turn, it is part of the even broader group of diseases called hematological **neoplasms**.

leukocyte: A nucleated, motile, colorless **cell** found in the **blood** and **lymph** of animals. It contains no respiratory **pigments**. It is a **lymphocyte**, a polymorph, or a **monocyte**. In humans, there are approximately 8000 **leukocytes** per cubic millimeter. They are formed like spheres with a diameter of 8–22 μm. See also **white blood cell (WBC)**.

leukoplakia: Condition in which thickened, white patches form on a subject's **gums**, on the inside of the cheeks, and sometimes on the **tongue**. These patches cannot be easily scraped off. The cause of **leukoplakia** is unknown, but it is considered to result from chronic **irritation**, caused by tobacco or long-term **alcohol** use. It is the most common of all chronic **mouth lesions**, more frequently appearing in older men.

light detection and ranging (LIDAR): Technique analogous to radar that uses **laser** pulses to measure distances to objects. It can be also used to monitor atmospheric pollutants and provide distant measurement of target motion based on the **Doppler effect** (Doppler **LIDAR** systems). See **laser Doppler anemometry (LDA)**.

lifetime of the excited state: Lifetime refers to the time that a molecule (atom) stays in its **excited state** before emitting a **photon**. The lifetime is related to the rates of **excited state** decay and to the facility of the relaxation pathway, radiative and nonradiative. If the rate of **spontaneous emission** or any of the other rates are fast, the lifetime is short. (For commonly used fluorescent compounds, typical **excited state** decay times are within the range of 0.5 to 20 ns.)

ligament: Band of **tissue**, usually white and **fibrous**, serving to connect **bones**, hold organs in place, and so on.

light: Common name of **electromagnetic radiation (EMR)** that we can see. Lamps, **lasers**, and **light-emitting diodes (LEDs)** that generate **light** can also emit **EMR** that is not **visible**; however, they have specific features characteristic to **visible light**, such as photochemical action for the shorter **wavelengths** (violet **color**) and thermal action for the longer ones (red **color**). Thus, two neighbor regions of **EMR**, i.e., **ultraviolet (UV)** and **infrared (IR)**, also belong to **light**. **UV** and **IR light** can be seen (visualized) with the help of matrix **photodetectors** such as **CCDs** or **infrared cameras**.

light beam: Slender stream of **light**. Often a user needs a so-called **collimated** beam in which all rays are parallel to each other. Such a beam, in some instances, can be provided automatically by using an appropriate **laser** (see **laser beam**) or can be formed by special optics (with possible significant loses of **light energy**) using conventional **light** sources, such as lamps.

light beam divergence: "Spreading" of a **light beam** in general, and in particular of a **laser beam** as it moves away from the **laser** or the **fiber tip**. The initial beam divergence of the **light** source is important for **light beam** focusing and providing of the required diameter of the **light** spot on the **tissue** surface. To control **light**-treatment effects, the **light beam** is focused onto the **tissue** surface by a **lens**, and the distance between output **lens** and **tissue** surface is varied to provide needed **light** spot size and **power density** within the area of treatment. The radius of the beam in the **focal plane** of the **lens** with a **focal length** f is given by $w = f \times q$, where q is the beam divergence. **Single-mode lasers** or **single-mode fibers** have a minimal beam divergence and can provide minimal **light** spot size. Minimal **light** spot size in the **focal plane** of the **aberration**-free optical system can be close to the **wavelength**. Various optic and **fiber optic probes** providing special configurations of **light beams** are available on the market.

light diode: See **light-emitting diode (LED)**.

light green SF: Other names include **light green SF** yellowish, or **light** green, acid green, Lissamine green SF, acid green 5, food green 2, FD&C green no. 2, green no. 205, acid brilliant green 5, pencil green SF, or C.I. 42095. This is a green triarylmethane dye, molecular formula $C_{37}H_{37}N_2O_9S_{3+}$, **molar mass** 749.893 g/mol (**Da**). It is used in **histology** for staining **collagen**. It is used as a counterstain to acid **fuchsine**. It is a critical component of **Papanicolaou stain** (**Pap stain**). It can be used to check the health of the anterior surfaces of the eye. It usually comes as a disodium salt. Its maximum **absorption** is at 630 nm.

light guide: In general, assembly of **optical fibers** that are bundled but not ordered and that are used for illumination.

light microscope: A device composed of an objective and imaging equipment, along with the appropriate lighting equipment, sample stage, and support. Typically, the image it produces is shown on a computer screen since the **CCD** camera is attached to it via a USB port. See **light microscopy**.

light microscopy (*Related term*: **microscopy**):   **Optical microscopy** or **light microscopy** involves passing **visible light** transmitted through or reflected from a sample through one or multiple **lenses** to provide a magnified view of the sample. The resulting image can be detected directly by the eye or captured digitally by a **CCD** via a **light microscope**. The major limitations of standard **light microscopy** (bright field **microscopy**): it can only image dark or strongly refracting objects effectively, **diffraction** limits resolution to approximately 200 nm, and out-of-focus **light** from points outside the **focal plane** reduces image clarity. Live **cells** in particular generally lack sufficient **contrast** to be studied successfully—the internal structures of **cells** are colorless and transparent. The most common way to increase **contrast** is to stain the different structures with selective dyes, but this involves killing and fixing the sample, and may introduce **artifacts**. These limitations have all been overcome to some extent by specific **microscopy** techniques that can noninvasively increase the **contrast**

of the image. In general, these techniques make use of differences in the **refractive index** of **cell** structures (see **phase-contrast microscopy**). With **dark-field illumination** in the **field of view** of the microscope on a dark background, bright images of the specimen particles that differ by their **refractive index** from the surrounding medium can be seen. The use of oblique (from the side) illumination gives the image a 3D appearance and can highlight otherwise invisible features.

lightness: Property of a **color**, or a dimension of a **color** space, that is defined to reflect the subjective **brightness** perception of a **color** for humans along a **lightness**–darkness axis. A color's **lightness** also corresponds to its amplitude.

light polarization: State, or the production of a state, in which rays of **light** exhibit different properties in different directions: linear (plane)—when the electric field vector of the **EMR** oscillates in a single, fixed plane all along the beam, the **light** is said to be linearly (plane) polarized; elliptical—when the plane of the electric field rotates, the **light** is said to be elliptically polarized, because the electric field vector traces out an ellipse at a fixed point in space as a function of time; and circular—when the ellipse is a circle, the **light** is said to be circularly polarized.

light refraction: Change in direction of a ray of **light** when passing obliquely from one medium into another in which the **speed of light** is different. **Light refraction** is characterized by the **index of refraction**.

light scattering: Change in direction of the propagation of **light** in a turbid medium caused by **reflection** and **refraction** by microscopic internal structures.

light wavelength range: Physicians who use **light** in **phototherapy** or vision science classify the whole **light spectrum** as from 100 nm to 1000 µm, depending of its major mechanism of interaction with **biological cells** and **tissues**. In particular, spectral

273

ranges of **light** are described as follows: **Ultraviolet (UV)**: **UVC** (100–280 nm), **UVB** (280–315 nm), **UVA** (315–400 nm); **Visible**: 400–780 nm (violet: 400–450 nm; blue: 450–480 nm; green: 510–560 nm; yellow: 560–590 nm; orange: 590–620 nm; red: 620–780 nm); and **Infrared (IR)**: IRA (0.78–1.4 μm), IRB (1.4–3.0 μm), IRC (3–1000 μm). Physicists who consider **light** interaction with and propagation in nonbiological **media** (atmosphere, ocean, etc.) classify **light** spectra as **near-infrared (NIR)**: 0.78–2.5 μm; **mid-infrared (MIR)**: 2.5–50 μm; and **far-infrared (FIR)**: 50–2000 μm. As **light** is increasingly and effectively used in medicine, both classifications and terminologies are used in the **biomedical optics** field. For example, because of a great success in **tissue spectroscopy** and imaging in the **near-infrared** range, the term **NIR** is often used now by physicians. Current interest in and future perspectives on the **terahertz** range of **electromagnetic radiation** in biomedical applications will spread the **light wavelength range** used in medicine to 2000 μm, which physicists use.

light-emitting diode (LED) (*Synonym*: light diode): **Semiconductor** device that emits **light** when the forward-directed current passes the *p–n* junction. **LEDs** are **light** sources with a wide range of selected **wavelengths** from **UV** to **IR**. The typical **wavelength** half-bandwidths are 10–20 nm for **LEDs** working on 255–890 nm and 50–100 nm for **LEDs** working above 900 nm. The **light power** of **LEDs** ranges from a few milliwatts to a few watts. Their **light beam divergence** is ±120 degrees for SMT chips and may range from ±60 degrees to ±5 degrees for special constructions. **LEDs** are very effective **light** sources for photomedicine because of their high efficiency (conversion of electrical to **light energy**), long lifetime (more than 10^5 hours), and ability to emit many different **wavelengths** (**colors**) from **UV** to **IR** with a high **brightness**. Examples: AlGaN/GaN **LEDs** emit **UV** (255–365 nm) **light** with **power** in the range from 10 μW to 10 mW. InGaN **LEDs** emit **UV** (370–400 nm) and violet blue (400–420 nm) **light** with **power** up to 50 mW. GaN/SiC **LEDs** emit violet-blue (425–450 nm) **light** with **power** up to 50 mW. InGaN/GaN **LEDs** emit blue (470 nm) and green (490–525 nm) **light** with **brightness** up to

20 cd per chip. GaP **LEDs** emit green (568 nm) **light** with **power** up to 500 mW. InGaAlP/GaAs **LEDs** emit green (572 nm), yellow (580–590 nm), orange (600–615 nm), and red (620–645 nm) **light** with **brightness** up to 20 cd per chip. GaAlAs **LEDs** emit red (650–700 nm) and **NIR** (710–850 nm) **light** with **power** up to 500 mW. GaAs **LEDs** emit **NIR** (880–980 nm) **light**. InGaAsP **LEDs** emit **NIR** (1000–1550 nm) **light**. **LEDs** with shorter (<200 nm, vacuum **UV**) and longer **wavelengths** (>2000 nm) have also been designed. Also available are arrays of **LEDs** with number of chips from 2 to 60 in a unit (for 365–1550 nm). There are multicolor **LEDs** [typically, bicolor and tricolor (**RGB**)] as well as white **LEDs**, in which **light** emitted by a short-**wavelength LED** is converted with the help of phosphors, **semiconductors**, and dyes to white **light**; their **brightness** can reach up to 20–30 **lumens**.

light-scattering matrix (LSM): (*Synonym*: intensity matrix) A 4 × 4 matrix that connects the **Stokes vector** of incident **light** with the **Stokes vector** of scattered **light**. It describes the **polarization** state of the scattered **light** in the far zone that is dependent on the **polarization** state of the incident **light** and structural and **optical properties** of the object. See also **Mueller matrix**.

light-scattering matrix (LSM) element: One of sixteen elements of the **light-scattering** matrix. Each element depends on the **scattering** angle, the **wavelength**, and the geometrical and **optical parameters** of the **scatterers** and their arrangement.

light-scattering spectroscopy (LSS): Techniques used to identify and characterize **pathological** changes in human **tissues** at the cellular and subcellular levels, based on quantification of **light scattering** spectra measured from superficial (**epithelial cell**) layers of **tissues**. These spectra are sensitive to the enlarging, crowding, and **hyperchromaticity** of **epithelium cell** nuclei that are common features to all types of **precancerous** and early **cancerous** conditions, and thus can be used for detection of early **cancerous** changes and other diseases in a variety of organs such as the **esophagus**, **colon**, **uterine cervix**, **oral cavity**, **lungs**, and **urinary bladder**.

limbus: Border, edge, or fringe of a part.

linear dynamic range (LDR): This term characterizes the range of linear response of a detector or a measuring system as a whole. The **LDR** will always be less than the total dynamic range of the instrument. The lowest measured signal (concentration) of the **LDR** is the minimum detectable signal (concentration) or the instrument sensitivity. The largest signal (concentration) is that where the response factor falls outside the linear range and the detected signal no longer linearly increases with a measured parameter increase. The **LDR** of a detector is the maximum linear response divided by the detector noise. In many biophotonic instruments and measuring techniques, such as **diffuse optical tomography (DOT)**, **optical coherence tomography (OCT)**, and **scattering phase function** measurements, **LDR** might reach up to 90–100 **dB**. **CMOS** cameras can provide **LDR** of more than 100 **dB**.

linear regression: Regression method that allows for the linear relationship between the dependent variable Y, the p independent variables X, and a random term ε.

line scan rate: Number of target lines scanned by an optical line scanner or imager in one second.

Linnik microscope: See **Linnik–Tolansky interferometer**.

Linnik–Tolansky interferometer: Dual-beam **interferometer** with a **beamsplitter**, two reflecting surfaces, and two **lenses** for focusing beams on the surfaces.

lipid: Any substance occurring in plants or animals that is soluble in **ether**, hot **ethanol**, and gasoline (i.e., **fat** solvents). The term includes true **fats**, waxes, sterols, steroids, phospholipids, and so on.

lipid bilayer: Also called a bilayer **lipid membrane**, a **membrane** or zone of a **membrane** composed of **lipid** molecules (usually phospholipids). The **lipid bilayer** is a critical component of all biological **membranes**, including **cell membranes**. The structure of a bilayer explains its function as a barrier: **Lipids** are **amphiphilic** molecules, since they consist of polar **head** groups and nonpolar acyl tails. The bilayer is composed of two opposing layers of **lipid** molecules arranged so that their hydrocarbon tails face one another to form an oily core, while their charged **heads** face the aqueous solutions on either side of the **membrane**. Thus, the bilayer consists of the **hydrophobic** core region formed by the acyl chains of the **lipids** and the **membrane** interfacial regions that are formed by the polar **head** groups of **lipids**. The **hydrophilic** interfacial regions are saturated with **water**, whereas the **hydrophobic** core region contains almost no **water**. Because of the oily core, a pure **lipid bilayer** is permeable only to small **hydrophobic** solutes but has a very low permeability to polar inorganic compounds and ionic molecules.

lipolysis: Process of decomposition of **fats** on free **fat** acids (FFAs) under action of lipase. As a result, the end-products of **lipolysis** are glycerin and FFAs. The hormone-initiated and **enzyme**-catalyzed reaction of **fat** released by a **fat cell** is **blood-flow** and temperature sensitive. In the temperature range of 36–43 °C, enhanced **fat cell lipolysis** is found. The opposite action renders **insulin**, which inhibits **lipolysis**.

lipophilic: Having affinity for **lipids**.

liposomes: Microscopic spherical vesicles prepared by adding a **water** solution to a phospholipid **gel**. A **liposome** is a good model of a **cell** organelle. **Liposome** diameters are usually in the range of 20–100 nm. They are used for drug delivery in medicine and **cosmetics**.

lips: **Visible** organ at the **mouth** of humans and many animals. Both **lips** are soft, protruding, and movable, and serve primarily for food intake, as a tactile sensory organ, and in articulation of speech. The external surface of **lips** is **skin**, which merges with the oral **mucosa** of the inner surface. The vermillion border is the transition zone on the lip between the lining oral **mucosa** of the **mouth** and **skin**, with a rich supply of sensory **nerves** and no **sweat glands** or **sebaceous glands** (it requires moistening by **saliva**). The oral **mucosa** side is typically lining **mucosa** with **salivary glands** in the **connective tissue**.

liquid-core waveguide (LCW): The principal desired characteristic of **LCW** is confinement of **light** rays within the liquid core when the **refractive index** n of the core is higher than the **refractive index** of the surrounding tubing. The three most common forms of **LCW** in use today are glass capillary cells, flexible Teflon AF-2400 ($n_T = 1.29$) tubing, and silica capillary cells coated with Teflon AF-2400 with a **water** core ($n_W = 1.335$). Teflon AF-2400 polymer ($n_P = 1.31$) is typically used as a coating for silica ($n_S = 1.46$) capillary cells. **LCW** exhibit low optical loss because of low **scattering** in pure **water**. Typical **LCW** core diameters are 2–8 mm, with lengths up to 5–30 m. **LCW** of different modifications cover the **wavelength** range from 300 to 2000 nm. Temperature range (long term) could be from −5 °C to +35 °C. **LCWs** are used to guide white **light** for medical **endoscopy** and blue **light** for dental curing. Some types have enhanced flexibility and are ethylene-oxide (ETO) sterilizable. For the commercial prototype adaptors available for all medical **light** sources and **endoscopes**, the typical **light** sources used for illumination via **LCW** are **halogen lamps**, **xenon arc lamps**, metal halide lamps, and **Nd:YAG** or **diode lasers**. **LCW** have outstanding photostability even in the **UVC** range, suitable for high-**power UV lasers** and deep-**UV mercury arc lamps**; they provide superior transmission of up to 5 W of **UV radiation**, as well as transmission of high-**power NIR radiation** in the multiwatt range.

liquid crystal (LC): An intermediate phase state of matter that has properties between those of a conventional liquid and those of a solid crystal. For instance, a liquid crystal may flow like a liquid, but have the molecules in the liquid arranged and/or oriented in a crystalline fashion. There are many different types of **LC** phases, which can be distinguished by their different **optical properties** (such as **birefringence**), and will appear to have distinct textures seen under a microscope. **LCs** can be classified as thermotropic, lyotropic, and metallotropic. The thermotropic and lyotropic **LCs** consist of organic molecules and exhibit a phase transition into the **LC** phase as the temperature or the temperature and concentration of the **LC** molecules in a solvent are changed. Metallotropic **LCs** are composed of both organic and inorganic molecules; their **LC** transition depends not only on temperature and concentration, but also on the inorganic-organic composition ratio. In **biophotonics**, **LCs** can be found in numerous applications. Lyotropic **LCs** are abundant in living systems; for example, many **proteins** and **cell membranes** are **LCs**.

liquid-crystal display (LCD): A flat-panel display in which **liquid crystals** change opacity when exposed to an electric field.

liquid-crystalline phase: Liquid having certain **crystalline** characteristics, especially different **optical properties** in different directions.

lithium niobate (LiNbO$_3$): Compound of niobium, lithium, and **oxygen**. It is a colorless solid material with trigonal crystal structure. It is transparent for **wavelengths** between 350 and 5200 **nanometers**. It is used for the manufacture of the optical modulators and **acoustic wave** devices.

liver: Large, reddish-brown, **glandular** organ located in the upper-right side of the abdominal cavity, divided by **fissures** into five **lobes**, and secretes **bile** and various **metabolic processes**.

lobe (*Synonym*: cerebral lobe): Each cerebral hemisphere is divided, more or less arbitrarily, into different regions, with each region being a **lobe**. The deeper **fissures** are used to distinguish the **lobes**. Each **lobe** is named for the part of the **skull** near which it is situated. They are terms of convenience, not of anatomical or physiological significance: frontal **lobe**, temporal **lobe**, occipital **lobe**, etc.

local oscillator (LO): **Radio**- (or **optical**) **frequency** oscillator used in heterodyne detecting systems. A local oscillator is stable in **frequency** and amplitude and has a slightly different **frequency** than the receiving signal. It is used to convert a high-**frequency** receiving signal to an intermediate **frequency** by mixing the local oscillator signal and the receiving signal at an electronic (or photo) detector.

lock-in amplifier: Low-**frequency** electronic device that provides synchronous detection of small signals that may have amplitudes a few orders less than the noise level. The lock-in circuit contains the selective **amplifier** and a phase detector tuned to the **modulation frequency** of the detecting signal.

Long–Evans rat: Strain of rats that was developed by Drs. Long and Evans in 1915. Rats are white with a black hood, or occasionally white with a brown hood. They are used as a multipurpose model organism, frequently in behavioral and **obesity** research.

long-pass filter: An optical **interference** or **absorptive filter** that attenuates shorter **wavelengths** and transmits (passes) longer **wavelengths** over the active range of the target **spectrum** (**UV**, **visible**, or **IR**). They can have a very sharp slope (referred to as edge filters) and are described by their cut-off **wavelength** at 50 percent of peak transmission. In **fluorescence microscopy**, they are frequently employed in **dichroic (dichromatic) mirrors (beamsplitters)** and barrier (emission) filters to prevent excitation **light** from mixing with emission **light** (see **epi-fluorescence interference and absorption filter combinations**).

Lorentz–Mie scattering theory: See **Mie scattering theory**.

low-level laser therapy (LLLT): Currently, low-level **laser** (or **light**) therapy (**LLLT**), also known as "cold **laser**," "soft **laser**," "biostimulation," or "photobiomodulation" is practiced as part of physical therapy in many clinics. In fact, **light** therapy is one of the oldest therapeutic methods used by humans. The use of **lasers** and **LEDs** as **light** sources was the next step in the technological development of **light** therapy, which is now applied to many thousands of people worldwide each day. To have any effect on a living biological system, the **photons** must be absorbed by electronic **absorption bands** belonging to some molecular **chromophore** or photoacceptor. The mechanism of **LLLT** at the cellular level is believed to be based on the **absorption** of monochromatic **visible** and **NIR radiation** by components of the cellular **respiratory chain. Cytochrome c oxidase (Cox)** is one of integral **membrane protein** complexes of mitochondrial **respiratory chain** of a **cell**. Its **absorption** spectra were found to be very similar to the action spectra for biological responses to **light**. Another class of cellular molecules that might act as **chromophores** are those of **porphyrins**, which are formed in **mitochondria** as part of the heme biosynthesis cycle. The **absorption spectrum** of **porphyrins** such as **protoporphyrin IX (Pp IX)** has five bands spanning the region between 400 and 630 nm. Another class of molecule that may act as a photoacceptor is that of flavoproteins such as **flavin adenine dinucleotide (FAD)** or **flavin mononucleotide (FMN)**. It is clear that signal transduction pathways must operate in **cells** in order to transduce the signal from the cellular **chromophores** or photoacceptors that absorb **photon energy** to the biochemical machinery that operates in **gene** transcription. Several classes of molecules such as **reactive oxygen species (ROS)** and **reactive nitrogen species (RNS)** are involved in the signaling pathways from **mitochondria** to nuclei. There is also a cyclic AMP-dependent signaling pathway and a **nitric oxide (NO)** signaling G-**protein** pathway. Although the underlying mechanisms of **LLLT** are still not clearly understood, *in vitro* and clinical experiments indicate **LLLT** can prevent **cell apoptosis** and improve **cell proliferation**, migration, and **adhesion. LLLT** can also activate **cell** secretion of different growth factors and can increase **collagen** synthesis by **fibroblasts**. It was found to be an effective lymphatic drainage in postmastectomy lymphedema patients, may enhance neovascularisation, promote **angiogenesis**, and increase **blood flow**. **LLLT** can also modulate matrix metalloproteinase activity and **gene expression** in aortic smooth **muscle cells**, stimulate reactivation and **proliferation** in isolated myofibers, and repair processes after **injury** or **ischemia** in skeletal and **heart muscles**. LLLT covers applications of the following broad areas of medicine: inflammatory disorders such as **burns** and **peritonitis**, stimulation of healing, relief of **pain**, and improvement of appearance. One very important application is to the **central nervous system**, involving repair of **spinal cord** injuries, reduction of **brain** damage after stroke and traumatic **brain injury**, and the treatment of degenerative **brain** conditions such as **Alzheimer's diseases** and Parkinson's disease. Both types—**CW** and **pulse lasers** and **LEDs**—are used in LLLT, such as 585-nm pulsed **dye lasers**, **He:Ne lasers** with **wavelength** 632.8 nm, and **diode lasers** with the following **wavelengths**: 635, 650, 655, 660, 670, 684, 725, 780, 810, 820, 830, and 904 nm. Typical mean **power** densities range from 1 mW/cm^2 to 250 mW/cm^2, and dosages could range from 0.5 to 160 J/cm^2.

low-pass filter (LPF):   Filter that rejects the high-**frequency** components in electronic devices.

low-step scattering: Scattering process in which, on average, each **photon** undertakes no more than a few **scattering** events (approximately less than five to ten).

lumen (lm):   **SI** unit of luminous flux, a measure of the perceived **power** of **light**. Luminous flux differs from radiant flux, which is the measure of the total **power** of **light** emitted, in that luminous flux is adjusted to reflect the varying sensitivity of the human eye to different **wavelengths** of **light**. The **lumen** is defined in relation to the **candela** by 1 lm = 1cd · sr. That is, a **light** source that uniformly radiates one **candela** in all directions radiates a total of 4π **lumens**. If the source is partially covered by an ideal absorbing hemisphere, that system would radiate half as much luminous flux—only 2π lm. The luminous **intensity** would still be one **candela** in those directions that are not obscured.

luminaire: Complete **light** fixture.

luminance: Photometric measure of the luminous **intensity** per unit area of **light** travelling in a given direction. It describes the amount of **light** that passes through or is emitted from a particular area, and falls within a given solid angle. The unit is **candela** per square meter (cd/m^2). It is often used to characterize emission or **reflection** from flat, diffuse surfaces. The **luminance** indicates how much luminous **power** will be perceived by an eye looking at the surface from a particular angle of view. **Luminance** is thus an indicator of how bright the surface will appear. In this case, the solid angle of interest is the solid angle subtended by the eye's **pupil**. **Luminance** is used to characterize the **brightness** of displays. A typical computer display emits between 50 and 300 cd/m^2. The sun has **luminance** of about 1.6×10^9 cd/m^2 at noon.

luminance (luminant) contrast: Refers to image **contrast**, the engineering concept that characterizes a particular stimulus's ability to stimulate the differential mechanisms of the human visual system (see **luminosity function**). Several statistics have been proposed for the measurement of **luminance contrast** and generally have two components, the first of which is the difference between the two luminances in question (e.g., of a symbol, L_s, and its background, L_b). If the state of adaptation of the visual system stays constant, larger **luminance** differences produce larger **brightness** differences (higher **brightness contrasts**). The second component of any **luminance contrast** statistic is some measure that describes the adaptation state of the eye. A **luminance** difference that produces a large **brightness** difference on a dim background will produce a smaller **brightness** difference on a brighter background due to visual adaptation. To capture this behavior, designers of **luminance contrast** statistics generally

283

divide a numerator that describes the **luminance** change by a denominator that describes the average **luminance** to which the eye is adapted. The variety of popular statistics for **luminance contrast** mostly reflects the fact that the adaptation state of the eye is affected differently by different kinds of stimulus pattern, such as small symbols on uniform backgrounds, dark symbols on **light** backgrounds, or **light** symbols on dark backgrounds. The Weber **contrast** is defined as $C_W = (L_s - L_b)/L_b$, where L_s is the **luminance** of the symbol and L_b is the **luminance** of the immediately adjacent background. The **luminance** ratio $CR = L_s/L_b$, its logarithm $\log CR = \log L_s - \log L_b$, or Michelson **contrast** (for simple periodic patterns) $C_M = (L_{max} - L_{min})/(L_{max} + L_{min})$ are often used for pattern description.

luminescence: **Light** not generated by high temperatures alone. It is different from incandescence, in that it usually occurs at low temperatures and is thus a form of cold-body **radiation**. It can be caused by, for example, chemical reactions, electrical **energy**, subatomic motions, or stress on a crystal. The following kinds of **luminescence** are known: photoluminescence (including **fluorescence**, **phosphorescence** and delayed **fluorescence**), **bioluminescence**, **sonoluminescence**, **chemiluminescence**, electroluminescence (in response to an electric current passed through), radioluminescence (in response to radioactive **radiation**), mechanoluminescence (resulting from any mechanical action on a solid), triboluminescence (resulting from friction of a solid), piezoluminescence (in response to mechanical compression), and thermoluminescence (in response to heat). The **absorption** of high-**energy** (short-**wavelength**) **photons** by a molecule raises an electron to a higher **energy** level, where it will remain until it relaxes to the lowest-vibrational level of the **excited state** by loss of thermal **energy**. It remains on this level for a short "lifetime" due to the large **bandgap**, but must return to the ground state by either direct **photon** emission (**fluorescence**) or via the "spin-forbidden" **triplet state** and subsequent emission at a longer **wavelength** (**phosphorescence**). The "forbidden" route has a longer lifetime ($\sim 10^{-5}$ s) due to its lower **probability**. These lifetimes can be shortened by interaction with other molecules.

luminescence lifetime spectroscopy: Spectroscopy that is based on **luminescence** (**fluorescence** or **phosphorescence**) quenching. The lifetimes of faster **fluorescence** or slower **phosphorescence** can be shortened by interaction with other molecules—for example, with **oxygen**, which has one of the lowest triplet energies occurring in the ground state and a low **energy singlet state**. The **diffusion**-limited process of collision with the luminescing molecules thus permits a measurement of **oxygen** tension pO_2, which can be extracted using the Stern–Volmer relation: $(\tau_o/\tau) = 1 + k_Q[pO_2]$, where τ_O and τ are the lifetimes in the presence and absence of **oxygen**, respectively, and k_Q is the quenching constant for which each probe must be calibrated. The luminescing dye is excited by a **xenon flash lamp** or blue **LED** (450 nm), and the longer **wavelength luminescence** is detected by a **photomultiplier tube (PMT)**. High-**frequency** excitation and phase-sensitive detection systems are used for measurements. Phase-fluorometric and phosphorometric instruments are available on the market. The immobilisation of the dyes can cause the detected lifetimes to exhibit multi-exponential decay characteristics complicating analysis. These techniques have great potential for measurement of other analytes, such as CO_2, or for **noninvasive spectroscopy** of naturally occurring luminescing compounds, such as **NADH** or **porphyrins** [see **fluorescence-lifetime imaging microscopy (FLIM)**].

luminosity function: Related to the standardized model of the sensitivity of the human eye. It is the curve that measures the **wavelength**-dependent response of the human eye to **light**. The human eye can only see **light** in the **visible spectrum** and has different sensitivities to **light** of different **wavelengths** within the **spectrum**. When adapted for bright conditions, the eye is most sensitive to greenish-yellow **light** at 555 nm. Light with the same **radiant intensity** at other **wavelengths** has a lower luminous **intensity**. This function, denoted $V(\lambda)$, is based on an average of widely differing experimental data from scientists using different measurement techniques.

luminous intensity: A photometric quantity; the measure of the **wavelength**-weighted (due to the human-eye **luminosity function**) **power** emitted by a **light** source in a particular direction per unit solid angle. The unit is **candela** (cd).

lung: Either of the two saclike respiratory organs in the thorax of humans. The **lungs** connect to the **larynx** via **trachea**, bronchi, and ramifications of bronchial tubes.

lycopene: Bright-red carotenoid **pigment** and phytochemical found in tomatoes and other red fruits and vegetables, such as red carrots, watermelons, and papayas (but not strawberries or cherries). In plants, algae, and other photosynthetic organisms, **lycopene** is an important intermediate in the biosynthesis of many carotenoids, including **beta-carotene**, responsible for yellow, orange, or red pigmentation, photosynthesis, and photoprotection. Structurally, it is a tetraterpene assembled from eight isoprene units, composed entirely of carbon and hydrogen, and is insoluble in **water**. Lycopene's eleven conjugated double bonds give it a deep red **color** and are responsible for its antioxidant activity. **Lycopene** is not an essential nutrient for humans but is commonly found in the diet, mainly from dishes prepared with tomato sauce. When absorbed from the **stomach**, **lycopene** is transported in the **blood** by various lipoproteins and accumulates in the **liver**, adrenal **glands**, and testes.

lymph: An alkaline colorless liquid obtained from **blood** by filtration through **capillary** walls. It contains a smaller amount of soluble **blood proteins** and **white blood cells** than **blood**, but more **lymphocytes**. Normally, it contains no **red blood cells**. **Lymph** is found between the **cells** of the human body. It enters the **lymphatic vessels** by filtration through pores in the walls of **capillaries**. The **lymph** then travels to at least one **lymph node** before emptying ultimately into the right or the left subclavian vein, where it mixes back with **blood**. The **lymph** that leaves a **lymph node** is richer in **lymphocytes**. Likewise, the **lymph** formed in the digestive system called chyle is rich in triglycerides (**fat**), and looks milky white. The purpose of **lymph** is to bathe the **cells** with **water** and nutrients.

lymph node: Small, circular, ball-shaped organ of the **lymphatic system** (immune system), distributed widely throughout the body and linked by **lymphatic vessels**. **Lymph nodes** containing **immune cells** are found all through the body and act as filters or traps for foreign particles. They are important in the proper functioning of the immune system. Their clinical significance is due to disease-related **inflammation** or enlargement, which is used even for **cancer** staging (see **sentinel lymph node**). **Lymph nodes** can also be diagnosed by **biopsy** whenever they are inflamed because certain diseases affect them with characteristic consistency and location.

lymphatic system: Network of conduits that carry **lymph**. It also includes the **lymphoid tissue** and **lymphatic vessels** through which the **lymph** travels one-way toward the **heart** as well as all the structures providing the circulation and production of **lymphocytes**. **Lymph** is formed when **interstitial fluid** enters the initial **lymphatic vessels** of the **lymphatic system**, which transport **lymph** back to the **blood** and ultimately replace the volume lost during the formation of the **interstitial fluid**. Unlike the cardiovascular system, the **lymphatic system** is not closed and has no central pump. **Lymph** transport, therefore, is slow and sporadic, like a shuttle-stream. **Lymph** movement occurs due to peristalsis (propulsion of the **lymph** due to alternate contraction and relaxation of smooth **muscle**), valves, and compression during contraction of adjacent skeletal **muscle** and arterial pulsation. If excessive **hydrostatic pressure** develops within the **lymphatic vessels**, though, some fluid can leak back into the **interstitial space** and contribute to the formation of **edema**. The **lymphatic system** is responsible for the removal of **interstitial fluid** from **tissues**. It absorbs and transports **fatty acids** and **fats** as chyle to the circulatory system, and it transports **immune cells** to and from the **lymph nodes**, where an **immune response** is stimulated. The study of lymphatic drainage of various organs is important in the diagnosis, prognosis, and treatment of **cancer**. The **lymphatic system**, because of its physical proximity to many **tissues** of the body, is responsible for carrying **cancerous cells** between the various parts of the body in a process called metastasis. The intervening **lymph nodes** can trap the **cancer cells**. If they are not successful in destroying the **cancer cells**, the nodes may become sites of secondary **tumors** (see **sentinel lymph node**). Diseases and other problems of the **lymphatic system** can cause swelling and other symptoms. Problems with the system can impair the body's ability to fight infections.

lymphatic vessel: Thin-walled tubular **vessel** resembling a vein in structure but with thinner walls and more valves. The walls are enclosed by smooth **muscle** and **connective tissue**. **Lymphatic vessels** drain into **lymph** ducts. **Lymphatic vessels** act as channels along which pathogens are conducted from infected areas of the body, the pathogens being unable to enter the **blood capillaries**. **Lymph nodes** are distributed along the **lymphatic vessels**. The **lymph** flow is maintained by peristaltic contractility of the **lymphatic vessels**, aided by the squeezing of the **vessels** by skeletal **muscles**, with the valves maintaining a flow in one direction only.

lymphocyte: Spherical **white blood cell** with one large **nucleus** and relatively little **cytoplasm**. Two types exist, small and large **lymphocytes**. They are produced continually in **lymphoid tissues**, such as **lymph nodes**, by **cell** division. The **cells** are nonphagocytic, exhibit amoeboid movement, and produce **antibodies** in the **blood**. They constitute about 25% of all **leukocytes** in the human body.

lymphoid tissue: Part of the **lymphatic system**. It consists of **connective tissue** with various types of **white blood cells** enmeshed in it, most numerous being the **lymphocytes**. The **thymus** and the **bone marrow** constitute the primary

lymphoid tissues involved in the production and early selection of **lymphocytes**. Secondary **lymphoid tissue** provides the environment for the foreign or altered native molecules (**antigens**) to interact with the **lymphocytes**. These are the **lymph nodes** and the lymphoid follicles in **tonsils**, **spleen**, adenoids, **skin**, etc. The tertiary **lymphoid tissue** typically contains far fewer **lymphocytes** and assumes an immune role only when challenged with **antigens** that result in **inflammation**. It achieves this by importing the **lymphocytes** from **blood** and **lymph**.

lymphotropic agent: An agent that influences the functioning of **lymphatic vessels**.

lyophilized: Related to **tissues**, or **blood**, or **serum**, or other biological substances that are dried by freezing in a high vacuum. Preserved samples are prevented from decaying or spoiling, and are prepared for future use.

lysed blood: Product of **blood** at its **hemolysis**.

lysosome: **Membrane**-bound particle, smaller than a **mitochondrion**, occurring in large numbers in the **cytoplasm** of **cells**. They contain hydrolytic **enzymes** that are released when the **cell** is damaged. These **enzymes** assist in the digestion and removal of dead **cells**, the digestion of food and other substances, and the destruction of redundant organelles.

Mach–Zehnder interferometer: Dual-beam four-mirror (two serve as the **beamsplitter** and beam **coupler**, and two as reflectors) **interferometer** usually used as a refractometer, especially for objects occupying a large space.

macromolecules: Pertaining to conventional polymers and biopolymers (such as **DNA**) as well as nonpolymeric molecules with large molecular mass, such as **lipids** or macrocycles.

macrophage: Large phagocytic **cell** with one **nucleus**. It moves by **membrane**-like pseudopodia. These **cells** are found in contact with **blood** and **lymph** at the sites of corpuscle formation (e.g., in **bone marrow**, **lymph nodes**, and the **spleen**). Their function is to remove foreign particles from **blood** and **lymph**. **Macrophages** are also found in all loose **connective tissue**, but they only become active when the **tissue** is damaged. Their function is to remove the debris from damaged **tissues**. They form the reticuloendothelial system. In the inactive state (i.e., in undamaged **tissue**), the resting form of the **cell** is called a "histiocyte." **Macrophages** are closely related to **monocytes**.

macroscopic polarization: See **dielectric-polarization density**.

magnesia: See **magnesium oxide (MgO)**.

magnesium oxide (MgO) (*Synonym*: magnesia): White solid mineral that occurs naturally as periclase and is a source of magnesium. It is formed by an ionic bond between one magnesium and one **oxygen** atom. It is used as a reference white **color** in photometry and **colorimetry**. The **emissivity** value is about 0.9. Pressed **MgO** is used as an optical material. It is transparent from 300 nm to 7 μm. The **refractive index** is 1.72 at 1 μm.

magnetic nanoparticles: Typically, Fe_2O_3-core spherical **nanoparticles** of around 30 nm in diameter. For example, such particles are well-recognized lymphographic tracers and were used as **photoacoustic contrast agents**. **Polyethylene glycol (PEG)** coating is typically used to reduce their interaction with **tissue** during delivery.

magnetic resonance imaging (MRI) [*Synonym*: magnetic resonance tomography (MRT)]: A **noninvasive** imaging technique that is based on magnetic resonance method [magnetism and **radio frequency (RF)** waves] and computer reconstruction of 2D and 3D images of body structures. It provides a wealth of information about inner structures in the body and in particular about **tumors**.

It is often used in clinical studies using optical instrumentation as a subsidiary technique.

malachite green: An organic compound being a member of the triphenylcarbenium salts, classified in the dyestuff industry as triarylmethane dyes. It often refers to the colored cation. The intense green **color** of the cation comes from an intense (extinction coefficient of 10^5 M^{-1} cm^{-1}) **absorption band** at 621 nm. It is used as a biological stain for microscopic analysis of **cell** biology and **tissue** samples. In the **Gimenez-stain** method, basic **fuchsine** stains **bacteria** red or magenta, and **malachite green** is used as a blue–green counterstain. It can also directly stain endospores within **cells**.

malignant: Clinical term that means to be severe and become progressively worse, as in **malignant** hypertension. In the context of **cancer**, a **malignant tumor** can invade and destroy nearby **tissue**, and may also spread (metastasize) to other parts of the body.

malignant tissue: An abnormally growing **tissue** having the tendency to spread to other parts of the body, even when the original growth is removed by surgery. It eventually causes death.

mammary gland: Large **gland** on the ventral surface of the mature female. It is thought to be a modified **sweat gland**. It consists of clusters of **gland cells** that can extract the necessary substances from **blood** to produce milk. The milk drains through ducts into a cistern. A canal leads from the cistern to a mammary papilla. The growth and activity of the **gland** is under the control of gonadal **hormones**, and the state of the **gland** is influenced by the estrous cycle. Milk production is stimulated by the pituitary lactogenic **hormone**.

mammogram: An image of a female **breast** obtained by **mammography**.

mammography: **X-ray** imaging, **magnetic resonance imaging (MRI)**, **ultrasound (US)**, and positron-emission imaging of a female **breast**, especially for screening or early detection of **cancer**.

mannitol: Hexan-1,2,3,4,5,6-hexol ($C_6H_8(OH)_6$) is an osmotic diuretic agent and a weak renal vasodilator. It is a sorbitol and is used clinically to reduce acutely raised intracranial **pressure**.

mast cell (*Synonym*: mastocyte): Resident **cell** of several types of **tissues** and contains many granules rich in histamine and heparin. **Mast cells** play an important protective role in allergies and anaphylaxis, and are also involved in **wound** healing and defense against pathogens. These **cells** are considered to be part of the immune system. Two types of **mast cells** are recognized, those from **connective tissue**, and a distinct set of mucosal **mast cells**. They are present in most **tissues** characteristically surrounding **blood vessels** and **nerves**, and especially in the **skin**, **mucosa** of the **lungs** and **digestive tract**, as well as in the **mouth**, **conjunctiva**, and nose.

mastocyte: See **mast cell**.

mastopathy: Any disease of the female **breast**.

matching substance: Substance used to reduce the boundary effects caused by the complex shape of a **scattering** object. The **scattering** properties of such a substance should be similar to the **scattering** properties of the object under study.

material dispersion: Describes the separation of the different **wavelengths** in a given medium (material) that occurs because the waves are traveling at different velocities in that medium.

Mathematica: Computational software program from Wolfram Research used in scientific, engineering, and mathematical fields, and other areas of technical computing.

MATLAB®:   High-level language and interactive environment that enables one to perform computationally intensive tasks faster than with traditional programming languages such as C, C++, and Fortran.

maxillary sinusitis: Pathophysiology of the disease is in the obstruction at the level of the ostiomeatal complex leading to stasis and infection of secretions within the maxillary sinus. Obstruction may occur secondary to any number of inciting factors including upper respiratory tract infection (viral, bacterial, or fungal), allergic rhinitis, **trauma**, or prior surgery. It produces purulent material that drips along the back of the **throat** onto the **tongue** (postnasal drip), which may cause **halitosis**.

meal tolerance test (MTT):   In medical practice, the complete nutrient test (**carbohydrate**, **fat**, and **protein** containing meals) that induces both **glucose** and **insulin** responses. The **MTT** is a more potent **insulin** stimulator than **glucose** alone (see **OGTT**).

mean blood glucose (MBG):   The **blood glucose** level (**blood sugar** concentration) is the amount of **glucose** (sugar) present in the **blood** of a human. The mean normal **blood glucose** level in humans is about 4 mM (4 mmol/L) or 72 mg/dL (milligrams/deciliter). However, the **glucose** level fluctuates during the day—it rises after meals for an hour or two and is usually lowest in the morning, before the first meal of the day (termed "the fasting level"). When **MBG** is outside the normal range, it may be an indicator of a medical condition. A high level above normal is referred to as **hyperglycemia**, or if low, as **hypoglycemia**. **Diabetes mellitus** is characterized by persistent **hyperglycemia** from any of several causes, and is the most prominent disease related to failure of **blood** sugar regulation. A temporarily elevated **blood**-sugar level may also result from severe stress, such as **trauma**, stroke, **myocardial infarction**, or surgery.

mean free path (MFP):   This is the mean distance between two successive interactions with **scattering** (μ_s) or **absorption**

(μ_a) that a **photon** traveling in a **scattering-absorption** medium experiences: **MFP** $\equiv l_{ph} = 1/\mu_t$, where $\mu_t = (\mu_s + \mu_a)$ is the **attenuation coefficient**.

mechanical stress: The action on a body of any system of balanced forces that results in strain or **deformation**.

media: Middle layer of an **artery** or lymphatic **vessel** wall.

medical fiber: Depending on application area, all types of **fibers** could be used in biomedicine: **single-mode fibers**; **multimode fibers** with a low **numerical aperture** as various physical, chemical, and biochemical **fiber optic sensors**; guided **optical imaging**; and remote monitoring, as well as multimode with a high **numerical aperture** and **fiber bundles** for guiding low-intensity and high-intensity **light** to internal organs and back. However, medical **fibers** are usually classified as non-toxic **fibers** for allowing easy sterilization of the distal end, their suitable flexibility and high **transmittance** for relatively short **fiber** lengths (1–10 m), and high degree of **radiation** resistance. As a rule, medical **fibers** have large core diameters, $2a = 100$–1000 μm. Biomedical applications use **light** of all **wavelength** ranges, from deep **UV** up to far **IR**. Silica **fibers** have an unique transparency in the **visible** and **NIR**, and are ideal for guiding **neodymium lasers** ($\lambda = 1060$ nm) and **diode lasers** (390–1560 nm) used in **endoscopy**, internal organ **laser** therapy, and surgery. For example, for a typical silica **fiber** with **attenuation** less than 6 **dB**/km at $\lambda = 1060$ nm and core diameter of 400 μm, it is possible to provide transmission of mean **laser power** up to 40 W during a few hours without noticeable optical degradation. Of specific interest for medicine are fibers that have two or more **wavelength** ranges, such as **UV** ($\lambda \leq 351$ nm), where pulse **excimer lasers** operate, and **IR** ($\lambda \geq 2000$ nm), where pulse and **CW holmium**, **erbium**, **CO**, and **CO$_2$** lasers operate. To guide pulse-periodic **UV radiation** of **excimer lasers**, silica **fibers** are used. For example, **radiation** of a **XeCl laser** ($\lambda = 308$ nm) with pulse duration of $\tau_p = 40$ ns and repetition rate of $f = 75$ Hz for more than 10^3 pulses, transmitted through a typical silica **fiber** with core diameter of 400 µm and length of 4 m, provides an output **energy density** of 6–7 J/cm^2—about four times larger than the **vessel** wall **tissue ablation** threshold and lower than the **energy density** limit for distal **fiber tip** damage caused by ablated **tissue** debris. The so-called "wet" or "superwet" silica **fibers** with a pure silica core and a high concentration of OH$^-$ groups have a comparatively low **attenuation** in **UV**, $\alpha \leq 0.17$ **dB**/m ($\lambda = 308$ nm) (see **fiber attenuation**). A precise layer-by-layer **tissue ablation** could also be realized by using **IR lasers** ($\lambda \geq 2000$ nm), which, in combination with **infrared fibers**, are applicable, for example, in cardiology for **angioplasty** and **heart** disease treatments. The commercially available silica-plastic **fibers** (core diameter of 400–600 µm) with typical **attenuation** $\lambda = 850$ nm of 8–10 **dB**/km can be used for the sufficiently effective transport ($\geq 50\%$) of **holmium laser** ($\lambda = 2090$ nm) **radiation** for 3–10 m. Accounting for coupling losses (10–13%) of the 3-m **fiber** delivers around 70% of **laser energy**, i.e., 6 J. Such energetic pulses with $\tau_p = 10$ ns and $f = 1$ Hz can be transported by silica **fiber** for a few hours ($\sim 10^4$ pulses) without causing damage, which is sufficient for many surgery and therapeutic treatments. One of the best **IR fibers** is a polycrystalline Ag-halide **fiber** (0.25 AgCl/0.75 AgBr) that allows one to transmit **CO$_2$ laser** ($\lambda = 10.6$ µm) **radiation** with a **power density** of 70 kW/cm^2 or highly energetic (up to 6.5 J/cm^2) short pulses ($\tau_p \sim 0.1$ µs) with a **power density** of 8 MW/cm^2. A flexible Ag-halide **fiber** cable transmitting ~ 1 W of **CW CO$_2$ laser radiation** can be used as a surgical instrument, for example, for welding **blood vessels**. Sapphire **fibers** are also widely used in medicine for the transportation of **erbium laser radiation** with high efficiency, 1.2 kJ/cm^2 for $\tau_p = 110$ µs. With active dopants, such as neodymium or erbium, **fibers** with an optical **gain** under optical pumping can be used as optical **amplifiers** and **fiber lasers**, opening up many new biomedical applications.

medical imaging: **Noninvasive** or least-**invasive** imaging techniques that are based on different physical principles and allow for getting morphological and/or functional information about **tissues** or organs within some area or volume—2D or 3D imaging. For example, well-established and commonly used **x-ray computed tomography** and **magnetic resonance imaging** provide a wealth of information about inner structures in the body and in particular about **tumors**. Much less invasive **optical imaging** techniques, such as optical **diffusion** tomography, **polarization** imaging, **OCT**, **optoacoustic** and **acousto-optic tomographies** are under intensive study and have good prospects for medical imaging (see **tomography**).

mediolateral projection: Pertaining to the medial and lateral planes of the body.

medulloblastomas: Most **brain tumors** are named after the type of **cells** from which they develop. **Medulloblastomas** are **malignant tumors** formed from poorly developed **cells** at a very early stage of their life. They develop in the **cerebellum**, in a part of the **brain** called the posterior fossa, but may spread to other parts of the **brain**. Very rarely, **medulloblastomas** may spread to other parts of the body. If they do spread to other parts of the **brain**, or to the **spinal cord**, this is usually through the **cerebrospinal fluid (CSF)**. They are more common in children.

meiosis: Process of reductional division in which the number of **chromosomes** per **cell** is cut in half. In animals, **meiosis** always results in the formation of gametes, while in other organisms it can give rise to spores. As with **mitosis**, before **meiosis** begins, the **DNA** in the original **cell** is replicated during the S-phase of the **cell** cycle. Two **cell** divisions separate the replicated **chromosomes** into four haploid gametes or spores. **Meiosis** is essential for sexual reproduction, and therefore occurs in all **eukaryotes** (including single-celled organisms) that reproduce sexually.

melanin: Dark-brown or black **pigment**. **Melanin** in **melanosomes** of normal **skin** is an extremely dense, virtually in-soluble polymer of high molecular weight and is always attached to a structural **protein**. Mammalian **melanin pigments** have one of two chemical compositions: eumelanin, a brown polymer, and pheomelanin, a yellow-reddish alkali-soluble **pigment**.

melanin granular (*Synonym*: melanosome): Cytoplasmic organelles on which **melanin pigments** are synthesized and deposited. Normal human **skin color** is primarily related to the size, type, **color**, and distribution of **melanosomes**. **Melanosomes** are the product of specialized exocrine **glands, melanocytes**.

melanocyte: Component of the **melanin** pigmentary system, which is made up of **melanocytes** distributed in various sites: the **eyeball** (retinal **pigment epithelium**, uveal tract), the **ear** (in the stria vascularis), the **central nervous system** (in leptomeninges), the **hair** (in the **hair** matrix), the **mucous membranes**, and the **skin** (at the dermoepidermal junction, where they rest on the **basement membrane**). In the **skin, melanocytes** project their **dendrites** into the **epidermis** where they transfer melanosomes to **keratinocytes**.

melanoma: Darkly pigmented **tumor** (typically **malignant**) of **melanocytes**, which are found predominantly in **skin** but also in the bowel and the eye. It is one of the less common types of **skin cancer** but causes the majority (75%) of **skin-cancer**-related deaths. A popular method for remembering the signs and symptoms of **melanoma** is the mnemonic "ABCDE": *A*symmetrical **skin lesion**, *B*order of the **lesion** is irregular, *C*olor (**melanomas** usually have multiple **colors**), *D*iameter (moles greater than 6 mm are more likely to be **melanomas** than smaller moles), and *E*nlarging or evolving. To identify high-risk **lesions** within a given patient, many new photonic technologies, such as OCT, allow pathologists to view 3D reconstructions of the **skin** and offers more resolution than other techniques could provide. *In vivo* **confocal microscopy**, fluorescently tagged **antibodies**, and **polarization**-imaging techniques are also proving to be valuable diagnostic tools. The treatment includes surgical removal of the **tumor**, adjuvant treatment, chemo- and immunotherapy, or **radiation** therapy. The **PDT** as a prospective technique for **melanoma** treatment is under intensive research.

melanoma maligna: Special kind of **melanoma** *in situ* that occurs on sun-damaged **skin**. On the face or **neck**, it may be described as lentigo maligna **melanoma**.

melanosome: See **melanin granular**.

membrane: (1) A very thin layer of **connective tissue** covering an organ; (2) **connective tissue** dividing **cells**; (3) a thin layer of **cells**.

meningiomas: Most common **benign tumors** of the **brain** (95% of **benign tumors**). However, they can also be **malignant**. They arise from the arachnoidal cap **cells** of the meninges and represent about 15% of all primary **brain tumors**. They are more common in females than in males (2:1) and have a peak incidence in the sixth and seventh decades.

meniscus: Disk of **cartilage** between the articulating ends of the **bones** in a joint.

menopause: The permanent cessation of menstruation in women.

mercury arc lamp: Discharge arc lamp filled with mercury vapor at high **pressure** that gives out a very bright **UV** and **visible light** at some **wavelengths** including 303, 312, 365, 405, 436, 546, and 578 nm.

mercury cadmium telluride (MCT) (HgCdTe): Material used for fast, sensitive, **infrared** photodetectors used in **infrared** sensors, scanners, and imagers that require cooled operation.

meridional plane: Plane that includes the optical axis. It is common to simplify problems in radially-symmetric optical systems by choosing object points in the vertical plane only. This plane is then sometimes referred to as the **meridional plane**.

mesentery: (1) Sheets of thin **connective tissue** by which the **stomach** and **intestines** are suspended from the **dorsal** wall of the **abdominal cavity**; (2) the **tissue** supporting the **intestines**. The mesenteries carry **blood, lymphatic vessels**, and **nerves** to the organs of the alimentary canal.

messenger ribonucleic acid (mRNA): A molecule of **RNA** encoding a chemical "blueprint" for a **protein** product. **mRNA** is transcribed from a **DNA** template and carries coding information to the sites of **protein** synthesis—the **ribosomes**, where the **nucleic acid** polymer is translated into a polymer of **amino acids**, a **protein**. In **mRNA**, as in **DNA**, genetic information is encoded in the sequence of **nucleotides** arranged into codons consisting of three bases each. Each codon encodes for a specific **amino acid**, except for the stop codons that terminate **protein** synthesis. This process requires **tRNA** and **rRNA**.

metabolic processes: See **metabolism**.

metabolism (*Synonym*: metabolic processes): Chemical processes that take place in a living organism or within part of a living organism (e.g., **cell**). **Metabolism** consists of **catabolism** and **anabolism**.

metabolite: Substance that takes part in a metabolic process. Those **metabolites** that the organism cannot manufacture have to be obtained from the environment. Some **metabolites** are supplied partly by the environment and partly by the organism. The majority of the **metabolites** in an organism are manufactured by the organism.

metachromasy: See **metachromasia**.

metachromasia (*Synonym*: metachromasy): Characteristic change in the **color** of staining carried out in biological **tissues**, exhibited by certain aniline dyes when they bind to particular substances present in these **tissues**, called chromotropes. For example, **toluidine blue O** becomes pink when bound to **cartilage**. The absence of **color** change in staining is named orthochromasy. **Metachromasy** is related to the quantitative determination of sulfate esters of high molecular weight.

metal organic vapor phase epitaxy (MOVPE): Method of depositing thin layers of **crystalline** materials used in the construction of **LEDs**.

metal-vapor laser: Atomic or ionic **laser** that uses vapor of a chemical element (Cu, Ag, Cd, Zn, Se, Te, Hg, etc.) mixed with a low-**pressure** helium or neon buffer gas to create gas-discharge **plasma** as a **laser-gain** medium. Atomic copper and **gold vapor lasers** and ionic He–Cd, He–Se and CO–Zn **lasers** are available on the market. White **laser radiation** at approximately equal **powers** on each line [441.6 nm, 533.7/537.8 nm and 615.0 nm (Hg)] can be provided by the **laser** with a combined active medium He–Cd–Hg. The powerful three-**color** (green–yellow–red) **lasers** on copper- and gold-vapor mixtures (510.5/578.2/627.8 nm) are designed, as well as special medical computer-aided **water**- and air-cooled **laser** systems. **Metal-vapor lasers** are used in photobiochemistry, dermatology, photodynamic therapy, and many other biomedical applications.

metamaterial: Synthetic artificial material designed to have specific **optical properties** such as a negative **refractive index**.

methemoglobin: Abbreviated as metHb. It is a form of **hemoglobin** in which the iron in the heme group is in the Fe_3^+ (ferric) state, not the Fe_2^+ (ferrous) of normal **hemoglobin**. **Methemoglobin** cannot carry **oxygen**. It is a bluish chocolate-brown in **color**. The **NADH**-dependent **enzyme methemoglobin** reductase (diaphorase I) is responsible for converting **methemoglobin** back to **hemoglobin**. Normally, 1–2% of **hemoglobin** in humans is **methemoglobin**. A higher percentage than this can be genetic or caused by exposure to various chemicals, and depending on the level, can cause health problems known as methemoglobinemia. A higher level of **methemoglobin** will tend to cause a **pulse oximeter** to read closer to 85% regardless of the true level of **oxygen** saturation. This occurs due to the differences in spectra of **oxyhemoglobin** and **methemoglobin**—**methemoglobin** in solution has a four-banded **absorption spectrum** with a strong band in the orange-red at 630 nm.

methylene blue (MB): Biological dye (stain) showing a phototoxic effect. Its **absorption bands** in the **visible** range are between 609 and 668 nm. It is used as a stain in bacteriology and as an oxidation–reduction indicator. It can be activated by **light** to an **excited state**, which in turn activates **oxygen** to yield oxidizing **radicals**; such **radicals** can cause cross-linking of **amino acid** residues on **proteins**, and hence achieve some degree of cross-linking. It is also used as a photodynamic dye for inflammatory disease treatment and bacteria killing using red **diode laser** or **LED** irradiation.

micelle: An aggregate of surfactant molecules dispersed in a liquid colloid. A typical **micelle** in aqueous solution forms an aggregate with the **hydrophilic** "**head**" regions in contact with surrounding solvent, sequestering the **hydrophobic** tail regions in the **micelle** center. This type of **micelle** is known as a normal-phase **micelle** (**oil-in-water micelle**). Inverse **micelles** have the head groups at the center with the tails extending out (**water-in-oil micelle**). **Micelles** are approximately spherical in shape. Other phases, including shapes such as ellipsoids, cylinders, and bilayers, are also possible. The shape and size of a **micelle** is a function of the molecular geometry of its surfactant molecules and solution conditions such as surfactant concentration, temperature, **pH**, and **ionic strength**. The process of forming **micelles** is known as micellization and forms part of the phase behavior of many **lipids** according to their polymorphism.

Michelson interferometer: Dual-beam **interferometer** with a **beamsplitter** and two reflecting surfaces. It allows one to realize various types of **interference** and is widely used in metrology for measurements of lengths, displacements, vibrations, and surface roughness; an integrated fiber optic prototype has become very popular (see **fiber optic single-mode X-coupler**). It is also widely used in **tissue spectroscopy** and imaging (see **dual-beam coherent interferometry** and **Doppler interferometry**).

microcirculation: Flow of **blood** from **arterioles** to **capillaries** or sinusoids (sinusoidal **capillaries**) to venules. Blood flows freely between an **arteriole** and a **venule** through a **vessel** channel called a thoroughfare channel. **Capillaries** extend from this channel, and structures called precapillary sphincters control the flow of **blood** between the **arteriole** and **capillaries**. The precapillary sphincters contain **muscle fibers** that allow them to contract. When the sphincters are open, **blood flows** freely to the **capillary** beds where gases and waste can be exchanged with body **tissue**. When the sphincters are closed, **blood** is not allowed to flow through the **capillary** beds and must flow directly from the **arteriole** to the **venule** through the thoroughfare channel. It is important to note that **blood** is supplied to all parts of the body at all times, but all **capillary** beds do not contain **blood** at all times.

micro-cooler: Small, palm-size cooler based on the Stirling cycle that cools an **infrared detector** or **focal plane array (FPA)** to liquid-nitrogen temperature (77 K).

micro-electromechanical system (MEMS): System made on the basis of the micro-scale technology. **MEMSs** are made up of components 1–100 μm in size, and **MEMS** devices generally range in size from 20 μm to 1 mm. They usually consist of a central unit that processes data, the microprocessor, and several components that interact with the outside, such as microsensors. At these size scales, the standard constructs of classical physics are not always useful. Because of the large surface area-to-volume ratio of **MEMS**, surface effects such as electrostatics and wetting dominate volume effects such as inertia or thermal mass. **MEMSs** became practical once they could be fabricated using modified

semiconductor-device-fabrication technologies, normally used to make electronics. These technologies include molding and plating, wet etching and dry etching, electro-discharge machining, and other technologies capable of manufacturing very small devices. For example, scanners fabricated with **MEMS** technology are well suited to meet the size and speed requirements for *in vivo* endoscopic **optical imaging** applications, where a fairly rapid scan rate is needed to overcome motion **artifacts** introduced by organ peristalsis, **heart** beating, and respiratory activity, requiring a frame rate of >4 per second.

microfibril: Very fine **fibril**, or **fiber**-like strand, consisting of glycoproteins. Its most frequently observed structural pattern is a 9 + 2 pattern in which two central protofibrils are surrounded by nine others. Cellulose inside plants is one example of a nonprotein compound that fits this description.

microfilament: Fine, thread-like **protein fibers** 3–6 nm in diameter. They are composed predominantly of a contractile **protein** called actin, which is the most abundant cellular **protein**. The association of **microfilaments** with the **protein** myosin is responsible for **muscle** contraction. **Microfilaments** can also carry out cellular movements including gliding, contraction, and cytokinesis.

microfluidics: Broad term that describes miniature hydrome-chanical flow control devices such as micro-capillaries, pumps and valves, or sensors like **flowmeters** and viscometers. They are widely used in optical **flow cytometry** and **cell optical transfection** systems, as well as in **lab-on-a-chip (LOC)** devices.

micrometer (μm) (*Synonym*: micron): Unit of length that is equal to 10^{-3} millimeters (mm) or 10^{-6} meters (m).

micron: See **micrometer**.

microphone: Device that transforms sound **energy** into electrical **energy**; various types include carbon **microphones**, crystal **microphones**, condenser **microphones**, and a moving coil or dynamic **microphone**.

microprofilometer: Device that measures the roughness of a surface.

microscopy: Any technique that produces **visible** images of structures or details too small to otherwise be seen by the human eye, by using a microscope or other magnification tool. There are three main branches of **microscopy**: optical, electronic, and scanning probe **microscopy**. Optical and **electronic microscopy** involve the **diffraction**, **reflection**, or **refraction** of **radiation** incident upon the subject of study, and the subsequent collection of this scattered **radiation** in order to build an image. This process may be carried out by wide-field irradiation of the sample (for example, standard **light microscopy** and transmission **electronic microscopy**) or by scanning a fine beam over the sample (for example, **confocal microscopy** and scanning **electronic microscopy**). Scanning probe **microscopy** involves the interaction of a scanning probe with the surface or object of interest.

microsecond (μsec or μs): Unit of time that is equal to 10^{-6} seconds (s).

micro-spectrophotometric technique: Technique that measures an object's **transmittance** or **reflectance** spectra with a high **spatial resolution**. Usually, a combination of a microscope and a **grating spectrograph** with an optical multichannel **analyzer** (**cooled CCD** or **photodiode array**) is used for such measurements.

micro total analysis system (μTAS): Related to **lab-on-a-chip** (**LOC**) technology, but mostly dedicated to the integration of the total sequence of lab processes to perform chemical analysis.

microtubules: Cylindrical tubes 20–25 nm in diameter. They are composed of subunits of the **protein** tubulin. They act as a scaffold to determine **cell** shape and provide a set of "tracks" for **cell** organelles and vesicles to move along. **Microtubules** also form the spindle **fibers** for separating **chromosomes** during **mitosis**. When arranged in geometric patterns inside flagella and **cilia**, they are used for locomotion.

microvessel: See **capillary**.

mid-infrared (MIR): See **light wavelength range**.

Mie scattering theory (*Synonym*: Lorentz–Mie scattering theory): An exact solution of Maxwell's electromagnetic field equations for a homogeneous sphere. Mie **scattering** relates to **scattering** by comparatively large spherical particles of the order of the **wavelength**.

milliradian (mrad): One thousandth (10^{-3}) of a **radian**. It is a unit used to express instrument angular **field of view**, and it is an angle whose tangent is equal to 0.001. One **mrad** = 0.05729578 deg.

millisecond (msec or ms): Unit of time that is equal to 10^{-3} sec (s).

mineralization: Process whereby a substance is converted from an organic substance to an inorganic substance, thus becoming mineralized.

minimal erythema dose (MED): The minimal single dose of **UV radiation**, expressed as **energy** per unit area J/cm^2, to produce a clearly marginated **erythema** at the irradiated **skin** site after 24 hours for **UVB** and 48 hours for **UVA**.

minimally-invasive technique: Least-**invasive** technique; any procedure (diagnostic, therapeutic or surgical) that inserts some invasiveness in comparison with a **noninvasive** technique or provides much less invasiveness than an open surgery used for the same purpose. Many medical procedures are described as minimally **invasive**, such as **hypodermic** injection, air-**pressure** injection, subdermal **implants**, **endoscopy**, **percutaneous** surgery, laparoscopic surgery, arthroscopic surgery, **cryosurgery** (**cryotherapy**), microsurgery, endovascular surgery (such as **angioplasty**), coronary catheterization, **laser tissue coagulation** and **ablation**, **laser heating**, **laser-induced interstitial thermotherapy (LITT)**, **photodynamic therapy**, and radioactivity-based medical imaging methods such as gamma camera, PET, and **single-photon emission computed tomography (SPECT)**.

minimum detectable temperature difference (MDTD): The **minimum resolvable temperature difference (MRTD)** of an extended source target, that is, a target large enough to be fully resolved by the instrument.

minimum resolvable temperature difference (MRTD): Smallest temperature difference that an instrument can clearly distinguish out of the noise, taking into account target size, the characteristics of the display, and the subjective interpretation of the operator. The limit of MRTD is the **minimum detectable temperature difference (MDTD)**.

mitochondrion (*Plural*: mitochondria): Threadlike or rodlike granular organelle in the **cytoplasm** of **cells**, about 0.5 μm in width and up to 10 μm in length for threadlike **mitochondria**. **Mitochondria** are bounded by a double **membrane**; the inner **membrane** is folded inward at a number of places to form cristae. **Mitochondria** contain phosphates and numerous **enzymes** that vary in different **tissues**. Their function is cellular respiration and the release of chemical **energy** in the form of **ATP** for use in most of the cell's biological functions. The **cells** of all organisms, except **bacteria** and blue–green algae, contain **mitochondria** in varying numbers; **mitochondria** are especially numerous in **cells** involved in significant metabolic activity, such as **liver cells**. **Mitochondria** are self-replicating, have dimensions of 1–2 μm, and their material has a **refractive index** that lies within a relatively narrow range (1.38–1.41).

mitosis: Process by which a **cell nucleus** usually divides into two. The process takes place in four phases: prophase, metaphase, anaphase, and telophase. The daughter nuclei are genetically identical to each other and to the parent **nucleus**.

M-mode OCT image: Image obtained from repeated **A-scans** without moving the incident beam, so one can easily visualize living object movement and time-dependent changes of **tissue** structure.

modal dispersion: Disperson that occurs because different modes in a **multimode fiber** propagate at different group velocities. To find the modal **dispersion**, the difference in **group refractive index** $n_g\beta$ between modes of different propagation constant β should be considered. This difference exists even when there is no intramode **chromatic dispersion**. In a **multimode fiber**, the **modal dispersion** between the fundamental mode (low) and the highest-order mode (high) supported by the **fiber** can be expressed as $(n_{g\ high}-n_{g\ low}) = n_{g1}[\Delta(\alpha-2-\delta)/(\alpha+2)+(\Delta^2/2)(3\alpha-2-2\delta)/(\alpha+2)]$, where $\Delta \cong (n_1 - n_2)/n_1$ is the normalized index difference (see **fiber numerical aperture**), α characterizes the **power**-law index profile of the **fiber** core of graded-index **fibers** (for a **step-index fiber**, $\alpha = \infty$), and $\delta = -(2n_1/n_{g1})(\lambda/\Delta)(d\Delta/d\lambda)$. When $\alpha > 2+\delta, n_{g\ high} > n_{g\ low}$, but $n_{g\ high} < n_{g\ low}$ when $\alpha < 2+\delta$. Because $v_g = c/n_g$, this **dispersion** represents the difference in the group velocity between different modes. It depends on many factors, including the **waveguide** structure, the index profile, the material properties, and how far away the modes are from **fiber** cutoff **wavelength**, and can be modified by choosing appropriate structure and material parameters.

mode-locked laser: **Multimode laser** with synchronously irradiating modes; the regime is obtained typically by applying an intracavity high-**frequency** optical modulator, with a typical pulse duration of up to a subpicosecond range and a repetition rate of dozens of megahertz. A **cavity-dumped mode-locked laser** is a **laser** that uses a specific technology for producing high-**energy** ultrashort pulses by decreasing the pulse repetition rate. Other modifications of **mode-locking** technology are used to provide generation of the **ultrashort laser pulses**.

mode-locking: Regime of a **multimode laser** with synchronously radiating modes that produce collectively an **ultrashort laser pulse**. The regime can be achieved spontaneously or induced by applying passive or active intracavity optical elements providing **frequency** equidistance between **laser** longitudinal modes.

modified amino resin (MAR):   Material used in preparation of **tissue phantoms**.

modulation: In general, the changes in one **wave** train caused by another. For example, the process of varying the characteristics of an optical **wave** motion by superimposing on it the characteristics of a second (audio- or **radio-frequency**) **wave** motion. There are three main types of **modulation:** amplitude **modulation**, **frequency modulation**, and phase **modulation**.

modulation frequency: **Frequency** of the modulating **wave**.

modulation transfer function (MTF):   Measure of the ability of an imaging system to reproduce the image of a target. A formalized procedure is used to measure **MTF**; it assesses the spatial **frequency** resolution of a scanning or imaging system as a function of distance to the target.

moisturizer: Complex mixtures of chemical agents specially designed to make the external layers of the **skin** (**epidermis**) softer and more pliable by increasing its **hydration**. It includes naturally occurring **skin lipids** and sterols as well as artificial or natural

oils, humectants, emollients, lubricants, etc. It may be part of the composition of commercial **skin moisturizers**. They are usually available as commercial products for cosmetic and therapeutic uses.

molality: Number of **moles** of solute dissolved in one kilogram of solvent. For example, to make a one molal aqueous (**water**) solution of sodium chloride (NaCl), measure out one kilogram of **water** and add one **mole** of the solute, NaCl, to it. The formula weight for NaCl, is equal to 58 = 23 (sodium) + 35 (chlorine); thus, 58 grams of NaCl dissolved in 1 kg **water** would result in a 1 molal (m) solution of NaCl.

molarity: Molar unit is probably the most commonly used chemical unit of measurement. It is the number of **moles** of a solute dissolved in a liter of solution. A molar solution of sodium chloride (NaCl) is made by placing 1 **mole** of a solute (58 grams) into a 1-liter volumetric flask. **Water** is then added to the volumetric flask up to the one-liter line. The result is a 1-molar (M) solution of sodium chloride.

molar mass: Mass of one **mole** of a chemical element or chemical compound.

mole: **SI** base unit of amount of substance n; the symbol is mol. It is defined as the amount of substance of a system that contains as many atoms, molecules, ions, or electrons as there are atoms in 12 g of carbon-12. A **mole** has $6.02214179(30) \times 10^{23}$ atoms or molecules of the pure substance being measured. A **mole** of a substance has mass in grams exactly equal to the substance's molecular or atomic weight, e.g., 1 mol of Calcium-40 is equal to 40 grams. One can measure the number of **moles** in a pure substance by weighing it and comparing the result to its molecular or atomic weight. It is commonly used in medicine to measure small amounts of a substance in **blood** or other liquids. Such units as millimoles per liter (mmol/L), micromoles per liter (μmol/L), or nanomoles per liter (nmol/L) are often used.

molecular beacon (molecular beacon probe): Oligonucleotide hybridization probe that can report the presence of specific **nucleic acids** in homogenous solutions. They are hairpin-shaped molecules with an internally quenched **fluorophore** whose **fluorescence** is restored when they bind to a target **nucleic-acid** sequence. This is a novel nonradioactive method for detecting specific sequences of **nucleic acids**. They are useful in situations where it is either not possible or desirable to isolate the probe-target hybrids from an excess of the hybridization probes. In **PDT/PDD**, **molecular beacons** allow one to provide quenching of molecular photoactivation until the molecules reach specific targets.

molecular hyperpolarizability: See **hyperpolarizability**.

monochromatic light: **Light** of one **color** (**wavelength**) only. It is ideally produced by a **CW**, single-**frequency** (single-longitudinal mode), well-stabilized **laser**.

monocyte: Spherical **white blood cell** with an oval **nucleus**. **Monocytes** are the largest of the **white blood cells**. The **cells** are voraciously phagocytic and exhibit amoeboid movement. They are produced in **lymphoid tissues** and constitute about 5% of all **leukocytes**.

monodisperse model: Model presenting a disperse medium as a monodisperse one, such as an ensemble of **scatterers** with an equal size and **refractive index** for each **scatterer**. Healthy eye **cornea** can be described well in the framework of a **monodisperse model**.

monodisperse system: Disperse system (medium) with a single value of characteristic parameter, such as an ensemble of **scatterers** with an equal size and **refractive index** for each **scatterer**. A healthy eye **cornea** is a good example of a **monodisperse system**, because it consists of dielectric rods with the same **refractive index** and radius dispersed in a homogeneous **ground substance**.

mono-L-aspartyl chlorine e6 (*Synonyms*: NPe6, LS11, talaporfin sodium, or MACE): A **photosensitizer** of the chloryn family with an excitation band around 664 nm. It is used in **cancer** diagnostics and photodynamic therapy. **Laserphyrin**® is the commercialized product. At **PDT**, typical **laser power** dose is 100 J/cm².

monomer (monomeric form): Original compound from which a polymer is formed, e.g., ethylene is the **monomer** from which polyethylene is formed.

mononucleotide (*Related term*: nucleotide): Unit in a long-chain molecule of **nucleic acid**. It is a chemical compound formed from one molecule of a sugar (ribose or deoxyribose), one molecule of phosphoric acid, and one molecule of a base (containing an amino group). **Nucleotides** are also found free in **cells** (see **DNA**).

monounsaturated fatty acid: **Fatty acid** with one double-bonded carbon in the molecule and the rest single-bonded carbons, in contrast to polyunsaturated **fatty acids**, which have more than one double bond.

Monte Carlo (MC) method: Numerical method of statistical modeling. In **tissue** studies, it provides the most accurate simulation of **photon** transport in samples with a complex geometry, accounting for the specificity of the measuring system and **light beam** configurations. The MC technique is employed as a method to solve the forward problem in the inverse **algorithm** for the determination of the **optical properties** of **tissues** (see **inverse Monte Carlo method**). It is based on the formalism of the RTT, where the **absorption coefficient** is defined as a **probability** of a **photon** to be absorbed per unit length, and the **scattering** coefficient is defined as the **probability** of a **photon** to be scattered per unit length. Using these probabilities, a random sampling of **photon** trajectories is generated. The basic **algorithm** for the generation of **photon** trajectories can be briefly described as follows: a photon described by three spatial coordinates and two angles $(x, y, z, \theta, \varphi)$ is assigned its weight $W = W_0$ and

311

placed in its initial position, depending on the **light** source characteristics. When an incident **photon** enters a **scattering** layer, it is allowed to travel a free pathlength l; the l value depends on the particle concentration ρ and extinction cross section σ_{ext}. The free pathlength l is a random quantity that takes any positive values with the **probability density function** $p(l) = \rho\sigma_{ext}e^{-\rho\sigma_{ext}l}$. The particular realization of the free pathlength l is dictated by the value of a random number ξ that is uniformly distributed over the interval $[0, 1]$:

$$\int_0^l p(l)dl = \xi, l = -(1/\rho\sigma_{ext})\ln\xi.$$

If the distance l is larger than the thickness of the **scattering** system, then this **photon** is detected as transmitted without any **scattering**. If, having passed the distance l, the **photon** remains within the **scattering** volume, then the possible events of **photon**-particle interaction (**scattering** or **absorption**) are randomly selected. The direction of the photon's next movement is determined by the **scattering phase function** substituted as the **probability density distribution**. Several approximations for the **scattering phase function** of **tissue** and **blood** have been used in MC simulations. These include the two empirical **phase functions** widely used to approximate the **scattering phase function** of **tissue** and **blood**, the **Henyey–Greenstein phase function (HGPF)** and the **Gegenbauer kernel phase function (GKPF)**, and the theoretical Mie **phase function**. When the **photon** reaches the boundary, part of its weight is transmitted according to the **Fresnel equations**. The amount transmitted through the boundary is added to the **reflectance** or **transmittance**. Since the **refraction** angle is determined by **Snell's law**, the angular distribution of the outgoing **light** can be calculated. The **photon** with the remaining part of the weight is specularly reflected and continues its random walk. When the photon's weight becomes lower than a predetermined minimal value, the **photon** can be terminated using a "Russian roulette" procedure; this procedure saves time since it does not make sense to continue the random walk of the **photon**, which will not essentially contribute to the measured signal. On the other **hand**, it ensures that the **energy** balance is maintained throughout the simulation process. The MC method has several advantages over other methods because it may take into account mismatched medium–glass and glass–air interfaces, losses of **light** at the edges of the sample, any **phase function** of the medium, and the finite size and arbitrary angular distribution of the incident beam. If the **collimated transmittance** is measured, then the contribution of scattered **light** into the measured **collimated** signal can be accounted for. The **standard deviation** of a quantity (**diffuse reflectance**, **transmittance**, etc.) approximated by the MC technique decreases proportionally to $1/\sqrt{N}$, where N is the total number of launched **photons**. It is notable that stable operation of the **algorithm** is maintained by the generation of $(1 - 5) \times 10^5$ **photons** per iteration. The only disadvantage of this method is the long time needed to ensure good statistical convergence, since it is a statistical approach.

motion tracking (*Synonym*: gating): Patient-body motions, i.e., motion of the **heart** or **tumor** due to respiration, **heart** beats, swallowing, and **muscle tremor**, may cause blurring **artifacts**, decreasing image resolution and consequently a limitation in pathology detection or **radiation**-beam treatment. All imaging modalities such as **x-ray computed tomography**, **magnetic resonance imaging (MRI)**, **positron emission tomography (PET)**, **single-photon-emission computed tomography (SPECT)**, **diffuse optical tomography**, **optical coherence tomography (OCT)**, **optical-projection tomography (OPT)**, **acousto-optic tomography (AOT)**, and **optoacoustic tomography (OAT)**—are affected by body movement. The use of advanced motion-**artifact**-reduction techniques, such as respiratory gating, can improve diagnostic image quality and precision of radiotherapy. Using real-time filtering, cardiac and respiratory variations can be separated and used for prospective triggering and gating; for example, this is the basis for a self-gated approach for time-efficient free-**breathing** cardiac imaging. For **MRI** and some other imaging techniques, the gating hardware can be immune to **electromagnetic radiation (EMR)** interferences, thus gating devices that employ acoustic and optical signals should be used.

mouse model: In **cancer** research, an experimental system in which mice are genetically manipulated or challenged with chemicals to develop malignancies in a particular organ or organ site. These models enable researchers to study the onset and progression of the disease, and understand in depth the molecular events that contribute to the development and spread of **cancer**. Ablation of a specific **gene** in mice causes development of **tumors**. For example, there are **mouse models** for colorectal **cancer** and intestinal **cancer**, such as familial **adenomatous** polyposis (FAP), multiple intestinal **neoplasia** (MIN); mouse models for hereditary nonpolyposis colorectal **cancer** (HNPCC); and an **inflammation**-related mouse model of colorectal carcinogenesis that combines azoxymethane (AOM—a genotoxic **colonic** carcinogen) and **dextran** sodium sulphate (DSS). The models allow for studying the development of gastrointestinal **tumors** in the **small intestine**, such as **adenomas**, **invasive adenocarcinomas**, and late-stage **carcinomas**, as well as **dysplastic** microadenomas in the proximal (but not in the distal) **colon** and **inflammation**-related **colon cancer**.

mouth: See **oral cavity**.

mucin: Mucoprotein that forms **mucus** in solution.

mucinous: Pertaining to **mucin** or containing **mucin**.

mucopolysaccharide: See **glycosaminoglycan**.

mucosa (*Synonym*: mucous membrane): **Membrane** consisting of moist **epithelium** and the **connective tissue** immediately beneath it. It usually consists of simple **epithelium** but is stratified near openings to the exterior. It is often ciliated and often contains goblet **cells**. **Mucosa** is found in the lining of the **gastrointestinal** and respiratory **tracts**, and in the urinogenital ducts. **Mucosa** is kept moist by **glandular** secretions.

mucus: Thin, slimy, viscous liquid secreted by **epithelial cells** in **tissues** or **glands**. It protects and lubricates the surface of structures, e.g., the internal surfaces of the greater part of the alimentary canal are lubricated with **mucus**.

Mueller matrix: 4×4 matrix that transforms an incident **Stokes vector** into the corresponding output **Stokes vector** of the sample. It fully characterizes the optical **polarization** properties of the sample. It can be experimentally obtained from measurements with different combinations of source **polarizers** and detection **analyzers**. At least 16 independent measurements must be acquired to determine a full **Mueller matrix**.

multicentered mode: Related to the arrangement of **optical fibers** to improve the imaging performance of **reflectance diffuse optical imaging (rDOI)**. In this mode, several **light** sources are located in the central area of the imaged object, and around these more detectors are placed. Significant improvements in overlapping measurements and image quality are provided. The **contrast**-to-noise ratio (CNR) analysis indicates that the best **spatial resolution** is 1 mm in radius. This method may advance the performance of **rDOI** both in image quality and practical convenience, and is appropriate for exploring activations in the human **brain**.

multichannel optoelectronic near-infrared system for time-re-solved image reconstruction (MONSTIR): Noninvasive imaging technique developed at University College London for studying infant **brain** function that is based on the detection of transmitted pulsed **NIR radiation**.

multichannel plate (MCP): An integrated optical system used for optical amplification (image intensification).

multichannel-plate photomultiplier tube (MCP-PMT): Photomultiplier tube that is integrated with a **multichannel plate (MCP)**.

315

multidimensional fluorescence imaging (MDFI): In general, when maximizing the **contrast** between different **fluorophores** or states of **fluorophores**, it is often useful to analyze **fluorescence** signals with respect to two or more spectral dimensions, as well as three spatial dimensions. For example, utilizing the **fluorescence excitation-emission map** or applying spectrally resolved lifetime measurements can improve the capability to unmix signals from different **fluorophores**, particularly for **autofluorescence**-based experiments, and to improve quantitation of changes to the local **fluorophore** environment. Applied to **microscopy**, **endoscopy** and assay technology imaging, a **MDFI** approach has the potential to add significant value for rapid imaging applications in biomedical diagnostics.

multiflux model: The simplest **multiflux model**, which describes the transportation of **radiation** in a **scattering** medium that employs only two fluxes, is the **Kubelka–Munk model**. A more general approach is the discrete-ordinates method (or many-flux theory) when the **radiation-transfer equation (RTE)** can be converted into a matrix differential equation by considering the **radiance** at many discrete angles. By increasing the number of angles, the matrix solution should approach the exact solution: for **laser beam** applications, the four-flux model makes use of two diffuse fluxes, and one forward and one backward coherent flux; a 3D six-flux model is also available.

multifrequency multiplex: Process in which measurements on many **modulation** frequencies are provided concurrently.

multilayer tissue: **Tissue** that consists of many layers with different structural and **optical properties**, such as **skin**, **blood vessel** wall, and wall of **bladder**. It is evident that all **tissues** are multi-layered, and to model their **optical properties**, one must account for all principle layers, their thicknesses, interfaces, and bulk **optical properties**. However, for some situations, a **tissue** model as a homogeneous **scattering** and **absorbing medium** with a semi-infinite geometry may be adequate, e.g., **breast** or **brain tissue** examined by a low-spatial-resolution optical probe.

multimodal imaging: Imaging approach based on the concurrent application of different imaging modalities in order to improve diagnostic significance of disease. **Optical imaging** techniques are often used together with **x-ray**, **MRI**, or **ultrasound** imaging techniques.

multimode fiber: Single **fiber** that allows the excitation (direction) of many modes (rays), e.g., for a silica **fiber** ($n_1 \approx 1.46$) with a core diameter of 50 μm, **numerical aperture** $NA = 0.2$, and an excitation **wavelength** of 633 nm, the number of excited modes $M \approx 4(V/\pi)^2$, where V is the **fiber waveguide parameter**, equal to 1250. **Multimode fibers**, in contrast to **single-mode fibers**, depolarize transmitted **radiation**. The output **radiation** of the **fiber** is unpolarized; however, for the individual **speckles** created by the **interference** of groups of waveguiding modes, it is polarized, but this **polarization** randomly changes from **speckle** to **speckle**, and thus the total output field is unpolarized.

multimode laser: **Laser** that produces more than one axial or transverse mode with different frequencies and different or similar transverse field distributions. A mode-locked **laser** is a typical **multimode laser** with many axial modes.

multiphoton absorption: Needs a very high density of **photons** (0.1–10 MW/cm^2) from a ps-to-fs-pulsed **light** source. This phenomenon occurs because the virtual **absorption** of a **photon** of nonresonant **energy** lasts only for a very short period (10^{-15}–10^{-18} s). During this time, a second **photon** must be absorbed to reach an **excited state**.

multiphoton fluorescence: Relies on the quasi-simultaneous **absorption** of two or more **photons** (of either the same or different **energy**) by a molecule. During the **absorption** process, an electron of the molecule is transferred to an excited-state molecular orbital. The molecule (i.e., the **fluorophore**) in the **excited state** has a high **probability** ($>10\%$) to emit a **photon** during relaxation to the ground state. Due to radiationless relaxation in vibrational levels, the **energy** of the emitted **photon** is lower compared to the sum of the **energy** of the absorbed **photons**.

multiphoton fluorescence scanning microscopy: Microscopy that employs detection of multiphoton **fluorescence** when the scanning of a **laser** beam induces the multiphoton signal (see also **two-photon fluorescence microscopy** and **laser scanning microscopy**).

multiple scattering: Scattering process in which on average each **photon** undertakes many **scattering** events (approximately more than five to ten).

multispectral imaging: Imaging technique based on the collection of several monochrome images of the same scene, each of them taken with a different sensor. A well-known multispectral (or multiband imaging) technique is **RGB color** imaging. The **wavelengths** may be separated by filters or by the use of instruments that are sensitive to particular **wavelengths**, including **light** beyond the **visible** range, such as **infrared (IR)**. This method allows for the extraction of additional information that the human eye fails to capture with its receptors for red, green, and blue. Multispectral images with more numerous bands, finer spectral resolution, or wider spectral coverage are called hyperspectral or ultraspectral. Multispectral **optical imaging** is a promising technique for biomedical imaging; however, new particular models and **algorithms** will need to be designed. The disadvantage is that the required computation time and memory increase significantly with the number of spectral bands.

multiwavelength multiplexing [*Synonym*: wavelength-division multiplexing (WDM)]: Process in which measurements on many **wavelengths** are provided concurrently.

muscle: Organ of movement that is highly contractile, extensible, and elastic. It is composed of **muscular tissue**. A **muscle** contracts and relaxes. It can also be stretched beyond its normal length and return to its original length and shape when stretching ceases.

muscular tissue: Tissue characterized by its ability to contract after being stimulated by a motor **nerve**. There are three main types of **muscular tissue**, forming three types of **muscle**: striped **muscle**, unstriped **muscle**, and cardiac **muscle**.

myelin: An electrically insulating phospholipid layer that surrounds the **axons** of many **neurons**. It is an outgrowth of glial **cells**.

myocard (myocardium): Muscular substance of the **heart**. It consists mostly of cardiac **muscle**, which is composed of **myofibrils** (about 1 μm in diameter) that in turn consist of cylindrical **myofilaments** (6–15 nm in diameter) and aspherical **mitochondria** (1–2 μm in diameter). Fibers in **myocardium** are oriented along two different axes. It is typically **birefringent** since the **refractive index** along the axis of the **muscle fiber** is different from that in the transverse direction.

myocardial infarction (MI) [*Related term*: acute myocardial infarction (AMI)]: Commonly known as a **heart attack**, it is the interruption of **blood** supply to part of the **heart**, causing **heart cells** to die. This is most often due to **occlusion** of a **coronary artery** following the rupture of a vulnerable **atherosclerotic plaque**. The resulting **ischemia** and **oxygen** shortage, if left untreated for a sufficient period of time, can cause damage or death (infarction) of **myocardium**.

myofibril: Cylindrical organelles found within **muscle cells**. They are bundles of filaments that run from one end of a **cell** to the other and are attached to the **cell** surface **membrane** at each end.

myofilament: Filaments of **myofibrils** constructed from **pro-teins**. They consist of two types, thick and thin. Thin filaments

319

consist primarily of the **protein** actin. Thick filaments consist primarily of the **protein** myosin. In striated **muscle**, such as skeletal and cardiac **muscle**, the actin and myosin filaments each have a specific and constant length.

myoglobin: Variety of **hemoglobin** found in voluntary **muscle fibers**. It has a higher affinity for **oxygen** than **hemoglobin**, and thus assists in the transfer of **oxygen** to **muscles**. Spectra of oxy-, deoxy-, and metmyoglobin are similar to those of **hemoglobin**. See **hemoglobin spectra**.

nailfold capillaroscopy: Capillaries in the nailfold area run in parallel with the **skin** surface and can be made clearly visible by **light microscopy** with a magnification of 200–600×. In spite of the high degree of magnification, movement artifacts can be reduced by fixing the position of the fingernail to the microscope **objective**, while the transparency of the **skin** can be increased by use of **optical clearing agents**. If a video camera is attached to the microscope, the motion of the **RBCs** can be examined in a frame-by-frame procedure, yielding velocity information that can aid the diagnosis of certain diseases. Application of cross-**correlation** techniques improves the **RBC** velocity calculations. Measured **capillary** density, diameter and structure are age-dependent, and the appearance of abnormal **vessels** is related to specific diseases. Some conditions can be detected very early, as **capillary deformations** can be observed before other symptoms occur.

nano-electromechanical system (NEMS): System based on a similarly principled engineering platform such as **micro-electromechanical system (MEMS)**, but using nanotechnology.

nanometer (nm): Unit of length equal to 10^{-9} meter (m).

nanoparticle (NP): A microscopic particle whose size is measured in **nanometers** (nm). It is defined as a particle with at least one dimension <100 nm.

nanosecond (nsec or ns): Unit of time that is equal to 10^{-9} sec (s).

nanosphere: **Fat** particles used to transport biologically active substances to the deep layers of **epidermis** and **hair follicles**. See **liposomes**.

narrow-band filter: Electronic device that selectively damps oscillations of frequencies outside of the narrow band while not affecting oscillations of frequencies within.

National Institute of Standards and Technology (NIST) traceability: A means of ensuring that reference standards remain valid and their **calibration** remains current.

near-field scanning optical microscopy (NSOM) [*Synonym*: scanning near-field optical microscopy (SNOM)]: To overcome the **diffraction limit**, a **light** source and/or a detector that is itself **nanometers** in scale (near-field effects) can be used. In conventional optical systems, the **light** from an aperture is the **Fourier transform** of the aperture in the far field, and optical resolution is **diffraction limited**. NSOM forces **light** through the tiny tip of a pulled **fiber**; the aperture can be on the order of tens of **nanometers**. When the tip is brought within **nanometers** of a molecule, the resolution is not limited by **diffraction** but by the size of the tip aperture (because only that one molecule will see the **light** coming out of the tip). An image can be built by a raster scan of the tip over the surface to create an image. The main drawback of **NSOM** is the limited number of **photons** forced out of the tip of the microscope, and the minuscule collection efficiency for molecule **fluorescence** detection. Apertureless **NSOM** (ANSOM), instead of forcing **photons** down a tiny tip, creates a local bright spot in an otherwise **diffraction**-limited spot and uses a tip very close to a **fluorophore** to enhance the local electric field that the **fluorophore** sees. The ANSOM tip is like a lightning rod that creates a hot spot of **light**. Bowtie nanoantennae have been used to greatly and reproducibly enhance the electric field in the **nanometer** gap between the tips of two gold triangles, trying to enhance a very small region of a **diffraction**-limited spot, and thus improving the mismatch between **light** and nanoscale objects and breaking the **diffraction** barrier.

near-infrared (NIR): See **light wavelength range**.

near-infrared spectroscopy (NIRS): Powerful method in **tissue** studies largely due to the optical window between 600 and 1400 nm (see **therapeutic/diagnostic window**) and the distinct variations in **absorption** by important **chromophores**, especially those involved in the **respiratory chain** (**hemoglobin** and **cytochrome** a) in this region, depending on whether they are bound to **oxygen**. Because both contain a heme moiety they have similar **absorption** spectra, but they can be resolved in the **NIR**. Furthermore, the oxidized form of **cytochrome** has a weak **absorption** peak in this region that changes depending on its **redox** state. Time-domain (time-of-flight) techniques and **frequency-domain** techniques are typically used for absolute measurements of **tissue chromophore** concentration in highly **scattering** and complex **tissues**, which is only possible if the actual optical pathlength of the **laser light** is known. Subsequent time-of-flight studies using **picosecond lasers** and a synchroscan streak camera demonstrated that this pathlength was a simple multiple of the geometric distance between source and detector (5.9 for **brain** and 3.6 for **forearm muscle**). Spatially resolved measurements, especially the **spatially resolved reflectance (SRR)** technique, are also widely used in **NIRS**.

neck: Supports the weight of the **head** and protects the **nerves** that travel from the **brain** down to the rest of the body. The cervical portion of the human spine comprises seven bony segments, typically referred to as C-1 to C-7, with cartilaginous disks between each vertebral body. In addition, the **neck** is highly flexible and allows the **head** to turn and flex in all directions.

necrosis: Death or decay of **tissue**.

necrotic: Pertaining to **necrosis**.

needle-free injection gun: Device that creates enough **pressure** to ensure that medicine penetrates **skin tissue** directly and with the correct distribution. Traditional systems use compressed gas or a spring device to create the **pressure** that triggers the injection. A novel gas-generator system that produces a few **milliseconds** of gas sparks with a pre-determined **pressure** profile at the moment of injection.

neodymium (Nd) glass laser: Silicate or phosphate glass matrix doped by neodymium is the working medium. Nd^{3+} ions provide **gain** at optical pumping. The **Laser wavelength** is 1061 nm for the silicate glass and 1054 nm for the phosphate. These are pulse **lasers** with a high pulse **energy** (up to 10^3 J), broadband generation of 26 and 19 nm, respectively, and a low pulse repetition rate of 1–2 Hz.

neodymium:yttrium aluminium garnet (Nd:YAG) laser: One of the most efficient **solid-state lasers**, whose lasing medium is the crystal Nd:YAG with emission in the **NIR** at 1064 nm; other less-intensive lines at 946, 1319, 1335, 1338, 1356, and 1833 nm are also available. This **laser** is often used at **optical frequency doubling**, 532 nm; the third harmonic of the **radiation** (355 nm) is also widely applicable in photomedicine. Both **CW** and pulsed regimes are available. The typical **power** of the main harmonic (1064 nm) ranges from a few watts to a few hundred watts in **CW** mode. Pulsed **lasers** are characterized by a high repetition rate, 25–300 Hz; their pulse duration varies from a few **nanoseconds** to a hundred **milliseconds**, and the pulse **energy** is 0.05–100 J. The pulse **power** amounts up to several megawatts, the **average power** up to 1000 W.

neodymium:yttrium aluminum perovskite (Nd:YAP) laser: **Solid-state laser** whose lasing medium is the yttrium aluminum perovskite crystal doped with neodymium emitting at **wavelengths** 1054 and 1341 nm, among others.

neoplasia: (1) **Tumor** growth; (2) the formation and growth of new **tissue**.

neoplasm: New growth of different or abnormal **tissue**. See also **tumor**.

neoplastic: Pertaining to **neoplasia**, **neoplasm**.

nerve: Bundle of parallel funiculi with associated **connective tissue** and **blood vessels**, enclosed in a **sheath** of **connective tissue** that forms a tough external coat called the "epineurium."

nerve fiber: See **axon**.

nervous system: An organ system containing a network of specialized **cells** called **neurons** that coordinate the actions of humans and animals, and transmit signals between different parts of the body. In humans and most animals, the **nervous system** consists of two parts, the **central nervous system** and the peripheral **nervous system**.

nervous tissue: **Tissue** that consists of **nerve cells** and their **fibers**, or of **nerve fibers** alone, together with accessory **cells** that surround the **cells** or **fibers**, and **connective tissues** with **blood vessels**.

network analyzer: Two-channel electronic system used to measure amplitude **frequency** characteristics of a four-terminal network, producing **modulation** swept in the wide-**frequency** range (for example, 0.3–1000 MHz) and analyzing the detected signal synchronously in the same **frequency** range.

neurofibromas: Aggregate of all sorts of **cells** and structural elements that **infiltrate** the **nerve** and splay apart the individual **nerve fibers**. Although usually benign, they can sometimes degenerate into **cancer**. Single **neurofibromas** often occur in middle and old age and grow at the margins of the peripheral

nerves, displacing the nerve's main body. The vestibulocochlear (acoustic) **nerve** is the most commonly affected. Other cranial **nerves** and spinal **nerves** are less commonly involved.

neuroglia: Delicate **connective tissue** elements of **nerve tissue** in the **central nervous system**.

neuron: Electrically excitable **cell** that processes and transmits information by electrical and chemical signaling. Chemical signaling occurs via synapses, specialized connections with other **cells**. **Neurons** connect to each other to form networks. They are the core components of the **nervous system**. There are a number of specialized types of **neurons**, such as sensory **neurons**, that respond to touch, sound, **light**, and numerous other stimuli that affect the **cells** of the sensory organs, which in turn send signals to the **spinal cord** and **brain**. Motor **neurons** receive signals from the **brain** and **spinal cord** that cause **muscle** contractions and affect **glands**. A typical **neuron** possesses a **cell** body (often called the soma), **dendrites**, and an **axon**. In the majority of synapses, signals are sent from the **axon** of one **neuron** to a **dendrite** of another. There are, however, many exceptions to these rules: **neurons** that lack **dendrites**, **neurons** that have no **axon**, synapses that connect an **axon** to another **axon** or a **dendrite** to another **dendrite**, etc. All **neurons** are electrically excitable, maintaining voltage gradients across their **membranes** by means of metabolically driven ion pumps that, combined with the **membrane** ion channel activity, generate an electrochemical pulse called action potential that travels rapidly along the cell's **axon** and activates synaptic connections with other **cells**. In general, **neurons** of the adult **brain** do not undergo **cell** division and usually cannot be replaced after being injured, although there are a few known exceptions. In most cases, **neurons** are generated by special types of **stem cells**. Astrocytes have been observed to turn into **neurons**, as they are sometimes pluripotent.

neutral density filters: Optical filters that have a constant **attenuation** across the range of **visible wavelengths** and are used to reduce the **intensity** of **light** by reflecting or absorbing a portion of it. They are specified by the **optical density (OD)** of the filter, and they can be reflective (in which case they look like partially-reflective mirrors) or absorptive (appearing grey or black).

neutral polymer: Polymer that has no electrical charge or ionizable groups such as polyethylene oxide, cellulose, sugar, **dextrans**, polyvinyl **alcohol**, or polystyrene, among others. Some neutral polymers are **water** soluble, others are not.

nevus: General term that refers to a number of different, usually benign, pigmented **lesions** of the **skin**. Most birthmarks and moles fall into this category.

nicotinamide adenine dinucleotide (NAD):   Important **coenzyme** found in **cells**, it plays a key role as the carrier of electrons in the transfer of reduction potential. **Cells** produce **NAD** from niacin and use it to transport electrons in **redox** reactions. During this process, **NAD** picks up a pair of electrons and a proton, and is thus reduced to **NADH**, releasing one proton (H^+): MH_2 + **NAD**$^+$ $\rightarrow$ **NADH** + H^+ + M + **energy**, where M is a **metabolite**. Two hydrogen atoms (a hydride ion and a proton H^+) are removed from the **metabolite**, and the proton is released into solution. From the hydride electron pair, one electron is transferred to the positively-charged nitrogen, and one hydrogen attaches to the carbon atom opposite to the nitrogen.

nicotinamide adenine dinucleotide, reduced (NADH):   The reducing potential stored in **NADH** can be converted to **ATP** through the aerobic electron-transport chain or used for anabolic **metabolism**. **ATP** is the universal **energy** currency of **cells**, and the contribution of **NADH** to the synthesis of **ATP** under aerobic conditions is substantial. However, under certain conditions (e.g., **hypoxia**), the aerobic regeneration of oxidized **NAD**$^+$ is unable to meet the cell's immediate demand for **ATP**. In contrast, glycolysis does not require **oxygen**, but it does require the **anaerobic** regeneration of **NAD**$^+$. The oxidation of **NADH** to **NAD**$^+$ in the absence of **oxygen** is called fermentation.

nicotinamide adenine dinucleotide phosphate, reduced (NADPH): Reduced form of **NADP**. In different types of organisms there are different mechanisms of **NADP** reduction. As an electron donor, **NADPH** is involved in biosynthetic reactions.

nicotinamide adenine dinucleotide phosphate, reduced (NADPH) oxidase: Membrane-bound **enzyme** complex. It can be found in the **plasma membrane** as well as in the **membrane** of **phagosome**. It generates **superoxide** by transferring electrons from **NADPH** inside the **cell** across the **membrane** and coupling these to molecular **oxygen** to produce the **superoxide**. **Superoxide** can be produced in **phagosomes**, which contain ingested **bacteria** and **fungi cells**, or it can be produced outside of the **cell**. In a **phagosome**, **superoxide** can spontaneously form hydrogen peroxide (H_2O_2) that will undergo further reactions to generate **reactive oxygen species (ROS)**.

nitric oxide (NO): Also called nitrogen monoxide, this gas is an important signaling molecule in the body of mammals, including humans. It is an important messenger molecule involved in many physiological and **pathological** processes within the mammalian body, both beneficial and detrimental. Appropriate levels of NO production are important to protect organs such as the **liver** from ischemic damage. However, sustained levels of NO production result in direct **tissue** toxicity and contribute to the **vascular collapse** associated with septic **shock**, whereas chronic expression of NO is associated with various **carcinomas** and inflammatory conditions including juvenile **diabetes**, multiple sclerosis, arthritis, and ulcerative colitis. The NO-signaling G-**protein** pathway is one of the possible mechanisms of **low-level laser therapy (LLLT)**.

nitrogen (N$_2$) laser: Molecular gas-discharge **laser** that works on electronic-**vibrational transitions** with generation in **UVA wavelength** range with the main line on 337.1 nm. **Nitrogen lasers** can only work in a pulse mode but with a high repetition rate up to 1 kHz, which for many biomedical applications is equivalent to a **CW**-mode. These **lasers** are superluminescent, i.e., their **radiation** is an enhanced **spontaneous emission** and **laser** mirrors serve only for reduction of the generation threshold and reduction of **light beam divergence**. The laser efficiency is not very high (0.01–1.00%); the **average power** ranges from a few milliwatts to a few watts; the pulse duration is 1–10 ns; and the pulse **power** is $1–10^3$ kW. **Nitrogen lasers** are good for photochemical applications and **fluorescence** excitation of **tissues**, **skin** in particular.

noise: A term with many contextual meanings; for example, acoustic or environmental **noise** differs from **electronic noise**, which is characteristic to both analog and digital electronics. Signal **noise** is heard as acoustic **noise** if played through a loudspeaker; it manifests as "snow" on a video image. Photon **noise** is characteristic to **photodetectors**. In signal processing or computer modeling, it can be considered unwanted data without meaning. In information theory, however, **noise** is still considered to be information. In biology, **noise** can describe the variability of a measurement around the mean; for example, transcriptional **noise** describes the variability in **gene** activity between **cells** in a population. **Noise** is often distinguished from signal **interference** (e.g., crosstalk) and distortion (unwanted alteration of the signal waveform). A **noise** signal is typically considered a linear addition to a useful information signal—typical signal quality measures of noise use a **signal-to-noise ratio (SNR)**. **Noise** is a random process, characterized by stochastic properties such as its **variance**, distribution, and spectral density. **Noise power** is measured in watts or **decibels (dB)** relative to a standard **power**; the spectral distribution of **noise** can vary with **frequency**, so its **power density** is measured in **watts** per **hertz** (W/Hz).

noise equivalent temperature (difference) [NET(D)]: Temperature difference that is equal to the **r.m.s. noise** signal. It is a measure of thermal resolution and sensitivity, but it does not take into account target size, characteristics of the display, or the subjective interpretation of the operator.

Nomarski polarizing interference microscope: An **optical microscope** with differential **interference contrast** (see **differential interference contrast (DIC) microscopy**) that incorporates a common-path **interferometer** based on a polarizing **prism**.

non-Gaussian statistics: Statistically nonuniform process in which the statistical characteristics of the scattered **light** essentially depend on the observation angle and the degree of nonuniformity of an object.

nongraybody: An object whose **emissivity** varies with **wavelength** over the **wavelength** interval of interest. It is a radiating object that does not have a spectral **radiation** distribution similar to a **blackbody**. Also called a "**colored body**" or "realbody," glass and plastic films are examples of **nongraybodies**. An object can be a **graybody** over one **wavelength** interval and a **nongraybody** over another.

noninvasive: Related to a diagnostic or therapeutic technique that avoids **trauma** to the **skin**, or involves insertion of an instrument through a body orifice, and is free of harmful **radiation**. Many photonics technologies can be counted as **noninvasive** procedures, such as **optical tomography**, **spectroscopy**, and **microscopy**, as well as **laser**-induced **hyperthermia** and **low-level laser therapy (LLLT)**.

nonionic: Not converted into ions.

nonlinear frequency conversion: The conversion of input **light** to **light** of other frequencies using optical nonlinearities. Not all **wavelength** regions of interest are directly accessible with **lasers**. Therefore, it is common to generate **visible light** by nonlinear conversion of **infrared light** from one or several **lasers**. Examples of nonlinear conversion processes: **optical frequency doubling** and sum and difference **frequency** generation in crystals with a $\chi^{(2)}$ nonlinearity parametric oscillation and amplification (also in nonlinear crystal materials); optical rectification, e.g., for generating **terahertz** pulses from optical **picosecond** or **femtosecond** pulses; Raman conversion in bulk crystals or in **optical fibers**, exploiting a $\chi^{(3)}$ nonlinearity (Raman **amplifier**, **Raman shifter**, Raman **laser**); **supercontinuum** generation, e.g., in **photonic crystal fibers**, where a range of different optical nonlinearities simultaneously contributes to the generation of new **frequency** components; and high harmonic generation in gases at extremely high optical intensities of the order of 10^{14} W/cm^2 or higher. Many but not all of these processes can be efficient only with phase matching and with **polarized light**. Laser **radiation** is usually polarized, but some devices (some high-**power fiber lasers** and **amplifiers**) do not emit with a stable linear **polarization** state and are therefore not suitable for **nonlinear frequency conversion**. As **nonlinear frequency conversion** can be efficient only at sufficiently high optical intensities, the **mode-locked** or **Q-switched lasers**, resonant enhancement cavities (resonant **optical frequency doubling**), and **laser** resonators (intracavity **optical frequency doubling**) are used. Waveguiding effects in LiNbO$_3$ **waveguides** or in **fibers** (for $\chi^{(3)}$ processes only) with a long interaction length are also used; **waveguides** with small effective-mode areas can lead to high conversion efficiencies even with low optical powers.

nonlinear optical imaging: Nonlinear **optical imaging** modalities for **cell** and **tissue** high-resolution imaging includes **second harmonic generation (SHG)** and sum **frequency** generation (SFG) techniques that combine **photons** of equal **energy** (SHG) or of different **energy** (SFG) to generate new **photons** with combined **energy**. SHG and SFG are sensitive to noncentrosymmetric biological structures, such as **collagen fibers** and **microtubules**. **Third-harmonic generation (THG)** combines **photons** of equal **energy** to form new **photons** with triple the **energy**. **THG**-based imaging is dependent on optical heterogeneities of probed objects, which include third-order **nonlinear susceptibility**, **refractive index**, and **refraction**. **Two-photon fluorescence (TPF)** combines **energy** of two **photons** to excite one molecule to an **excited state** that subsequently proceeds along the **fluorescence**-emission pathway. TPF is widely used to image fluorescently labeled molecules.

CARS is a four-**wave** mixing process in which a pump optical field $E_p(\omega_p)$ and a Stokes field $E_s(\omega_s)$ synchronously interact with a sample to generate an anti-Stokes field $E_{as}(2\omega_p - \omega_s)$. Because the **CARS** signal is significantly enhanced when $(\omega_p - \omega_s)$ is tuned to a Raman-active vibration band, it allows for chemically selective imaging; this process is a label-free and highly sensitive imaging technique with intrinsic 3D **spatial resolution** and relatively high **penetration depth**. A unique advantage of **CARS microscopy** is its intrinsic capability for multimodal nonlinear **optical imaging**, including SFG and TPF. See also **endoscopic nonlinear optical imaging**.

nonlinear optics: A field of optics that describes the behavior of **light** in nonlinear **media**, that is, **media** in which the **dielectric-polarization density** P responds nonlinearly to the electric field E of the **light** (see **nonlinear polarization density** and **nonlinear susceptibility**). Media include nonlinear crystal materials, **optical fibers**, and structured materials such as **tissues**. For applications, a field of particular importance is nonlinear **frequency** conversion, which generates new optical frequencies. Another wide area is concerned with the effects of optical nonlinearities in various situations, e.g., for the propagation of intense ultrashort pulses in **optical fibers**, biological **tissues**, in **supercontinuum** generation, or for optical signal processing. These nonlinearities are typically only observed at very high **light** intensities such as those provided by pulsed **lasers**. The length of **light beam** interaction is also important. The unique feature of **optical fibers** is that both the high **intensity** and long interaction length needed for efficient nonlinear optical interactions are simultaneously fulfilled at a modest **power** level due to the small core diameter of a **single-mode fiber** and its high optical **transmittance** (see **fiber nonlinear optics**). There are a great number of nonlinear effects successfully used in **biophotonics** for designing unique **light** sources with a number of frequencies (**wavelengths**)—**frequency** tuning and ultrashort pulse generation, **laser light beam modulation** and detection—as well as for designing unique new nonlinear spectroscopic and imaging methods with a superhigh spatial (much lower than **diffraction limit**) and temporal resolution allowing for molecular background-free lifetime and label-free **cell** and **tissue** imaging. See **optical frequency doubling, second harmonic generation, third-harmonic generation, Q-switching, mode-locking, mode-locked laser, mode-locked femtosecond lasers, Kerr lens mode-locking, optical frequency converters, optical parametric conversion, optical parametric oscillator (OPO), pump-beam (pulse), two-photon fluorescence, three-photon fluorescence microscopy, resonance Raman scattering (RRS), surface-enhanced Raman scattering (SERS), stimulated Raman scattering, coherent anti-Stokes Raman scattering (CARS), Raman amplifier, Raman shifter, stimulated Brillouin-Mandelshtam scattering, fiber nonlinear optics, fiber lasers, fiber pulse compressors, photonic crystal, photonic crystal fiber (PCF), supercontinuum, multiphoton fluorescence scanning microscopy, two-photon fluorescence microscopy, three-photon fluorescence microscopy, stimulated emission depletion microscopy (STED-microscopy), fluorescence-lifetime imaging microscopy (FLIM), fluorescence recovery after photobleaching (FRAP), structured illumination microscopy (SIM), endoscopic nonlinear optical imaging heterodyne microscopy, near-field scanning optical microscopy (NSOM), photo-activated localization microscopy (PALM), 4Pi-microscope,** and **ablation by femtosecond NIR lasers**.

nonlinear polarization density: If the **dielectric-polarization density** (**dipole moment** per unit volume) P is not linearly proportional to the electric field E, the medium (material) is termed nonlinear and is described by the field of nonlinear optics. To a good approximation (for sufficiently weak fields, assuming no permanent **dipole moments** are present), P is usually given by a Taylor series in E whose coefficients are the linear and **nonlinear susceptibilities**.

nonlinear regression technique: Related to a model $y = f(x, \theta) + \varepsilon$, based on multidimensional x, y data, where f is some nonlinear function with respect to unknown parameters θ. At a minimum, one may like to obtain the parameter values associated with the best-**fitting** curve.

nonlinear susceptibility: This is the **electric susceptibility** of a dielectric material, which is a measure of how easily it polarizes in response to an electric field. Linear susceptibility is defined as the constant of proportionality relating an electric field E, and nonlinear—relating to E^2, E^3, etc.—to the induced **dielectric-polarization density**; $P = \chi^{(1)} \cdot \vec{E} + \chi^{(2)} \cdot \vec{E}\vec{E} + \chi^{(3)} \cdot \vec{E}\vec{E}\vec{E}, \chi^{(n)}$ is the susceptibility tensor of rank n, which is a property of matter.

nonmonochromatic light: Light that has a broad **wavelength bandwidth** and can be presented as many groups of monochromatic waves with different **wavelengths**. For conventional white **light** sources, such as incandescent lamps, or for **LEDs**, generated **light** has a limited **spatial coherence**, and thus cannot be effectively guided by single-mode **fibers**. Other kinds of non-monochromatic **light** sources, such as **superluminescent light diodes (SLDs)**, **mode-locked femtosecond lasers**, and **laser** systems that generate a **supercontinuum** using single-mode **fiber**- or **photonic crystal fiber (PCF)**-based setups, generate spatially coherent nonmonochromatic **radiation** with a very broad **wavelength** range from 50 to more than 1000 nm around the central **wavelength**.

non-Newtonian flow: Flow of a fluid in which the viscosity changes with the applied strain rate. As a result, non-Newtonian fluids may not have a well-defined viscosity.

nonradiative energy transfer (*Synonym*: nonradiative relaxation): Relaxation of an excited molecule (losing **energy**) without emission of **light** when the molecule's **energy** is transformed into heat, which raises the temperature of the body absorbing the **energy** by increasing the kinetic **energy** of the particles composing the body.

nonradiative relaxation: See **nonradiative energy transfer**.

nonuniform medium: See **inhomogeneous medium**.

normal distribution: See **Gaussian distribution**.

normalization: Normalization is any process that makes something more normal, which typically means conforming to some regularity or rule. In image processing, it is a process that changes the range of **pixel intensity** values, for example, to improve poor **contrast** due to glare. Sometimes **normalization** is referred to as **contrast** stretching or dynamic range expansion in digital signal processing. The purpose of dynamic range expansion is usually to bring an image or other type of signal into a range that is more familiar or normal to the senses. Auto-normalization in image-processing software typically normalizes to the full dynamic range of the number system specified in the image file format. The **normalization** model in medical science is an influential model of responses, for example, of **neurons** in the primary visual **cortex**, where the numerator is the output of the classical receptive field and the denominator is a constant plus a measure of local stimulus **contrast**. The concept of a normalizing constant arises in **probability** theory and a variety of other areas of mathematics. In **probability** theory, a normalizing constant is a constant by which an everywhere nonnegative function must be multiplied so the area under its graph is unity, e.g., to make it a **probability density function (PDF)** or a **probability mass function (PMF)**. In the field of relational database design, **normalization** is a systematic way of ensuring that a database structure is suitable for general-purpose querying and free of certain undesirable characteristics—insertion, update, and deletion anomalies—that could lead to a loss of data integrity.

nourishing (nutritive) cream: Used in **skin cosmetics** for preventing **transepidermal water loss (TEWL)**. These creams easily penetrate to the deep layers of **epidermis**. Skin **hydration** can be provided by two mechanisms—osmotic or physiological. As hydrating substances, **sodium lactate**, **pyrrolidonecarboxylic acid**, and derivatives of **amino acids**, sugars, **proteins**, and

mucopolysaccharides are usually used. As a **hygroscopic** component, **glycerol** is often used (usually less than 10% in composition); however, at present, **glycerol** is usually replaced by a **propylene glycol**.

nuclear envelope: Main structural elements of the **nucleus**. It is a double **membrane** that encloses the entire organelle and keeps its contents separated from the cellular **cytoplasm**.

nuclear pore: Because the nuclear envelope is impermeable to most molecules, pores are required to allow movement of molecules across the envelope. These pores cross both **membranes** of the envelope, providing a channel that allows for free movement of small molecules and ions. Movement through the pores is required for both **gene expression** and chromosomal maintenance.

nucleic acid: Complex, high-molecular-weight biochemical **macromolecule** composed of **nucleotide** chains that convey genetic information. The most common **nucleic acids** are **DNA** and **RNA**. **Nucleic acids** are found in all living **cells** and **viruses**.

nucleolus: A "suborganelle" of the **cell nucleus**, which itself is an organelle. A main function of the **nucleolus** is to synthesize **rRNA** and assemble **ribosomes**. The **nucleolus** is roughly spherical occupying around 20% of the **cell nucleus**, and is surrounded by a layer of condensed **chromatin**. No **membrane** separates the **nucleolus** from the nucleoplasm.

nucleus: Membrane-enclosed organelle found in most eukaryotic **cells**. It contains most of the cell's genetic material, organized as multiple long linear **DNA** molecules in complex with a large variety of **proteins** such as histones to form **chromosomes**. The **genes** within these **chromosomes** make up the cell's nuclear **genome**. The function of the **nucleus** is to maintain the integrity of these **genes** and to control the activities of the **cell** by regulating **gene expression**. In healthy **tissues, cell** nuclei are on the order of 5–10 μm in diameter and have **refractive indices** that lie within a relatively narrow range (1.38–1.41). In **dysplastic epithelium, cells** proliferate and their nuclei enlarge and appear darker (hyperchromatic) when stained. Enlarged nuclei are primary indicators of **cancer, dysplasia,** and **cell** regeneration in most human **tissues.** For example, in healthy **mucosa,** the **cell**-to-**nucleus** area ratio is 5:12; for **carcinoma [carcinoma *in situ* (CIS)]**, it is only 3:4.

numerical aperture (NA): Light-gathering **power** of an **objective** or **optical fiber.** It is proportional to the sine of the **acceptance angle** θ_a, $NA = n \times \sin \theta_a$, where n is the **refractive index** of the medium in which the **lens** or **fiber** operates. A higher NA allows more **light** to be collected by a **lens** or a **fiber.**

obesity: A disease characterized by superfluous development of a **fatty tissue.** A major factor leading to the development of **obesity** is the infringement of **power** balance consisting of a discrepancy between **power** receipts in an organism and their expenses. In other words, processes of lipogenesis prevail over processes of **lipolysis.** Normally, **fat** accumulation occurs only by an increase in the sizes of already existing fatty **cells.** Such growth of a **fatty tissue** is called hypertrophic. However, no **cell** can increase indefinitely. When the quantity of **fat** in a **cell** reaches a critical weight, the cell's predecessors receive a signal and start to breed, giving growth to new **fatty cells.** Such growth of a **fatty tissue,** at the expense of an increase in quantity of **fatty cells,** is called hyperplastic. This phenomenon can take place at any age. Again, formed **fatty cells** are not subject to reverse development and thus remain indefinitely. If the person loses weight, the **cells** only decrease in size. The type most resistant to treatment is hyperplastic **obesity.** Excess weight is associated with two areas: central and peripheral. At the central location of **obesity, fat** is stored mainly in a belly cavity (so-called **abdominal fat**); with peripheral **obesity,** it is stored more under the **skin.** These two types of **fat** do not appear identical in their effect on health. Almost all health problems are connected to central **obesity. Diabetes,** hypertension, and atherosclerosis as

obesity complications are connected to **abdominal fat**. Besides **obesity**, undesirable changes of shape of a human body are caused by **cellulitis**.

objective: The **lens** or mirror in a microscope, telescope, camera, or other optical instrument that gathers the **light** coming from the object being observed and focuses the rays to produce a real image. The **objective** is also called the object **lens**, object glass, and **objective** glass. Microscope **objectives** are typically designed to be parfocal, which means that when one changes from one **lens** to another on a microscope, the sample stays in focus. Microscope **objectives** are characterized by two parameters, namely, magnification and **numerical aperture**. The former typically ranges from 5× to 100×, while the latter ranges from 0.14 to 0.7, corresponding to **focal lengths** of about 40 to 2 mm, respectively. For high-magnification applications, specially designed **objectives** are used with **refractive-index**-matching **oil** or **water** filling the air gap between the front element and the object to allow for the **numerical aperture** to exceed 1, and thus provide greater resolution at high magnification. **Numerical apertures** as high as 1.6 can be achieved with **oil** immersion. Usually the interchangeable **lens** defines the total **field of view** of the optical system.

objective speckle: **Speckles** formed in free space and usually observed on a screen placed at a certain distance from an object.

occlusion: Term indicating that the state of something that is normally open is now totally closed. In medicine, the term is often used to refer to **blood vessels**, **arteries**, or veins that have become totally blocked to any **blood flow**. (For issues of **artery occlusion**, see **stenosis** and **atheroma**.) In dentistry, **occlusion** refers to the manner in which teeth from the upper and lower arches come together when the **mouth** is closed.

occlusion spectroscopy: Most important **blood** parameters such as **hemoglobin**, **glucose**, **oxygen** saturation, etc., influence the optical transmission growth following over-systolic **occlusion** and, therefore, may be extracted from the detailed analysis of the time evolution of optical transmission. This forms a basis for a kind of **noninvasive** measurements, i.e., **occlusion spectroscopy.**

oil: Neutral liquid, soluble in **ether**, hot **ethanol**, and gasoline, but not in **water**. It contains carbon and hydrogen, is capable of combustion, and has a marked viscosity. The main types of **oils** are essential **oils**, fixed **oils**, and mineral **oils**. **Oils** are esters of **glycerol** with **unsaturated fatty acids**, of which the most usually occurring are **oleic acid**, linoleic acid, and linolenic acid. **Oleic acid** has one double bond, linoleic has two double bonds, and linolenic has three double bonds. A neutral **fat**, liquid below 20 °C is usually called an **oil**. It contains a higher proportion of **unsaturated fatty acids** than a solid **fat**.

ointment: Viscous semisolid preparation used topically on a variety of body surfaces. These include the **skin** and the **mucous membrane.**

oleic acid: **Monounsaturated fatty acid** found in various animal and vegetable sources. It has the formula $C_{18}H_{34}O_2$ (or $CH_3(CH_2)_7CH=CH(CH_2)_7COOH$). It comprises 55–80% of olive **oil**.

olfactory tract: Narrow white band, triangular on coronal section (the apex being directed upward), that lies in the olfactory sulcus on the inferior surface of the frontal **lobe** of the **brain**, and divides posteriorly into two striae, a medial and a lateral.

oncotic pressure: The **osmotic pressure** of a **colloid** in solution. For example, a higher concentration of **protein** in the **plasma** on one side of a **cell membrane** than in the neighboring **interstitial fluid** provides **oncotic pressure**. In **plasma**, it is relatively small (~0.5% of the total **osmotic pressure**), but because **colloids** cannot cross the **cell** or **capillary membrane** easily, **oncotic pressure** is extremely important in transmembrane and transcapillary fluid dynamics.

opacity: Characterizes opaque materials (**tissue**).

opaque: In optics and **biophotonics**, an opaque material (**tissue**) is one that does not (or does so poorly) transmit optical **energy**, i.e., **collimated transmittance** T_c and/or **total transmittance** T_t are equal to zero (not detectable). For example, in thermography, an opaque material is one that does not transmit thermal **infrared energy**.

open circuit: In electronics, the absence of a load through which electric current would otherwise flow. This can be represented by an infinitely large resistance or **impedance**.

open-path Fourier transform infrared spectroscopy (OP-FTIR): Spectroscopic technique for detecting molecules in air by their **absorption** of an **infrared** beam.

optic (optical) nerve: Second cranial **nerve**. It is connected to the **retina** and simulated by **light**, and it is the sensory **nerve** of sight.

optical activity: Ability of a substance to rotate the plane of **polarization** of plane- (linear) **polarized light** (see **chirality**). Many **tissue** components show **optical activity**. In **polarized light** research, the molecule's **chirality**, which stems from its asymmetric molecular structure, results in a number of characteristic effects generically called **optical activity**. The amount of rotation depends on the chiral molecular concentration, the pathlength through the medium, and the **light wavelength**. For instance, chiral asymmetry encoded in the **polarization** properties of **light** transmitted through a transparent biological **media** (**aqueous humor** of the eye) enables very sensitive and accurate determination of **glucose** concentration. Interest in chiral turbid **tissues** is driven by the attractive possibility of **noninvasive** *in situ* optical monitoring of the **glucose** in diabetic patients. Within turbid **tissues**, however, where the **scattering** effects dominate, the loss of **polarization** information is significant, and the chiral effects due to the small amount of dissolved **glucose** are difficult to detect.

optical amplifier: See **amplifier.**

optical anisotropy: Difference of **optical properties** of materials caused by the dependence of **light** velocity (**refractive index**) on the direction of **light** propagation and **polarization** of **light** (see **anisotropic crystal**). Manifests as **birefringence, dichroism,** and **optical activity,** as well as **depolarization** at **light scattering** in a medium, polarized **fluorescence,** etc. **Optical anisotropy** may be induced in an optically isotropic medium at external action (mechanical, electrical, magnetic, etc.) that changes its local symmetry. Related effects are **photoelasticity, Kerr effect,** Faraday effect, Cotton–Mouton effect, and nonlinear **optical activity.**

optical attenuator: Device for decreasing the **intensity** of **light.** Optically neutral or **color** filters are usually used as attenuators with a fixed or stepwise-variable **attenuation;** for **polarized light,** an attenuator with a continuously variable **attenuation** of the rotating **polarizer** (**analyzer**) is used.

optical autocorrelator: Device for measuring the **autocorrelation function** of **intensity** fluctuations of a scattered optical field.

optical axis: Direction along which there is some degree of rotational symmetry. The term can be used in several contexts. In an optical system, the optical axis is an imaginary line that defines the path along which **light** propagates through the system. For a system composed of simple lenses and mirrors, the axis passes through the center of curvature of each surface, and coincides with the axis of rotational symmetry. The **optical axis** is often coincident with the system's mechanical axis, but not always, as in the case of off-axis optical systems. An uniaxial **birefringent** material is isotropic within the plane orthogonal to the optical axis of the crystal. Light propagates along that axis with a speed independent of its polarization. For an **optical fiber**, the **optical axis** is along the center of the **fiber** core, and is also known as the **fiber** axis.

optical bench (*Synonym*: optical rail): Piece of equipment used for relatively simple optical measurements, especially for classroom demonstrations. It is a long, straight, sturdy rail of steel or aluminium with a specific profile onto which **light** sources, **lenses**, **pinholes**, **photodetectors**, and other optical and optoelectronic components can be bolted down and easily shifted along the length of the rail. Shorter optical benches can be exploited together with **optical tables** and **optical breadboards** as specific optical mounts.

optical biopsy: Measurement of the localized **optical properties** of **tissues** for diagnostic purpose, it is an analog to ordinary **biopsy**, characterizing *in situ* localized optical **spectroscopy** with typically elastic **light scattering**, **fluorescence** or Raman, which is provided to get information noninvasively or least-invasively on a tissue's health state, in particular its **malignancy**. Endoscopic and confocal geometries as well as **OCT** systems are applicable.

optical birefringence: See **birefringence**.

optical breadboard: A cheaper alternative to an **optical table**, it is a honeycomb panel with $1/4''$-20 or M6 threaded holes that can be placed on an ordinary table or workbench. An **optical breadboard** is not as effective as an **optical table**, but it is adequate for many optical measurements that do not require extremely low levels of vibration. However, its low weight enables one to use simpler approaches to dampen vibrations coming from the floor. The standard top skin is made of ferromagnetic steel. An **optical breadboard** allows one to provide more flexibility and variability in optical scheme design—one can bolt a breadboard onto an **optical table**, build up a module of the experiment on it, and then transfer the module as a whole onto another table without the need to realign the components on the breadboard.

When solidly attached to a dynamically rigid **optical table**, the performance of the resulting working surface becomes comparable to that of the table itself. Simpler and cheaper 15-mm-thick aluminium **optical breadboards** are sometimes used.

optical breakdown: Breakdown in air (and in other transparent **media**) that is initiated by intense **light**. The required **intensity** for **optical breakdown** depends on the pulse duration. For example, for 1-ps pulses, an optical **intensity** of $\approx 2 \times 10^{13}$ W/cm^2 is required. The high optical intensities can be reached in pulses as generated, e.g., in a **Q-switched laser** (with **nanosecond** durations) or in a **mode-locked laser** and amplified in a regenerative **amplifier** (for pulse durations of **picoseconds** or **femtoseconds**).

optical calorimetry: Measuring technique based on detection of a temperature rise in a sample induced by **light beam absorption**.

optical clearing: Controlling the **optical properties** of a **scattering** medium to increase its optical **transmittance** and decrease **backscattering**. Control of **tissue optical properties** *in vivo* is very important for many medical applications. A number of **laser** surgery, therapy, and diagnostic technologies include **tissue** compression and stretching for better transportation of a **laser beam** to underlying layers of **tissue**. The human-eye compression technique allows one to perform **transscleral laser coagulation** of the **ciliary body** and **retina/choroid**. The possibility of selective translucence of the upper **tissue** layers is very useful for developing eye-globe imaging techniques and for detecting local inhomogeneities hidden by a highly **scattering** medium in functional **tomography**. In general, the **scattering coefficient** μ_s and **scattering anisotropy factor** g of a **tissue** is dependent on **refractive index** mismatch between cellular **tissue** components: **cell membrane, cytoplasm, cell nucleus, cell organelles, melanin** granules, and the **extracellular fluid**. For **fibrous** (connective) **tissue** (eye scleral **stroma**, corneal **stroma**, **skin dermis**, cerebral **membrane**, **muscle**, **vessel** wall noncellular matrix, female **breast fibrous** component, **cartilage**, **tendon**, etc.), index mismatch of interstitial medium and long strands of scleroprotein (**collagen**-, **elastin**-, or **reticulin**-forming **fibers**) defines its turbidity due to strong **light scattering**. The **refractive index** matching, which can be provided by **tissue** impregnation by a suitable **optical clearing agent (OCA)**, is manifested in the reduction of the **scattering** coefficient ($\mu_s \to 0$) and the increase of **single-scattering** directness ($g \to 1$). For **skin dermis**, **eye sclera**, **cerebral membrane**, **muscle**, **gastrointestinal** and **vascular tissue**, **cartilage**, and **tendon** in the **visible** and **NIR wavelength** range μ_s, reduction can be very high, followed by up to 90% increase in **collimated transmittance**. **X-ray contrast agents** (verografin, **trazograph**-60 and -76, and **hypaque**-60 and -76), **glucose**, **propylene glycol**, **polypropylene glycol (PPG)**-based polymers, **polyethylene glycol (PEG)**, **PEG**-based polymers, **glycerol**, and other solutions have been tested as effective **optical clearing agents (OCAs)**. Osmotic and diffusive processes that occur in **tissues** treated with **OCAs** are also important. Evidently, the loss of **water** by **tissue** seriously influences its **optical properties** due to less thickness and closer packing of **tissue** compounds. One of the major reasons for **tissue dehydration** *in vivo* is the action of **endogenous** or **exogenous** osmotic liquids. In *in vitro* conditions, spontaneous **water evaporation** from **tissue**, **tissue** sample heating at noncoagulating temperature, or its freezing in a refrigerator will push **tissue** into loose **water**. It is possible to significantly increase transmission through a **soft tissue** by squeezing (compressing) or stretching it. The optical clarity of living **tissue** in that case is due to its optical homogeneity, which is achieved through the removal of **blood** and interstitial liquid (**water**) from the compressed site; this results in a higher **refractive index** of the ground matter, whose value becomes close to that of **scatterers** (**cell membrane**, **muscle**, or **collagen fibers**). Closer packing of **tissue** components at external compression and dehydration makes the **tissue** a redundant, more-organized system that produces less **scattering** due to cooperative (**interference**) effects. As a particle system, **whole blood** shows pronounced clearing effects with the application of the **optical immersion technique**, which may be accompanied by induced or spontaneous **aggregation** and **disaggregation** processes as well as **RBC** swelling or shrinkage following the application of **biocompatible OCAs** with certain osmotic properties.

optical clearing agent (OCA): Chemical agent used to control the **optical properties** of **cells** and **tissues** to decrease **light scattering**, increase **tissue** optical **transmittance**, and reduce backreflectance. Typical OCAs include the following: **x-ray contrast agents** (verografin, **trazograph**-60 and -76, and **hypaque**-60 and -76), **glucose, propylene glycol, polypropylene glycol (PPG)**-based polymers, **polyethylene glycol (PEG)**, PEG-based polymers, **glycerol**, 1, 4- and 1, 3-**butanediol**, among other solutions.

optical clearing potential (OCP): The ratio of values of the **tissue-reduced scattering coefficient** before and after agent action, **OCP** $\equiv \mu'_s$ (before)/ μ'_s (after). **OCP** is measured *in vitro* at agent application to the **dermis** side of human **skin** using a Franz **diffusion** chamber after 20 min application time. There has been no **correlation** found between **OCP** and **refractive index** for agents used with indices from 1.43 to 1.48. Furthermore, there has been no **correlation** with osmolality in a wide range from 1,643 to 26,900 mOsm/kg, but the highest values of **OCP** from 2.4 to 2.9 are provided by agents with both the highest **refractive index** and osmolality, such as **glycerol**, 1, 4-**butanediol**, and 1, 3-**butanediol**.

optical coherence interferometry (OCI): See **Doppler interferometry** and **dual-beam coherent interferometry**.

optical coherence microscopy (OCM): Biomedical modality for cross-sectional subsurface imaging of **tissue**, combining the ultimate sectioning abilities of **optical coherence tomography (OCT)** and **confocal microscopy (CM)**. In **OCM**, spatial sectioning due to tight focusing of the probing beam and **pinhole** rejection provided by **CM** is enhanced by additional longitudinal sectioning provided by **OCT** coherence gating. The significantly better quality of the reconstructed images can be obtained with full-field **OCM** rather than **CM**. A typical compact **OCM** with a flexible sample **arm** and a remote optical probe for laboratory and clinical environment provides an axial resolution of the cellular level when used with a **light** source with an effective **bandwidth** of 100 nm. A **light** source comprising two **SLDs** based on one-layer quantum-dimensional (GaAl)As-**heterostructures** with shifted spectra can be used. Radiation from both **SLDs** can be coupled into a **polarization-maintaining (PM) fiber** by means of a multiplexer that is spectrally adjusted in order to achieve the minimum width of the **autocorrelation function**. Dynamic focusing can be achieved by scanning the output **lens** of the **objective** located at the very end of the sample **arm**; the **lens** movement can be controlled by the electronic system, and it is possible to align the **focal spot** with the coherence gating during scanning up to a depth of 0.5–0.8 mm into a **tissue**. The spectral sidelobes, caused by nonuniformity of the **light** source **spectrum**, should be suppressed for high-quality images.

optical coherence tomography (OCT) (*Synonym*: optical coherence reflectometry): A technique that is based on **Doppler interferometry** with a partially **coherent light** source. In addition to the reference beam pathlength scanning (**z-scan**) that provides in-depth profiling of an object, transverse (*x*–*y*) scanning for 3D images is used. This method is widely used for subsurface **tomography** of **tissues**, and a large number of schemes of **OCTs** for the investigation of **tissues** have been described. The typical time-domain (conventional) tomographic schemes are based on a **superluminescent diode (SLD)** ($\Delta\lambda$ = 30–60 nm) as a **light** source and a **single-mode fiber-optic Michelson interferometer**. The **interference** signal at the **Doppler frequency**, which is determined by the scanning rate of a mirror in the reference arm, is proportional to the coefficient of **reflection** of the nonscattered component from an optical inhomogeneity inside the **tissue**. One can localize an inhomogeneity in the longitudinal direction by equalizing the lengths of the signal and reference arms of the **interferometer** within the limits of the **coherence length** of the **light** source (~10 μm). The transverse resolution of beam scanning along the surface of a sample is determined by the radius w_0 of the **focal spot** of probing **radiation** (usually $w_0 \leq$ 20 μm, which should be consistent with the required length of the probed area in the longitudinal direction and determined by the length of the beam waist, $2n\pi w_0^2/\lambda_0$). Typically, a scanning velocity of 50 cm/s is needed to acquire images with a size of 2.5 × 4 mm^2, (axial size × lateral size), resolution of 20 × 20 μm^2, and **acquisition rate** of 1 image/sec. The scanning velocity should be kept constant with an accuracy of at least of 1% to confine the **Doppler frequency** signal within the detection band. Resonance properties of currently available mechanical scanning systems cannot guarantee constant velocity with required accuracy throughout the **modulation** period. A longitudinal-scanning system based on the **fiber**-optical piezoelectric converter is capable of scanning the pathlength difference between the **interferometer** arms at the rate of 50 cm/s up to 4 mm in depth.

optical coherence reflectometry: See **optical coherence tomography (OCT)**.

optical conjugate: Two optical points, lines, etc., that are so related as to be interchangeable in certain optical properties. The term describes an optical system that provides two points so that a source at one is brought to focus at the other, and vice versa.

optical darkening effect: Controlling the **optical properties** of a **scattering** medium to decrease its optical **transmittance** mostly due to a rearrangement of spatial distribution of **scatterers**, resulting in an increase of **scattering** ability.

optical density (OD): See **absorbance**.

optical depth: Measure of transparency defined as the fraction of **radiation** that is scattered and/or absorbed on a path. The **optical depth** τ expresses the quantity of **light** removed from a beam by **scattering** and/or **absorption** during its path through a medium.

optical detector: Refers mostly to **photodetectors**, but not necessarily because the detection of optical **radiation** and not only the direct conversion of optical **energy** to an electric signal, is possible. Some other phenomena may also be included, such as an optoacoustic effect (detected acoustically by hearing) or **fluorescence** (detected visually by eye).

optical diaphragm: The opening (hole) in a screen that is otherwise nontransparent for **light**, i.e., **light** is allowed to pass through this hole. **Optical diaphragms** vary in size (diameter) and typically have a circular form, although different forms are possible. **Optical diaphragms** are widely used for spatial filtering of **light beams**. See **aperture** and **pinhole**.

optical diffusion tomography: See **diffuse optical tomography (DOT)**.

optical element: Any element that collects, transmits, restricts, or reflects optical **energy** as part of an optical sensing or imaging instrument.

optical fiber: See **fiber**.

optical filter: Device that selectively transmits **light** having certain properties, such as a particular range of **wavelengths** or **polarization** state (see **polarizer**), while blocking the remainder. Attenuating **optical filters**, generally, belong to one of two categories, the **absorptive filters** and **interference** or **dichroic (dichromatic) filters**. They are widely used in photography, **microscopy**, and many other types of optical instrumentation, including biomedical applications. To filter a high-**power light beam**, **light scattering** and multi-reflecting **polarization** stacked-glass-plate filters could be used. For a super-monochromatic filter, a **prism** or **diffraction**-grating monochromator (see **grating spectrograph**) can be used.

optical Fourier transform: Transform when spatial variations in the **optical density** of the object plane are converted into spatial **frequency** variations in the **Fourier transform** plane in the rear **focal plane** of a **lens**.

optical frequency converter: Device based on nonlinear optical **frequency** conversion. For 3-**wave** nonlinear processes, this is the conversion of **electromagnetic radiation** from one **frequency** into two other frequencies, or from two into one. **Second-harmonic generation** is a special case in which two **photons** of the same **frequency** are combined into a single **photon** of twice the **frequency**. Other 3-**wave** nonlinear optical processes include difference-**frequency** generation, sum-**frequency** generation, optical parametric generation, and optical parametric oscillation (see **optical parametric oscillator**). Optical **frequency** conversion can occur when an intense beam of **light** passes through a nonlinear optical material, such as KDP or BBO. By properly aligning the beam with respect to the crystal lattice, it is possible to greatly enhance the **frequency** conversion effect through a phenomenon known as phase matching. This occurs when the interacting **light** travels through the material with the same velocity and phase, extending the interaction distance and increasing the conversion efficiency.

optical frequency doubling: A term in nonlinear optics that describes the behavior of **light** in nonlinear **media**, that is, **media** in which the **dielectric-polarization density** P responds nonlinearly to the electric field E of the **light**. This nonlinearity is typically only observed at very high **light** intensities, such as those provided by pulsed **lasers**. **Optical frequency doubling** or **second harmonic generation** is the generation of **light** with a doubled **frequency** (half the **wavelength**).

optical image: Reconstructed image of an object expressed in terms of local **optical parameters** such as **absorption** and/or **scattering coefficients**.

optical imaging: Application of **light** for the imaging of **cell** and/or **tissue** morphology and functioning (**blood** and **lymph** flow, **metabolism**, etc.). Spectroscopic and nonlinear techniques allow for chemical and molecular imaging. **Optical imaging** methods are divided into diffuse and **ballistic imaging**.

optical immersion technique: Based on impregnation of a **tissue** by a **biocompatible** chemical agent with a **refractive index** higher than the interstitial **refractive index** or by **topical** application of a **hyperosmotic** agent that induces **tissue dehydration**. Both processes cause an increase in the **refractive index** of the **interstitial space** relating to other **tissue** compartments and make **tissue** more optically transparent (less **scattering**). For **cell** systems, such as **blood**, adding a **biocompatible** chemical agent with a **refractive index** higher than **plasma** causes an increase of **blood** optical **transmittance**.

optical injection: Use of **light** to transiently increase the permeability of mammalian **cells** to allow **membrane**-impermeable substances to cross the **plasma membrane** (or more specifically, **optical transfection**), when genetic material is introduced into and expressed by a **cell**. The term **optical injection** is related to the introduction of other molecules into **cells** such as **membrane**-impermeable drugs, impermeable **fluorophores**, or even **antibodies**. There are two categories of **optical injection** (**transfection**)—targeted and untargeted. In targeted **optical injection**, the **focal point** of the **laser** is aimed at the **plasma membrane**, and a tiny hole or pore is generated. Only the targeted **cell** is injected (transfected), while neighboring **cells** remain completely unaffected. An acute reaction to the exposure of the **laser** is often observed under bright field **microscopy**. This reaction depends on the dose of exposure, the **laser** source, and in some cases the presence of chemical absorbers placed in the medium. Typical **laser** sources for targeted **optical injection** and **transfection** include the 800-nm **femtosecond**-(fs) pulsed **titanium sapphire laser**, or **CW light** sources such as a 405-nm violet **diode laser** or 488-nm **argon laser**. The 1064-nm **nanosecond**-(ns) pulsed **Nd:YAG lasers** have also been reported to produce a targeted injection (transfection); however, this **laser** is more often used for untargeted **optical injection** (**transfection**) where groups of 10 to 1000 **cells** are **membrane** permeabilized by direct or indirect **laser** dosing. This may be achieved directly by simply raster scanning a region of interest with a highly focused **laser beam**. The direct method involves dosing a large population with an unfocused **nanosecond**-pulsed beam, whereas the indirect method involves creating a **laser**-induced **shock wave**. In **shock-wave**-mediated injection (transfection), a **laser**-induced **pressure** gradient transiently permeabilizes the **plasma** and/or nuclear **membrane**. This **pressure** gradient is formed by hitting a **membrane** target or the glass-solution interface of the **cell culture** dish upon which the **cells** are sitting.

optical Kerr effect: **Light birefringence** in certain substances that is produced by an external electric field, including high-**frequency** fields up to the frequencies of **IR light**.

optical Kerr gate: Transparent cell filled with a substance showing an **optical Kerr effect** and containing two electrodes placed between two **polarizers**. The cell serves as a high-speed optical shutter.

optical length (*Synonym*: optical pathlength): In a medium of constant **refractive index**, the product of the geometric distance and the **refractive index**. In a medium of varying **refractive index**, the term refers to the integral of the product of an element of length along the path and the local **refractive index**. **Optical length** is proportional to the **phase shift** that a **light wave** undergoes along a path.

optical lens: See **lens**.

optical line scanner: An instrument that scans a **field of view** along a straight line at the target plane in order to collect optical radiant **energy** from a line on the target surface, usually by incorporating one scanning element within the instrument. If the target moves at a fixed rate normal to the line scan direction, the result can be displayed as an image.

optical mean free path (MFP): See **mean free path (MFP) length**.

optical medical tomography: See **medical imaging**, **optical diffusion tomography**, and **optical coherence tomography (OCT)**.

optical microangiography (OMAG): Combination of Doppler and **Fourier-domain OCT**. This is a very powerful imaging modality that images the volumetric microcirculations within **tissue** beds up to 2 mm beneath the surface *in vivo*. The imaging **contrast** of **blood perfusion** in **OMAG** is based on **endogenous light scattering** from the moving **blood cells** within biological **tissue**. Thus, no **exogenous contrast agents** are necessary for imaging. It is applicable for 3D imaging of dynamic **blood flow**, down to **capillary** level resolution, within the cerebral **cortex** in small **animal models** and within the **retina** in humans.

optical microscope: See **light microscope**.

optical microscopy: See **light microscopy**.

optical modulator: Device providing sinusoidal or pulsed **modulation intensity** of a **light** source. It can be internal or external to the **light** source. Many different physical principles are used; the simplest ones are based on **modulation** of electrical current of **power** supply of the **light** source (internal) or on **light-beam** chopping using an electrically driven, rotating, nontransparent disc with **pinholes** periodically drilled on the disc (external). More fast and complex modulators are designed and widely used, such as **acousto-optic modulators (AOMs)** on the basis of the **acousto-optic effect** and electro-optic modulators on the basis of the electrically induced **birefringence** in crystals (see **Pockels cell**). The latter two can also be used to provide phase and **polarization modulation** of **light**.

351

optical mount: Mechanical devices used to place, fix, and join different optical and optoelectronic components to assemble an optical system; for example, to join a camera and another optical instrument, such as a microscope. Optical mounts are used extensively in scientific imaging applications in **biomedical optics** and **biophotonics**. Many companies are designing and producing numerous types of optical mounts from the simplest classical models to modern, comprehensive motor-driven and computer-aided devices. There are plenty of optical mounts on the market that may provide very precise optical measurements with **tissues** and **cells**: holders for self-centering and adjustable **lenses**; variable **lenses**; optical plates; filters; **objectives**; **beamsplitters**; **prisms**; **polarizers** and **lasers**; table clamps and plate, bar, spring, and miniature clamps; base plates with eccentric and rotary clamps; miniature tilt/rotation mount of side control; gimbal mounts (defined as a mount whose axes of rotation are orthogonal and fixed in space. Also, when the axes are made to intersect at the center of the front surface of the optic in the mount, this allows for simple noncoupled rotation adjustment of the optic without translation); round optics, platform, mirror, **prism**, and polarizing cube adapters; precision spatial filters; self-made **pinholes**; y–z mounts; translation (x, x–y, and x–y–z) and five-axis optical mounts; y–z positioners for **lens, pinholes,** and **objectives**; continuously variable attenuators/**beamsplitters**; kinematic mirror and **beamsplitter** mounts; kinematic double optical mounts of side drive; variable wheel attenuators; adjustable **polarizer** holders of side drive; multi-axis tilt platforms; mini rail system ball slide positioners; **fiber** coupling stages; **laser beam** dumps; precise and **micrometer** screws; motorized micro- and nano-positioners, mirror mounts, translation stages, long-travel linear stages, delay lines, rotation stages, closed variable wheel attenuators, goniometers, screws, actuators and **fiber** coupling stages; and power supplies, stepper motor controllers, and software options.

optical multichannel analyzer (OMA): Spectrometric instrument that senses incident **radiation** in several channels at the same time, sorts the **radiation** from deep **UV** to the **IR**, and then digitizes and stores the information so that it can be processed and analyzed individually by the channel.

optical parameters: Physical parameters that characterize the **optical properties** of an object. In **tissues** and **cells**, they are **index of refraction**, **absorption** and **scattering coefficients**, **albedo**, **scattering anisotropy factor**, linear and circular (**optical activity**) **birefringence**, and **dichroism (diattenuation)**.

optical parametric conversion: Crystal materials lacking inversion symmetry can exhibit a so-called $\chi^{(2)}$ nonlinearity (see **nonlinear polarization density** and **nonlinear susceptibility**). Apart from **frequency** doubling and sum-and-difference **frequency** generation, this property allows for parametric amplification (see **nonlinear frequency conversion**) when the signal beam propagates through the crystal together with a pump beam of shorter **wavelength**. **Photons** of the pump **wave** are then converted into (lower-**energy**) signal **photons** and the same number of so-called idler **photons**. The **photon energy** of the idler **wave** is the difference between the **photon** energies of the pump and signal **wave**. As the pump **energy** is fully converted into the **energy** of signal and idler beams, the crystal material is not heated in this process. In the usual nondegenerate case, signal and idler waves constitute physically separate beams. Parametric **amplifiers** are particularly attractive for the generation of **wavelengths** that are very hard to access directly with **lasers** or when properties such as a large tuning range or a high **gain** in a short length are required. Tuning in a very wide **wavelength** range is often achieved simply by rotating the critically phase-matched nonlinear crystal.

optical parametric oscillator (OPO): Parametric oscillator that oscillates at optical frequencies; it converts an input **laser wave** (called a "pump") into two output waves of lower **frequency** (ω_s, ω_i) by means of nonlinear optical interaction. The sum of the output wave frequencies is equal to the input **wave frequency**: $\Omega_s + \omega_i = \omega_p$. The **OPO** consists essentially of an optical resonator and a nonlinear optical crystal. The optical resonator serves to resonate at least one of the output waves. Thus, this is a **light** source similar to a **laser**, but it is based on optical **gain** from parametric amplification in a nonlinear crystal rather than from **stimulated emission**. A main attraction of **OPOs** is that the signal and idler **wavelengths**, which are determined by a phase-matching condition, can be varied in wide ranges. Thus, it is possible to access **wavelengths** (e.g., in the **mid-infrared**, **far-infrared**, or **terahertz** spectral region) that are difficult or impossible to obtain from any **laser**, and wide **wavelength** tunability is also often possible. A limitation is that any **OPO** requires a pump source with high optical **intensity** and relatively high **spatial coherence**. Therefore, a **laser** is essentially always required for pumping an **OPO**, and since the direct use of a **laser diode** is in most cases not possible, the system becomes relatively complex, e.g., consisting of **laser diodes**, a **diode-pumped solid-state (DPSS) laser**, and the actual **OPO**.

optical pathlength: See **optical length**.

optical phase conjugation (OPC): Using nonlinear optical processes, it is possible to exactly reverse the propagation direction and phase variation of a beam of **light**. The reversed beam is called a conjugate beam, hence the name of the technique (also called time reversal, wavefront reversal, and retroreflection). One can consider this nonlinear optical interaction as being analogous to a real-time holographic process. In this case, the interacting beams interact simultaneously in a nonlinear optical material to form a dynamic **hologram** (two of the three input beams), or real-time **diffraction** pattern, in the material. The third incident beam diffracts off this dynamic **hologram**, and, in the process, reads out the phase-conjugate **wave**. In effect, all three incident beams interact (essentially) simultaneously to form several real-time **holograms**, resulting in a set of diffracted output waves that phase up as the time-reversed beam. In the language of **nonlinear optics**, the interacting beams result in a nonlinear **polarization** within the material, which coherently radiates to form the phase-conjugate **wave**. The most common way of producing **optical phase conjugation** is to use a four-**wave** mixing technique, though it is also possible to use processes such as **stimulated Brillouin–Mandelshtam scattering**. A device producing the **OPC** effect is known as a **phase conjugate mirror (PCM)**. In **tissues, turbidity suppression by optical phase conjugation (TSOPC)** is possible.

optical-projection tomography (OPT): Tomography based on detection **of ballistic photons** and/or **quasi-ballistic photons**, which allows for imaging inhomogeneities and quantifying **optical properties** of biological **tissues** with thicknesses from tens of microns to centimeters. Major applications are in developmental embryology and **gene expression** studies, as well as in 3D imaging and quantification within organs of small animals and xenograft **tumors**. Typically, **light** from a uniform backlight traverses the sample to form either projection images captured by a **CCD** camera or **fluorescence** from **fluorophores** distributed in biological **tissue** and excited by a **light** orthogonal to the imaging axis, detected during rotation of the sample around its axis. There have been substantial developments in modeling, reconstructing **algorithms, reflection, refraction,** and **scattering** reduction, and in enhancements of the optical systems used in **OPT**. Several applications of **OPT** would benefit from quantitative reconstructions, that is, reconstructions in which, for example, the intensities of two areas of **gene expression** could be reliably compared; thus, they describe methods of accounting for the quantitative effects of the isotropic emission and blurring in a **fluorescence OPT** imaging system.

optical properties: See **optical parameters**.

optical properties of blood (measurements): Fresh human **blood** placed in a calibrated thin cuvette (thickness from 0.01 to 0.5 mm, slab geometry) is usually used for the determination of **blood optical parameters**. Before the optical measurements, standard clinical tests are necessary to determine the concentration of **red** and **white blood cells**, concentration of **platelets**,

hematocrit, mean corpuscular volume and **hemoglobin content**, and the other parameters of interest. If **blood** sample oxygenation level is of interest, it may be controlled using a conventional **blood** gas **analyzer**. In most cases, the experiments are performed with either completely oxygenated or completely deoxygenated **blood**. To obtain complete **oxygen** saturation, the sample is exposed to air or O_2. To completely deoxygenate **blood**, sodium dithionite ($Na_2S_2O_4$) is added. To be sure that neither the volume nor the surface area of the **blood** particles changes during the experiments, the **pH** of the samples should be maintained in the range of physiological values, at approximately 7.4. In reality, **blood** is flowing through the **blood vessels** and, therefore, it is preferable to study the **optical properties** of flowing **blood**. The **red blood cells (RBCs)** in flow are subject to **deformation** and orientation. At lower shear rates, reversible **aggregation** occurs. While under the higher shear rates, **erythrocytes** are deformed into ellipsoids.

optical rail: See **optical bench**.

optical reflectance (reflection coefficient): Ratio of the **intensity** of **light** reflected from a surface to the incident **intensity**. It is a dimensionless quantity.

optical reflection: Phenomenon of incident **light** going back from a surface without a change to its **wavelength**. It is described in terms of the outgoing **intensity** and angular distribution. See **backscattering** and **remittance**.

optical retarder: Device that provides an optical retardation, **phase shift**, or optical path difference. **Retarders** such as the half- or the quarter-**wavelength** plates provide, respectively, the half-**wave** or the quarter-**wave phase difference**.

optical sectioning (slicing): Process of extracting the optical image of a thin layer of **tissue**. The image is used for tomographic reconstruction of a whole body organ.

optical table: Piece of equipment used for optical experiments requiring the alignment of components with precision down to a fraction of a **wavelength**, typically a few hundred **nanometers**, especially those involving interferometry-based measurements and sharply-focused **laser beam** measurements and treatments. It is protected from environmental vibrations and strains to provide potential sensitivity and **reproducibility** of optical measurements. A modern **optical table** typically consists of a 5-mm-thick, ferromagnetic, stainless-steel top skin and a 3–6 mm-thick bottom skin, both bound under high **pressure** to a honeycomb core by a special epoxy resin. The thickness of the skins depends on the dimensions of the table top. The top skin has a pattern (grid) of $1/4''$-20 or M6 threaded holes that allow the components to be bolted down so that they cannot move even a few **nanometers**. The surface of the top skin is ground to a flatness of ± 0.1 mm over any 1 m^2 area across the entire surface, allowing precision optical mounts to make good contact with the table. Standard honeycomb core is made of 0.25 mm corrosion-resistant coated sheet steel. A special composition of epoxy resin guarantees **adhesion**, rigidity, stability, and damping corresponding to optical measurements requirements. The side walls of the table top are made of a special acoustically hollow plastic that damps acoustic vibrations. Components may also be held to the steel surface by magnets in the base of the optical mounts. Often, the legs of the table are pneumatic vibration dampers. Active isolation systems offer a solution that combines stiffness with a very short settling time; the most useful active systems employ inertial velocity in a feedback loop.

optical thickness: Depth of a material or medium in which the **intensity** of **light** of a given **wavelength** is reduced by a factor of $1/e$ because of **absorption** and/or **scattering** [see **attenuation**]. A sample with high thickness and/or high **turbidity** that correspond to a few **optical thickness** depths is an optically thick sample, whereas a sample with a low thickness and/or low **turbidity** that correspond to one or less than one **optical thickness** depth is an optically thin (transparent) sample.

optical tomography: General term characterizing any kind of **tomography** that uses **light** as a probing **radiation**. Examples include **acousto-optic tomography (AOT)**, **diffuse optical tomography**, **fluorescence diffuse optical tomography (fDOT)**, **fluorescence molecular tomography (FMT)**, **optical coherence tomography (OCT)**, **optical projection tomography (OPT)**, **optoacoustic tomography (OAT)**, **polarization optical tomography**, **sonoluminescence tomography (SLT)**, and **time-resolved optical absorption and scattering tomography (TOAST)**.

optical transfection: Technology where genetic material is introduced into and expressed by a **cell**. Transfection by **optical injection** is now an established technology. It can provide a performance comparable to or better than existing nonviral transfection techniques, with one of its key advantages being the ability to treat individual **cells** in a targeted fashion under aseptic conditions. It is compatibile with other optical technologies such as confocal **laser scanning microscopy (LSM)**, **optical tweezers**, and microfluidic systems.

optical transition: Typically, an **electronic transition** where **energy** is given out as **electromagnetic radiation** in the optical range.

optical transition lifetime: Radiative lifetime, which is determined by the emission cross section for transition to a lower-lying **energy** level.

optical transmittance: Ratio of the **light intensity** transmitted through a sample to the incident **intensity**. It is a dimensionless quantity.

optical tweezer: Scientific instrument based on optical trapping that uses a focused **laser beam** to provide an attractive or repulsive force (typically on the order of piconewtons), depending on the **refractive index** mismatch, to physically hold and move microscopic dielectric objects. Within the **laser beam** waist, a very strong electric field gradient exists to which dielectric particles are attracted along the gradient to the region of the strongest electric field. The **laser light** also tends to apply a force on particles in the beam along the direction of beam propagation. Optical traps are very sensitive instruments and are able to manipulate and detect subnanometer displacements for submicrometer dielectric particles. For this reason, they are often used to manipulate and study single molecules by interacting with a bead that has been attached to that molecule. **DNA** and the **proteins** and **enzymes** that interact with it are commonly studied in this way. **Micron**-sized **cells** such as living **erythrocytes** can be optically manipulated noninvasively without damage. For example, by using two **optical tweezers**, a single **erythrocyte** can be trapped and stretched to investigate its Raman or other spectral properties of mechanical force action. Optical trapping of **gold nanoparticles** has also been demonstrated; however, the extension of the **optical tweezer** technique to **nanoparticles** is not straightforward. The gradient forces responsible for trapping decrease with the particle size, and moreover, non-negligible **absorption** of **nanoparticles** causes dramatic heating at high **laser power**, making the single-beam optical traps unstable. In addition, optical observation of **nanoparticles** that are approximately ten times smaller than the **wavelength** of **visible light** is quite difficult and can be performed only using dark-field **microscopy**. Another approach to **nanoparticle** manipulation uses **light pressure** forces to organize flows of **nanoparticles** in colloidal solutions. The potential applications of **laser**-driven **nanoparticles** are micro- and nanofluidics, where **laser light pressure** forces can be used as a "pump" to drive flows containing **nanoparticles**, even for local submerged-flow organization.

optical waveguide: General term for any optical system that provides optical waveguiding with a low loss. Many types of **optical waveguides** are available. The major principle for low-loss waveguiding is the **total internal reflection** of the propagating **light**. **Optical fibers** are typical **waveguides** that are widely used in **biomedical optics** and **biophotonics**; planar **waveguides**

are typically used in biosensors. Complex holey **fibers** and **photonic crystal fibers** (**PCFs**) are also very promising for optical waveguiding and nonlinear transforming of **radiation**. Holey **fibers** containing a central empty channel of around 50 μm in diameter are potential **waveguides** for biosensing. **Fresnel reflection** from metal surfaces (gold and silver) that is relatively high in the **IR** is used to guide a high-**power IR laser light** for short distances, around 1 m; such **hollow waveguides** with their internal surface covered by a metal layer are used in **laser** systems for **laser** surgery and therapy.

optical-fiber cladding: See **fiber**.

optical-fiber connector: See **fiber connector**.

optical-fiber core: See **fiber**.

optical-fiber coupler: See **fiber coupler**.

optical-fiber dispersion: In optics, **dispersion** is a phenomenon that causes the separation of a **wave** into spectral components with different **wavelengths** due to a dependence of the wave's speed on its **wavelength**. **Dispersion** is sometimes called **chromatic dispersion** to emphasize its **wavelength**-dependent nature. There are generally two sources of **dispersion**: material **dispersion**, which comes from a **frequency**-dependent response of a material to waves, and **waveguide dispersion**, which occurs when the speed of a **wave** in a **waveguide** (**optical fiber**) depends on its **frequency**. The transverse modes for waves confined laterally within a finite **waveguide** generally have different speeds (and field patterns) depending upon the **frequency** (the relative size of the **wave**—the **wavelength**—compared to the size of the **waveguide**). **Dispersion** in an **optical fiber** results in signal degradation because the varying delay in arrival time between different components of a signal "smears out" the signal in time. A similar phenomenon is **modal dispersion**, caused by a **waveguide** having multiple modes at a given **frequency**, each with a different speed. A special case of this is **polarization** mode **dispersion**, which comes from a superposition of two modes that travel at different speeds due to random imperfections that break the symmetry of the **waveguide**.

optical-fiber divider: See **fiber divider**.

optical-fiber multiplexer: See **fiber multiplexer**.

optically pumped gas lasers: These **lasers** work on vapors of high molecular compounds that are optically pumped by another **laser** to produce inverse population. For example, a **laser** on the vapor of formic acid (HCOOH) pumped by the **radiation** of a CO_2 **laser** with $\lambda = 9.27$ μm (25 W) generates a **frequency** with the **wavenumber** of $\tilde{v} = 1/\lambda = 23.13$ cm^{-1} ($\lambda \sim 0.5$ mm) with the **power** of a few milliwatts. For therapeutic purposes, other submillimeter **lasers** may be of interest: CH_3OH (118.8 μm), CH_3I (447.2 and 1250.0 μm), and CH_3OH (570.0 μm), with the output **power** up to a few tenths of milliwatts. Other chemical compounds are also used as **laser media**: CH_3Br (545 and 1582 μm), CD_3Br (351 and 554 μm), CD_3Cl (791 μm), and DCOOH (362 and 528 μm). Submillimeter **lasers** with optical pumping cover a wide range of **wavelengths** from 70 to 1990 μm.

optically thick sample: See **optical thickness**.

optically thin (transparent) sample: See **optical thickness**.

optical-resolution photoacoustic microscopy (OR-PAM): Optical illumination and ultrasonic detection are configured coaxially and confocally in **OR-PAM**. The lateral resolution is determined by the product of the two **point spread functions (PSFs)** of the optical illumination and acoustic detection. Since lateral resolution is difficult to push further acoustically, a more feasible alternative is to use fine optical focusing to provide the lateral resolution while still deriving the axial resolution from time-resolved ultrasonic detection. Within the acoustic focus, only an optically **diffraction-**

limited spot is illuminated by the focused **laser beam**, so the detected **photoacoustic** signal is exclusively generated within the optical focus. **OR-PAM** provides the lateral resolution of **PAM** from 50 μm to 5 μm or even finer. Although having a depth-penetration limit of the same order of magnitude as that of existing high-resolution **optical imaging** modalities—including optical **confocal microscopy**, **multi-photon microscopy**, and **optical coherence tomography (OCT)**—**OR-PAM** is primarily sensitive to optical **absorption contrast**, whereas all of the other modalities are dominantly sensitive to optical **scattering** or **fluorescence contrast**.

optoacoustic flow cytometry: The **flow cytometry** technique that uses optoacoustic signal detection abilities. The major advantage is the possibility to provide *in vivo* studies. It is used for monitoring and **quantitative measurements** of **cells**, including stem and metastatic **cancer cells**, **nanoparticles**, and other absorbing components within the **blood** and **lymph** streams (see *in vivo* **flow cytometry**).

optoacoustic interaction: Generation of **acoustic waves** by the interaction of pulsed or **intensity**-modulated optical **radiation** with a sample. Several effects can be responsible for such interaction, e.g., the optical inverse piezoelectric effect, optical electrostriction, or **optothermal** effect.

optoacoustic (OA) method: Detection of **acoustic waves** generated via **optoacoustic interaction** with a sample (initially the term **OA** referred primarily to the time-resolved technique utilizing pulsed **lasers** and measuring profiles of **pressure** in **tissue**; now the term **photoacoustic** is widely used instead).

optoacoustic (OA) microscopy: **Microscopy** based on the detection of an **OA** signal induced by a sharply focused **laser beam**. See **photoacoustic microscopy (PAM)** and **optical-resolution photoacoustic microscopy (OR-PAM)**.

optoacoustic (OA) spectroscopy: Spectroscopy based on detection of an **OA** signal induced by a monochromatic **light** source (**laser**) with a tuned **wavelength**.

optoacoustic tomography (OAT): Tomography that is based on the **optoacoustic method** or thermoelastic effect. **OA** imaging combines optical **absorption contrast** with ultrasonic detection. **Endogenous** optical **absorption**, for example, oxy- and **deoxyhemoglobin absorption**, is physiologically specific, and thus, in many practical cases, **OAT** does not need specific labeling. Ultrasonic detection enables better resolution in the optical quasi-diffusive or diffusive regime because ultrasonic **scattering** per unit pathlength in biological **tissues** is 2–3 orders of magnitude weaker than optical **scattering**. Combining these two attractive features generates a high-resolution **functional imaging** tool. **Absorption** of pulsed **laser radiation** by the biological **tissue** leads to its heating and subsequent thermal expansion that in turn results in the excitation of the acoustic (or **OA**) pulse. The waveform of the **OA** signal contains information on the distribution of **laser**-induced heat release that in turn depends on the distribution of the optical **absorption coefficient** in **tissue**. Therefore, detection of the **OA** signals by an array of **piezoelectric transducers** allows one to reconstruct the distribution of heat release and to deduce the information on the distribution of absorbing inclusions in **tissue**. **OAT** is applicable in any diagnostic procedure that involves imaging of objects that possess a higher **absorption coefficient** than the surrounding medium. Such applications include, firstly, the image of **blood vessels**, because **blood** is the strongest absorber among biological **tissue** components in the **visible** and **NIR** range. Enhanced **angiogenesis** is typical for **malignant tumors** from the very beginning of their development; therefore, **OAT** shows promise for early **tumor** detection and diagnosis. A number of array designs, employing both optical and piezoelectric detection of the **OA** signals, are available.

optode: Transducer that is attached to the distal tip of a **fiber optic sensor**. The interaction between the optode and the body is monitored by the **fiber optic sensor**.

optogeometric technique: Detection of surface **deformation** in solids and volume changes in fluids induced by an **optothermal interaction**.

optothermal (OT): Related to the process of heat generation by **light**.

optothermal interaction: Generation of heat waves by the interaction of pulsed or **intensity**-modulated optical **radiation** with a sample.

optothermal method: Detection of heat waves generated via interaction of pulsed or **intensity**-modulated optical **radiation** with a sample.

optothermal radiometry (OTR): Detection of time-dependent **infrared** thermal emissions induced by the **optothermal interaction** of **light** with a sample.

oral cavity: The major structures of the **oral cavity** (**mouth**) are teeth. Supporting structures of teeth include **periodontal ligament** and **bone**. Oral mucosal **tissue** and organs include **gingiva** (**gums**), **palate**, lining **mucosa**, **tongue**, **salivary glands**, and **lips**.

oral glucose tolerance test (OGTT): See **glucose tolerance test**.

oral mucosa: The entire **oral cavity** is lined by oral **mucosa**. There are three types of oral **mucosa**: (1) masticatory **mucosa** (hard **palate** and **gingival** with **keratin** on surface), (2) lining **mucosa** (lining of **lips** and cheeks, floor of **mouth**, bottom of **tongue**, soft **palate**), and (3) specialized **mucosa** (covers surface of **tongue**).

oral pain: Pain that originates in soft or hard oral **tissues**, may be localized or generalized; different combinations are also possible. In **soft tissues**, possible pain sources include infection (e.g., abscesses, herpetic **lesions**), mechanical/chemical **trauma**

(e.g., traumatic **ulcer**, aspirin **burn**), immune dysregulation (e.g., recurrent aphthous **ulcers**), hormones (e.g., pregnancy, **gingivitis**), surgery, **cancer** with ulceration, etc. In **hard tissues**, causes of **pain** are mostly **tooth** related due to **inflammation/irritation** of pulpal **tissues** (pulpitis), usually from infection (**caries**). Other causes include: (1) a leaky restoration, (2) a crack in a **tooth**, or (3) **dentinal hypersensitivity. Bone pain** may be caused by dry socket, a painful **bone** condition that can occur 3–5 days after **tooth** extraction, especially after traumatic extractions. **Blood** clotting ceases, resulting in exposure of **bone** to the oral environment. If a stimulus can reach **dentin**, there can be transmission of the stimulus to the dental **pulp** through the dentinal tubules; **pain** results as the **nerve** endings in the **pulp** are stimulated, e.g., at **caries**, bacterial toxins reach the **pulp** through the **dentin**—this causes an inflammatory response that results in **pain**. Other conditions, such as **maxillary sinusitis** and temporomandibular joint disorders, can feel like dental **pain**.

oral submucosa: Loose layer of **tissue** that contains **connective tissue cells, collagen, fat**, and small **salivary glands**. In areas where there is **bone**, e.g., hard **palate, lamina propria** is connected to **bone** by a thin **fibrous submucosa**.

orange G: Synthetic azo dye used in **histology** in many staining formulations. It usually exists as a disodium salt and has the appearance of orange crystals or powder. Its molecular formula is $C_{16}H_{10}N_2Na_2O_7S_2$, with **molar mass** 452.38 g/mol (**Da**). When exposed to **UV light**, it shows a light blue **fluorescence**. The main use of the dye is the **Papanicolaou stain (Pap stain)** to stain **keratin**; it is often combined with other yellow dyes and used to stain **erythrocytes** in the trichrome methods (the major component of the test for pollen staining), and can be used as a **color** marker to monitor the process of **agarose gel electrophoresis** and polyacrylamide **gel electrophoresis**.

organelle: Part of a **cell** that is a structural and functional unit, e.g., a **mitochondrion** is a respiratory organelle. **Organelles** in a **cell** correspond to organs in an organism.

organic light-emitting diode (OLED): LED that employs a small organic molecule compound or organic polymer film as an emissive electroluminescent layer. This layer of organic **semiconductor** material is formed between two electrodes, where at least one of the electrodes is transparent. Such devices can be used in computer displays, as screens of portable systems, and large-area **light**-emitting elements. Currently, **OLEDs** typically emit less **light** per unit area than inorganic solid-state-based **LEDs** that are usually designed for use as point **lights**; however, they can display deep black levels, achieve higher **contrast** ratios, and can be thinner and lighter than **LCD** panels.

Ornstein–Zernice equation: Equation for the **radial distribution function** $g(r)$ of classical many-particle systems. Thermodynamic properties of such systems are determined by the interaction between the particles from which the system is built up. If one knows the **radial distribution function** $g(r)$, one can calculate all thermodynamic properties of the considered system. **Light scattering** properties of such systems also can be calculated.

orthogonal polarization spectroscopy (OPS): OPS can be employed as a single **wavelength** (for example, 548 nm constituting an **isobestic point** of **hemoglobin**) in combination with video **microscopy** (for instance, operating at 30 frames per second), thereby increasing **contrast** and detail by accepting only depolarized backscattered **light** from the **tissue** into the probe achieved by **polarization** filtering. Single microscopic **blood vessels** are imaged *in vivo* at a typical depth of 0.2 mm and magnification of 10× between target and image, and information about **vessel** diameter and **RBC** velocity can be obtained. **OPS** in human studies is limited only to easily accessible surfaces but can produce similar values for **RBC** velocity and **vessel** diameter as conventional **capillary microscopy** at the human nailfold plexus. **OPS** has also been applied to study superficial and deep **burns** to the **skin**, adult **brain microcirculation**, and preterm infant **microcirculation**.

osmolality: The concentration of osmotically active particles in solution expressed in terms of **osmoles** of solute per kilogram or liter of solvent. Normal **serum osmolality** is 270–300 mOsm/kg water. A low **serum osmolality** indicates an abnormally high amount of **water** in relation to the number of particles dissolved in it, which accompanies **edema**. The normal **urine osmolality** is 500–800 mOsm/L, a useful parameter in diagnosing renal disorders.

osmolarity: A measure of the **osmoles** of solute per liter of solution. If the concentration is very low, **osmolarity** and **osmolality** are considered equivalent. In calculations for these two measurements, salts are presumed to dissociate into their component ions. For example, a **mole** of **glucose** in solution is one **osmole**, whereas a **mole** of sodium chloride in solution is two **osmoles** (one **mole** of sodium and one **mole** of chloride), both sodium and chloride ions affect the **osmotic pressure** of the solution.

osmole (Osm): Unit of measurement that defines the number of **moles** of a chemical compound that contribute to a solution's **osmotic stress** (**pressure**).

osmolyte: An osmotically active liquid (molecules).

osmolytic: Pertaining to **osmolyte**.

osmotic phenomenon: Tendency of a fluid to pass through a semipermeable **membrane** into a solution where its concentration is lower, thus equalizing the conditions on either side of the **membrane**.

osmotic pressure: The **hydrostatic pressure** produced by a solution in a space divided by a differentially permeable **membrane** due to a differential in the concentrations of solute.

osmotic stress: Force that a dissolved substance exerts on a semipermeable **membrane** through which it cannot penetrate when it is separated from a pure solvent by the **membrane**.

osteoblast: Mononucleate **cell** that is responsible for **bone** formation. **Osteoblasts** produce osteoid, which is composed mainly of **Type I collagen**. They are also responsible for **mineralization** of the osteoid matrix. **Bone** is a dynamic **tissue** that is constantly being reshaped by **osteoblasts**, which build **bone**, and **osteoclasts**, which resorb **bone**. **Osteoblast cells** tend to decrease as individuals age, thus decreasing the natural renovation of the **bone tissue**.

osteoclast: Type of **bone cell** that removes **bone tissue** by removing its mineralized matrix and breaking up the organic **bone** (organic dry weight is 90% collagen). This process is known as **bone** resorption. **Osteoclasts** and **osteoblasts** are instrumental in controlling the amount of **bone tissue: osteoblasts** mostly form **bone, osteoclasts** resorb **bone**. **Osteoclasts** are formed by the fusion of **cells** of the **monocyte–macrophage cell** line.

osteoporosis: **Bone** disease that leads to an increased risk of fracture. In **osteoporosis**, the **bone** mineral density is reduced, **bone** microarchitecture is disrupted, and the amount and variety of noncollagenous **proteins** in **bone** is altered. It is most common in women after menopause, but it may also develop in men, in anyone with particular hormonal disorders or other chronic diseases, or as a result of medications—specifically glucocorticoids—in which case the disease is called steroid- or glucocorticoid-induced **osteoporosis**.

ovalbumin: Main **protein** found in egg white, making up 60%–65% of the total **protein**. It is composed of 385 **amino acids**, and its relative molecular mass is 45 kD. It is a glycoprotein with 4 sites of glycosylation.

oversampling: Collecting samples (information) at a rate higher than the Nyquist critical **frequency**, $f_c = 1/(2D)$, where D is the sampling interval. It applies to both time and spatial domains.

overtone: Sinusoidal component of a waveform, of greater **frequency** than its fundamental **frequency**. The term is usually used in acoustics.

oxidase: Type of dehydrogenase. The hydrogen removed from the substrate combines with molecular **oxygen**.

oxidative stress: Caused by an imbalance between the production of reactive **oxygen** and a biological system's ability to readily detoxify the reactive intermediates or easily repair the resulting damage. All forms of living systems maintain a reducing environment within their **cells**. The cellular **redox** environment is preserved by **enzymes** that maintain the reduced state through a constant input of metabolic **energy**. Disturbances in this normal **redox** state can cause toxic effects through the production of peroxides and **free radicals** that damage all components of the **cell**, including **proteins**, **lipids**, and **DNA**. In humans, **oxidative stress** is involved in many diseases, such as atherosclerosis, Parkinson's disease, and **Alzheimer's disease**, and it may also be important in aging. However, **reactive oxygen species (ROS)** can be beneficial, as they are used by the immune system as a way to attack and kill pathogens and as a form of **cell** signaling.

oxygen: Chemical element with the chemical symbol O and atomic number 8. It is usually bonded to other elements covalently or ionically. An important example of a common **oxygen**-containing compound is **water** (H_2O). Dioxygen (O_2) is the second most common component of the atmosphere (about 21% by volume) and is produced predominantly through photolysis (**light**-driven splitting of **water**) during photosynthesis in cyanobacteria, green algae, and plants. **Oxygen** is essential for cellular respiration in all aerobic organisms. The diamagnetic form of molecular **oxygen** (O_2) is a **singlet oxygen** ($^1O_2$), which is less stable than the normal triplet **oxygen**. See also **reactive oxygen species (ROS)**. Triatomic **oxygen** (ozone, O_3) forms through **radiation** in the upper layers of the atmosphere and acts as a shield against **UV radiation**.

oxygenation: The combination (binding) of biological molecules in **tissue** and **blood** with **oxygen**, e.g., production of **oxyhemoglobin (HbO$_2$)**.

oxyhemoglobin (HbO$_2$) [oxygenated hemoglobin]: Hemoglobin combined with **oxygen**, it has its strongest **absorption band** at 415 nm (**Soret band**), two secondary **absorption bands** at 542 and 577 nm (Q-bands), and exhibits the lowest **absorption** at **wavelengths** longer than 620 nm.

oxyhemoglobin dissociation curve: Underpins the relationship between **oxygen** partial **pressure** pO_2 and **oxygen saturation** (SaO$_2$). Normally about 97% of the **oxygen** is carried by **hemoglobin**, whereas only 3% is carried dissolved in the **blood**. As the pO_2 increases, the amount of **oxygen** that is bound to **hemoglobin**, or the percent **saturation** of **hemoglobin**, also increases. Normally, at a pO_2 of about 95 mmHg, the **saturation** of **hemoglobin** is nearly 97%. Each gram of **hemoglobin** can carry nearly 1.34 ml of O_2; at 97%–98% **saturation** it actually carries about 19.4 ml of **oxygen**. In the **capillaries**, the **hemoglobin** is only around 75% saturated; thus, about 14.4 ml of **oxygen** is carried, i.e., the **blood** normally delivers about 5 ml of **oxygen** per 100 ml of **blood** to the **tissues**. Shifting of the **oxyhemoglobin** curve in response to physiological changes is called the Bohr effect. Normal **oxygen dissociation curve, saturation** point (plateau on the curve) is defined as $pO_2 = 80$ mmHg:

pO_2, mmHg	100	90	80	70	60	50	40	30
SaO$_2$, %	98	97	95	93	89	84	75	57

In **tissues, hemoglobin oxygenation saturation** is calculated as stO$_2$ = (ctO$_2$Hb/ctTHb) × 100%, where ctO$_2$Hb is the measured concentration of **oxyhemoglobin** and ctTHb is the **total hemoglobin** concentration in **tissue**.

oxymetry: Measurement of **tissue** or **blood oxygenation**.

pacemaker: Local rhythm driver. The region of the **heart** or the skeletal **muscles** around a **vessel** where the nervous impulse that starts the contraction of the **heart** or **blood vessel muscles** is sent out.

pachymeninx: See *dura mater*.

packing dimension: One of the most important notions of **fractal dimension**.

packing factor: The fraction of volume in a medium structure that is occupied by particles. It is dimensionless and always less than unity. For practical purposes, often a medium structure is determined by assuming that particles are rigid spheres.

packing function: An analytical expression for molecular (particle) overlap as a function of position. It can be calculated by means of a **Fourier transform**. Overlap functions between pairs of symmetry elements can be combined to give a crystallographic **packing function**.

pain: Subjective experience caused by system that carries information about **inflammation**, damage, or near-damage in **tissue** to the **spinal cord** and **brain**.

palate: The roof of the **mouth** in humans and vertebrate animals. It separates the **oral cavity** from the nasal cavity and is divided into two parts, the anterior bony hard **palate** and the posterior fleshy soft **palate** or velum. The maxillary **nerve** branch of the trigeminal **nerve** supplies sensory innervation to the **palate**.

pancreas: **Gland** organ in the digestive and endocrine system of vertebrates. It is both an endocrine **gland** producing several important **hormones**, including **insulin**, glucagon, and somatostatin, as well as an exocrine **gland**, secreting pancreatic juice containing digestive **enzymes** that pass to the **small intestine**. These **enzymes** help in the further breakdown of the **carbohydrates**, **protein**, and **fat** in the **chyme**.

Papanicolaou (Pap) stain: Multichromatic staining histological technique. It is used to differentiate **cells** in smear preparations of various body secretions. The specimens can be **gynecological smears**, sputum, brushings, washings, urine, **cerebrospinal fluid**, **abdominal fluid**, **pleural fluid**, synovial fluid, **seminal fluid**, fine needle aspiration material, **tumor** touch samples, or other materials containing **cells**. In gynecology it is used for **cervical cancer** screening (**Pap smears**). The classic form of **Pap stain** involves five dyes: **hematoxylin** (used to stain **cell** nuclei), **orange G (keratin)**, **eosin** Y and **azure** B (counterstaining where **eosin** Y stains the superficial **epithelial squamous cells**, nucleoli, **cilia**, and **red blood cells**), and **light green SF** (yellowish stains for the **cytoplasm** of all other **cells**). When performed properly, the stained specimen should display **hues** from the entire **spectrum**: red, orange, yellow, green, blue, and violet. The **chromatin** patterns are easily **visible**, the **cells** from borderline **lesions** are easier to interpret, and the photomicrographs are good. The **cell** nuclei are stained blue to black. **Cells** with high content of **keratin** are yellow, and **glycogen** stains yellow as well. Superficial **cells** are orange to pink, and intermediate and parabasal **cells** are turquoise green to blue. **Pap stain** is not fully standardized; it comes in several versions, slightly differing in the exact dyes used, their ratios, and timing of the process.

papillary: Related to papilla. **Papillary dermis** is the part of the **dermis** that lies immediately below the **epidermis**; it has vertically oriented **connective tissue fibers** and a rich supply of **blood vessels**. The **papillary muscles** of the **heart** limit the movements of the mitral and tricuspid valves. **Papillary tumors** are **tumors** shaped like small mushrooms, with their stems attached to the **epithelial cell** layer (inner lining) of an organ. Papillary **tumors** are the most common of all **thyroid cancers** (>70%). **Papillary thyroid cancer** forms in **cells** in the **thyroid** and grows in small finger-like shapes—it grows slowly, is more common in women than in men, and often occurs before age 40. **Papillary carcinoma** typically arises as an irregular, solid, or cystic mass that arises from otherwise normal **thyroid tissue**. **Papillary** serous **carcinoma** is an aggressive **cancer** that usually affects the **uterus**/endometrium, peritoneum, or ovary.

Papanicolaou (Pap) smear: **Gynecological smear** technique. This is a screening test that checks for abnormal changes in a woman's cervical **cells** that can sometimes turn into **cancerous cells**. The **Pap smear** test is done during a pelvic exam where the doctor uses a swab to collect a sample of **cells** from the **cervix**. The **cells** are sent to a laboratory to check for abnormalities using the **Papanicolaou (Pap) stain** technique.

parakeratosis: Disorder of the horny layer of the **skin epidermis** manifested by the appearance of **cell** nuclei in this layer. It can be seen in chronic **dermatitis**, such as **psoriasis**.

parakeratotic: Pertaining to **parakeratosis** (e.g., **parakeratotic** focus). The **cell** structure near such a focus is substantially disordered or consists of **parakeratotic** scales.

paraxial approximation: An approximation used in ray tracing **light** through an optical system, where only paraxial rays, lying close to the **optical axis** of an optical system, are accounted for.

paraxial region: Region where paraxial rays, lying close to the **optical axis** of an optical system, propagate. See **paraxial approximation**.

parenchymal cell: Pertains to the main functional **cells** of an organ or **tissue** in contrast to stromal **cells** (nonparenchymal **cells**) that provide supporting structural elements such as **cells** that form the **connective tissue**, **blood vessels**, and **nerves**. For example, hepatic **parenchymal cells** refer to the main functional **cells** of the **liver**, i.e., hepatocytes.

pars conv: Pars (partes) convalescent; a part of convalescent **tissue**.

partial coherence interferometry: See **Doppler interferometry**, **dual-beam coherent interferometry**, **optical coherence interferometry (OCI)**.

partial coherence tomography: See **optical coherence tomography (OCT)**.

partially permeable membrane (*Synonyms*: semi-permeable membrane, selectively permeable membrane, differentially permeable membrane): A **membrane** that allows certain molecules or ions to pass through it by **diffusion** and occasionally by specialized "facilitated **diffusion**." The rate of passage depends on the **pressure**, concentration, and temperature of the molecules or solutes on either side, as well as the permeability of the **membrane** to each solute. Based on the **membrane** and the solute, permeability may vary due to solute molecule size, solubility, other physical properties, or chemistry. An example of a semi-permeable **membrane** is a **lipid bilayer**, on which is based the **plasma membrane** that surrounds all **biological cells**.

particle image velocimetry (PIV): Technique for imaging the velocity distribution of **micron**-sized particles. The most common mode of **PIV** is to record two successive images of moving particles separated by a known time delay. Then, typically, both images are divided into uniformly separated interrogation regions that are cross-correlated to determine the most probable local displacement of the particles. A first-order estimate of the local particle velocity is then obtained by dividing the measured displacement by time delay. When the interrogation region does not contain enough particle images or the noise level is too high, the averaged **correlation** technique may be used for **laminar flow** analysis. A large number of image pairs are acquired, and then the corresponding interrogation regions are cross-correlated for each pair. The average local particle velocity is determined using the average cross-**correlation**. This technique has also been applied to **nanoparticles** moving along the **laser beam** under **light pressure** forces.

partition coefficient: See **permeability coefficient**.

pathological: Pertaining to pathology, the study and diagnosis of disease through examination of organs, **tissues**, **cells**, and body fluids. The term encompasses both the medical specialty, which uses **tissues** and body fluids to obtain clinically useful information, as well as the related scientific study of disease processes.

peak hold: Feature of an instrument whereby an output signal is maintained at the peak instantaneous measurement for a specified duration.

peak power: Power of the individual pulse.

peeling: Body treatment technique used to improve and smooth the texture of facial **skin** using physical (mechanical, acoustic, **laser**, etc.) or chemical action. For instance, a chemical solution causes **skin** to **blister** and eventually peel off. The regenerated **skin** is usually smoother and less wrinkled than the old **skin**. **Alpha (α)-hydroxy acids (AHAs)** are naturally occurring organic carboxylic acids such as glycolic acid, a natural constituent of sugar cane juice, and **lactic acid**, found in sour milk and tomato juices. The mildest of the peel formulas produces **light** peels for treatment of fine **wrinkles**, areas of dryness, uneven pigmentation, and acne.

pellicle: Thin layer of **proteins** from **saliva** that deposit on the **tooth** surface almost immediately after the **tooth** is cleaned. It has protective functions due to its containing calcium and phosphate (which can be taken up by a **tooth**), fluoride (which can aid in **enamel remineralization**), and **proteins** (which kill **bacteria**).

pelvic: Pertaining to the pelvis.

pelvic organs: Includes the **urinary bladder**, ureters and urethra, and the rectum. In males, the prostate, seminal vesicles, and vas deferens are also **pelvic organs**; in females, the fallopian tubes, **uterus**, and ovaries.

penetration depth: Depth in a biological material (**tissue**) to which **light** penetrates. It is defined by the **absorption** and **scattering** properties of a **tissue**. In the **diffusion approximation**, the **light penetration depth** $\delta = 1/\sqrt{3\mu_a (\mu_a + \mu'_s)}$, where μ_a is the **absorption coefficient** and μ'_s is the **reduced scattering coefficient**. This is an important parameter for the correct determination of the irradiation dose in **photothermal** and **photodynamic therapy** of various diseases as well as for the interpretation of **tissue** spectroscopic data. For example, certain phototherapeutic and diagnostic modalities take advantage of the dependence of **transdermal** penetration of **visible** and **NIR light** inside the body in the **wavelength** region corresponding to the therapeutic/diagnostic window (600–1600 nm).

percolation: The movement and filtering of fluids through porous materials. Recent **percolation** theory, an extensive mathematical model of **percolation**, has brought new understanding and techniques to a broad range of topics in physics and materials science.

Percus–Yevick approximation: In statistical mechanics this approximation is a closure relation to solve the **Ornstein–Zernike equation**. Also referred to as the Percus–Yevick equation, it is commonly used in fluid theory to obtain, e.g., expressions for the **radial distribution function** $g(r)$.

percutaneous: Pertains to any medical procedure where access to inner organs or other **tissue** is done through the **skin**, for instance, via needle-puncture of the **skin**, rather than by using an "open" approach where inner organs or **tissue** are exposed. **Phototherapy** is another example of **percutaneous** treatment.

perfusion: In physiology, **perfusion** is the process of nutritive delivery of arterial **blood** to a **capillary** bed in the **biological tissue**. See **blood perfusion**.

perfusion pump: Fluid propulsion systems for providing, for instance, long-term controlled-rate delivery of drugs such as chemotherapeutic agents or analgesics.

periodic acid-Schiff (PAS): Staining method used to detect **glycogen** in **tissues**. The reaction of periodic acid selectively oxidizes the **glucose** residues, creates aldehydes that react with the **Schiff base** reagent, and develops a purple-magenta **color**. A suitable basic stain is often used as a counterstain. **PAS** staining is mainly used for staining structures that contain a high proportion of **carbohydrate macromolecules** (**glycogen**, glycoprotein, **proteoglycans**), typically found in **connective tissues**, **mucus**, and **basal laminae**.

periodontal: A **fibrous connective tissue** attachment anchoring **tooth** to surrounding **bone**. **Collagen fibers** are embedded on the **tooth** side in **cementum** and on the **bone** side in lamina dura. **Periodontal** tissue is composed of **fibers** made by **fibroblasts** (mainly **collagen** with minor amounts of **elastin**) and **ground substance**—**proteoglycans** and **water**. It contains **cells** such as **fibroblasts**, **osteoblasts** and **cementoblasts**, and **immune cells** (e.g., **macrophages**, **lymphocytes**). The tissue is supplied by **blood** via **blood vessels** and contains **nerves**. **Periodontal** tissue has the following functions: supporting teeth in their sockets and absorbing forces of chewing, providing nutrition through **blood** supply to **cells** such as **osteoblasts** and **cementoblasts**, and serving a sensory function through **nerves** that relay signals to the **brain** during chewing.

periodontal ligament: See **periodontal**.

periodontitis: Disease that, due to **inflammation** of the **periodontium**, leads to destruction of the **periodontal ligament**

and surrounding **alveolar bone**, and further **tooth** loss. Types of **periodontitis** include juvenile, aggressive, and chronic. It may or may not have obvious signs and symptoms such as **gingival inflammation** and **pain**. Dental examination, whereby **periodontal** probes are placed under the gumline, can reveal the presence of "pockets" or areas of disease with **tissue** loss that will allow the probe to slide further down the **gingival sulcus** 2–3 mm and cause bleeding during probing, **bone** loss on radiographs, and **tooth** mobility. In accordance with current theory, the disease is the result of interplay between bacterial infection and the host's **immune response**. Only 5–10% of the population suffers from severe **periodontal** disease and ~20% from a moderate form. No simple single bacterium–disease link has been determined, but multiple microorganisms are implicated. Behavioral systemic and genetic factors may determine onset and progression of disease. The disease at each site goes through periods of activity, inactivity, and even regression—pockets in the patient's **mouth** can be at different stages of activity. Undisturbed plaque will, over time, result in **gingivitis**, but not all cases lead inevitably to **periodontitis**—factors related to the host are key in disease onset and progression. **Bacteria** are able to colonize, evade host immune defenses, and cause **inflammation** and **tissue** damage. **Tissue** destruction is due to the action of **enzymes** produced both by **bacteria** and the host's **immune cells**. Unlike **gingivitis**, **periodontitis** is not easily controlled by plaque removal, as the disease is dependent on both microbial and host factors. Composition of **bacteria** in pockets can vary between individuals and, in an individual, between disease sites. Cultures have shown about 300 types of **bacteria** in **periodontal** pockets. The challenge when identifying which specific **bacteria** are actually causing the disease is that certain types of **bacteria** have shown positive **correlation** with **periodontal** disease progression. **Bacteria** associated with **periodontal** disease include *Porphyromonas gingivalis*, *Prevotella intermedia*, and *Actinobacillus actinomycetemcomitans*. Host factors that have an impact on the **immune response** are genetic [variations in **gene** coding for certain immune **proteins** (e.g., IL-1) may be associated with more severe disease], systemic (diseases such as **diabetes** and HIV affect immune function), and behavioral (smoking has been closely tied with **periodontal** disease due to disruption of the immune function and healing). Systemic-link evidence exists from studies of a possible connection between **periodontitis** and cardiovascular events, **diabetes**, preterm low birth weight, and bacterial pneumonia.

periodontium: Refers to the specialized **tissues** that both surround and support the teeth, maintaining them in the maxillary and mandibular **bones**. The following four **tissues** make up the **periodontium: alveolar bone**, **cementum**, **gingiva** or **gums**, and **periodontal ligament**.

peripapillary: Surrounding a papilla. Papilla is a projection occurring in various animal **tissues** and organs.

peripheral nervous system: Consists of sensory **neurons**, ganglia, and **nerves** that connect to each other and to the **central nervous system**. These regions are all interconnected by means of complex neural pathways.

peritoneum: Serous **membrane** that lines part of the **abdominal cavity** and some of the viscera it contains. A fold of **peritoneum** may completely cover certain organs, whereas it may cover only one side of organs that usually lie closer to the **abdominal** wall.

peritonitis: Defined as **inflammation** of the **peritoneum**. It may be localized or generalized, generally has an acute course, and may depend on either infection (often due to rupture of a hollow organ, as may occur in **abdominal trauma**) or on a noninfectious process.

perivascular: Around the **blood vessels**, e.g., **perivascular lymphatics**.

permeability coefficient: Permeability (P) of molecules across a biological (**cell**) **membrane** can be expressed as $P = KD/\Delta x$, where K is the partition coefficient, D is the **diffusion coefficient**, and Δx is the thickness of the **membrane**. The **diffusion coefficient** (D) is a measure of the rate of entry into the **cell cytoplasm** depending on the weight or size of a molecule. K is a measure of the solubility of the substance in **lipids**. A low value of K describes a molecule like **water** that is not soluble in **lipids**.

permittivity: In electromagnetic theory, it is a measure of how an electric field affects, and is affected by, a dielectric medium. It is determined by the ability of a material to polarize in response to the field and thereby reduce the total electric field inside the material. Thus, it relates to a material's ability to transmit (or "permit") an electric field. It is directly related to **electric susceptibility**, which is a measure of how easily a dielectric may polarize in response to an electric field. **Permittivity** ε is measured in farads per meter (F/m), and **electric susceptibility** χ is dimensionless; they are related to each other through $\varepsilon = \varepsilon_r \varepsilon_0 = (1 + \chi)\varepsilon_0$, where ε_r is the relative **permittivity** of the material, and $\varepsilon_0 = 8.8541878 \cdots \times 10^{-12}$ F/m is the vacuum **permittivity**.

perovskite laser: See **Nd:YAP laser**.

peroxisome: Specialized organelle containing the oxidizing **enzymes** that degrade peroxides.

perturbation method: Used to find an approximate solution to a problem that cannot be solved exactly by starting from the exact solution of a related problem. It is applicable if the problem at hand can be formulated by adding a "small" term to the mathematical description of the exactly solvable problem. This method leads to an expression for the desired solution in terms of a power series in some "small" parameter that quantifies the deviation from the exactly solvable problem.

petrolatum: Semi-solid mixture of hydrocarbons obtained from petroleum. It is used in medicinal ointments and for lubrication.

pH: It is formally dependent upon the activity of hydrogen ions (H^+) but for very pure dilute solutions. Being a measure of the acidity or alkalinity of a solution, solutions with a **pH** less than 7 are considered acidic, while those with a **pH** greater than 7 are considered basic (alkaline); **pH** 7 is defined as neutral because it is the **pH** of pure **water** at 25 °C.

phagocyte: **White blood cell** that engulfs foreign bodies, particularly pathogens, by enclosing the body in **cytoplasm** through a process of extending pseudopodia around it (the amoeboid movement for engulfing). In mammals, polymorphs, **monocytes**, and **macrophages** are **phagocytes**. **Macrophages** can be **phagocytes** of other **WBCs**. **Phagocytes** are an important part of the defense mechanism of most animals against invading pathogens.

phagosome: **Vacuole** formed around a particle absorbed by a phagocyte. The **vacuole** is formed by the fusion of the **cell membrane** around the particle. A **phagosome** is a cellular compartment in which pathogenic micro-organisms can be killed and digested.

phantom: Standard experimental **tissue** model (see **tissue phantom**).

pharynx (*Plural*: pharynges)**:** The part of the **neck** and **throat** situated immediately posterior to (behind) the **mouth** and nasal cavity, and cranial (superior) to the **esophagus**, **larynx**, and **trachea**.

phase-cancellation method (*Related term*: amplitude cancellation method)**:** The basis for this method is the **interference** of **photon-density waves** [see **interference of photon-density waves (intensity waves)** and **photon-density wave**]. It uses either duplicate sources and a single detector, or duplicate detectors and a single source so that the phase characteristics can be nulled and the system becomes a differential.

phase conjugate mirror (PCM): Device producing the **optical phase conjugation (OPC)** effect. With the **PCM**, the object image is not deformed when passing twice through an element with **aberrations**.

phase difference: See **phase shift**.

phase fluctuations of the scattered field: Fluctuations that are induced by different optical paths for different parts or time periods of a wavefront interacting with an inhomogeneous generally dynamic medium.

phase function: See **scattering phase function**.

phase lag: Phase shift relative to the incident **light modulation** phase.

phase object: An object that introduces the difference in phase of the **light** transmitted through or reflected by an object.

phase plate: See **lambda (λ)/4-phase plate** and **optical retarder**.

phase retardation in tissues: Form **birefringence** arises when the relative optical phase between the orthogonal **polarization** components is nonzero for forward-scattered **light**. After multiple forward-**scattering** events, a relative **phase difference** accumulates, and a delay (δ_{oe}) similar to that observed in **birefringent crystalline** materials is introduced between orthogonal **polarization** components. For organized linear structures, an increase in phase delay may be characterized by a difference (Δn_{oe}) in the effective **refractive index** for **light** polarized along, and perpendicular to, the long axis of the linear structures. The effect of **tissue birefringence** on the propagation of linearly **polarized light** is dependent on the angle between the incident **polarization** orientation and the **tissue** axis. Phase retardation δ_{oe} between orthogonal **polarization** components is proportional to the distance d traveled through the **birefringent** medium $\delta_{oe} = (2\pi d \Delta n_{oe})/\lambda_0$. A medium of parallel cylinders is a positive uniaxial **birefringent** medium $[\Delta n_{oe} = (n_e - n_o) > 0]$ with its optic axis parallel to the cylinder axes. Therefore, a case defined by an incident electrical field directed parallel to the cylinder axes will be called "extraordinary," and a case with the incident electrical field perpendicular to the cylinder axes will be called "ordinary." The difference $(n_e - n_o)$ between the extraordinary index and the ordinary index is a measure of the **birefringence** of a medium comprised of cylinders.

phase screen: An optical model of an object or a real object providing fixed or controlled spatial variations of the **refractive index** that induce corresponding variations in the **phase shift** of the optical **wave** transmitted through or reflected by the screen. See **random phase screen** and **adaptive optics**.

phase shift (*Synonym*: phase difference): Difference in phase between two **wave** forms. The **phase difference** is measured by the phase angle between the waves: when two waves have a **phase shift** of 90 deg (or $\pi/2$ **radians**), one **wave** is at maximum amplitude when the other **wave** is at zero amplitude. With a **phase difference** of 180 deg (π **radians**), both waves have zero amplitude at the same time, but one **wave** is at a crest while the other **wave** is at a trough.

phase-contrast microscopy: **Microscopy** that translates the difference in the phase of **light** transmitted through or reflected by an object into a difference of **intensity** in the image. It does not require staining to view the object. This type of microscope made it possible to study the cell cycle. The system consists of a circular annulus in the condenser that produces a cone of **light**. This cone is superimposed on a similarly sized ring within the phase-**objective**. Every **objective** has a different size ring, so for every **objective**, another condenser setting must be chosen. The ring in the **objective** has special optical properties: it reduces the direct **light** in **intensity** and creates an artificial **phase difference**

of about a quarter **wavelength**. As the physical properties of this direct **light** have changed, **interference** with the diffracted **light** occurs, resulting in the phase **contrast** image. Phase **contrast** is a widely used technique that shows differences in **refractive index** as difference in **contrast**. The **nucleus** in a **cell**, for example, will show up darkly against the surrounding **cytoplasm**; **contrast** is excellent. However, **phase-contrast microscopy** is not for use with thick objects. Frequently, a halo is formed even around small objects, which obscures details.

phased-array technique: See **phase cancellation method**.

phase-delay measurement device (PDMD): See **cross-correlation measurement device** and **heterodyne phase system**.

phase-sensitive optical low-coherence reflectometer (PS OLCR): See **differential phase-sensitive OCT (DPS OCT)**.

phase-velocity dispersion: Phase velocity of the **wave** is defined as $v_p = dz/dt = \omega/k$, where ω is the **frequency** and k is the **propagation constant** of an **electromagnetic wave (EMW)**. The phase velocity is a function of optical **frequency** because the **refractive index** of a medium, where **EMW** propagates, is a function of **frequency** (**wavelength**), $n(\omega) \equiv n(\lambda); k = (\omega/c)n(\omega) = 2\pi n(\lambda)/\lambda$. There is **phase-velocity dispersion** due to the fact that $dn/d\omega \neq 0$. In the case of normal **light dispersion**, $dn/d\omega > 0$ and $dn/d\lambda < 0$. In the case of anomalous **light dispersion**, $dn/d\omega < 0$ and $dn/d\lambda > 0$.

phenol: Class of chemical compounds consisting of a hydroxyl group (–OH) attached to an aromatic hydrocarbon group. The simplest of the class is **phenol** (C_6H_5OH).

phenotype: Any observable characteristic or trait of an organism, such as its morphology, development, biochemical or physiological properties, or behavior. **Phenotypes** result from the **gene expression** of an organism as well as the influence of environmental factors and the interactions between the two.

phenylalanine: An essential alpha-**amino acid**. It exists in two forms, a *D* and an *L* form, both of which are enantiomers (mirror-image molecules) of each other. Phenylalanine has a benzyl side chain; its name comes from its chemical structures consisting of a phenyl group substituted for one of the hydrogens in the side chain of alanine. Because of its phenyl group, **phenylalanine** is an aromatic compound.

Philly mice: New model for genetic **cataracts** in which there is an apparent defect in **lens membrane** permeability.

phonon: Quantized mode of vibration occurring in a rigid crystal lattice, such as the atomic lattice of a solid. The study of **phonons** is an important part of solid state physics, because **phonons** play a major role in many of the physical properties of solids, including a material's thermal and electrical conductivities. In particular, the properties of long-**wavelength phonons** give rise to sound in solids — hence the name **phonon**, i.e., voice in Greek. In insulating solids, **phonons** are also the primary mechanism by which heat conduction takes place.

phonophoresis: Use of **ultrasound** to enhance the delivery of topically applied drugs.

phosphate-buffered saline (PBS):   Saline solution with phosphates added to keep the **pH** approximately constant. As an **isotonic** and nontoxic-to-**cells** solution, it can be used to dilute biological substances containing **cells**, to rinse containers with **cells**, to provide *in vitro* studies of **tissue** samples put in **PBS** bath, etc.

phospholipids: A class of **lipids** and a major component of all biological **membranes**, along with glycolipids, **cholesterol**, and **proteins**. Study of the **aggregation** properties of these molecules is known as **lipid polymorphism**.

phosphorescence: **Luminescence** that is delayed with respect to the excitation of a sample.

photoacoustic: Related to **photoacoustic (PA) method**.

photoacoustic flow cytometry: See **optoacoustic flow cytometry**.

photoacoustic (PA) method: The term **PA** was originally used to describe primarily spectroscopic experiments with **CW**-modulated **light** and a **photoacoustic** cell. It is now used more broadly as an equivalent to the term **optoacoustic (OA)**. The use of **endogenous chromophores** (e.g., **melanin** or **hemoglobin**) or **exogenous nanoparticles (NPs)** as **PA contrast agents** has demonstrated tremendous potential for imaging **tumors** *in vivo* with higher resolution in deeper **tissues** (up to 3–5 cm) compared to other optical modalities. In particular, **carbon nanotubes (CNTs)**, **quantum dots (QDs)**, and golden **carbon nanotubes** (GNTs) and their clusters with red-shift effects are used as **PA contrast agents**. **PA** detection schematics are also successfully used in *in vivo* **flow cytometry** for real-time counting of circulating **tumor cells** targeted by advanced NPs. The possibility of using the **PA** method for assessing **sentinel lymph nodes (SLNs)** and multicolor **PA** detection of disseminated **tumor cells** (DTCs) in **lymphatics** have been demonstrated. A **PA** imaging technique with microscopic schematic was successfully applied to mapping **lymph nodes** with depths up to ~3 cm in **animal models** using blue dyes and NPs as **contrast agents**. It is important to note **PA** detection of metastasis in **SLNs** can be integrated with their **photothermal (PT)** purging using a **fiber**-based multimodal diagnostic-therapeutic platform with time-resolved multicolor **PA** lymphography, **PA lymph flow cytometry**, and **photothermal therapy**. See also **optoacoustic (OA) method**.

photoacoustic microscopy (PAM): **Microscopy** utilizing the **photoacoustic method** and sometimes a **photoacoustic** cell for signal detection. **PAM** can overcome many limitations characteristic of other microscopies, including confocal and multi-photon, as it relies on **endogenous** optical **absorption contrast** and works in **reflection** mode noninvasively with time-resolved depth detection. With multi-**wavelength** measurements, **PAM** can accurately assess **hemoglobin oxygenation** within each single **vessel**, providing a convenient and robust tool for **functional imaging**. However, the **spatial resolution** in the **PAM** design is limited by ultrasonic parameters, making it blind to **capillaries** as well as small **arterioles** and venules (<50 μm).

photoacoustic tomography (PAT): See **optoacoustic tomography (OAT)**.

photo-activated localization microscopy (PALM): Also called **stochastic optical reconstruction microscopy (STORM)**. The basis of the technique is to fill the imaging area with many dark **fluorophores** that can be photoactivated into a fluorescing state by a flash of **light**. Because photoactivation is stochastic, only a few well-separated molecules "turn on." Gaussians are then fit to their **PSFs** with high precision. After the few bright dots photobleach, another flash of the photoactivating **light** activates random **fluorophores** again, and the **PSFs** are fit of these different well-spaced objects. This process is repeated many times, building up an image molecule by molecule. Because the molecules were localized at different times, the "resolution" (inverse distance between objects) of the final image can be much higher than that limited by **diffraction**. To collect the data for good images, time on the order of hours is needed.

photo-aging: This condition is most noticeable in women who have spent hours in the sun without the benefit of **sunscreen**. The most obvious symptoms of **photo-aging** are dark age spots on the face and décolleté, deep **wrinkles** around the eyes, fine lines, leathery **skin**, a gradual thickening of the **skin**, and uneven complexion.

photobleaching: Removing **color** from a sample by irradiating it with **light** of a certain **wavelength** and **intensity**. In photochemotherapy, the **photosensitizer** can be photobleached, either permanently or transiently, by the treatment **light**. The term "**photobleaching**" is variously used to denote actual photochemical destruction of the **photosensitizer** or simply decreased optical **absorbance** and/or **fluorescence**, which may not be equal and which does not necessarily involve molecular decomposition. For example, the irreversible decomposition (formation of nonfluorescent product) of fluorescent molecules in the **excited state** before **fluorescence** emission may occur because of their interaction with molecular **oxygen** (or impurities in the solution). The average number of excitation and emission cycles that occur for a particular **fluorophore** before **photobleaching** is dependent upon its molecular structure and the local environment. Some **fluorophores** bleach quickly after emitting only a few **photons**, while others can undergo thousands or millions of cycles before bleaching occurs. Several mechanisms could lead to **photobleaching** of a **fluorophore**, typically involving long-lived **triplet states** and/or radical states. At different experimental conditions, **oxygen** can either enhance or reduce **photobleaching** affecting the equilibrium between triplet quenching and radical formation. The **photobleaching** effect can also be utilized to obtain specific information that would not be otherwise be available, for example, in **FRAP** measurements.

photocatalytic effect: The basis for so-called advanced oxidation technologies that produces free hydroxyl **radicals** •OH, which have a highly oxidizing **power** superior to other oxidants. When the •OH **radicals** are generated by either illumination of **semiconductors** with lamps, **LEDs**, and **lasers** or sunlight in **water**, **bacteria** suspensions, or **tissues**, this is termed photocatalysis. The photocatalytic degradation of various toxic organic compounds (particularly organochlorides and nitrogenous compounds) has been proposed as a viable process to detoxify drinking **water**. Irradiating pulverulent **semiconductors** like titanium dioxide (TiO_2) in suspension (or fixed to various supports in aqueous solutions containing organic pollutants) creates a **redox** environment able to destroy these pollutants. TiO_2 has been demonstrated to be an excellent photocatalyst, and the EPA (US Environmental Protection Agency) made an inventory of more than 800 molecules that can be degraded by this process, including **bacteria** killing. The basic process of photocatalysis consists of ejecting an electron from the valence band to the conduction band of the TiO_2 semiconductor and creating a hole in the valence band. This is due to **UV** irradiation of TiO_2 with an **energy** equal or superior to the **bandgap** (>3.2 eV). This is followed by the formation of extremely reactive **radicals** (like •OH) at the **semiconductor** surface and/or a direct oxidation of the polluting species (R). The ejected electrons react with electron acceptors such as **oxygen** adsorbed or dissolved in **water**. Also, the electrons and holes may recombine without electron donors or acceptors. While mechanisms involved in these phenomena are not yet perfectly known, a few technological applications have been developed and have shown their feasibility to detoxify drinking **water**, to destroy pollutants, and **bacteria**, and for the **photobleaching** of plant **cell** mass and human teeth.

photocathode: **Cathode** that emits electrons when activated by **light** or other **radiation**. It is used in **photodetectors**, **PMTs** in particular.

photochemical (photobiochemical) reaction: Chemical reaction in a living organism that is induced by **light**. It causes the change of chemical bonds and forms toxic **radicals**, such as the release of **singlet oxygen**, leading to the death of organized **tissues**, as in the case of **photodynamic therapy**. Photochemical interaction of **light** and **tissue** is of great interest for the understanding of **tissue** damage induced by solar **radiation**, in particular in the **skin**-aging process, as well as for the designing of controllable technologies for **tissue** repair and rejuvenation. Such interaction depends on the type of **endogenous** or **exogenous chromophore** (**photosensitizer**) involved in photochemical reaction, **oxygen** tension, and **light wavelength**, **intensity**, and exposure. To characterize a photochemical reaction, a **quantum yield** is introduced.

photochemical therapy: Branch of therapy that deals with the biochemical action of **light** on a **tissue** photosensitized by the

389

appropriate chemical or a chemical that induces the photosensitive agent in **tissue**, e.g., **photodynamic therapy**, **PUVA therapy**.

photocoagulation: **Coagulation** (clotting) of **tissue** using a **laser** (or lamp) that produces **light** in the **visible** (green) **wavelength** that is selectively absorbed by **hemoglobin**, the **pigment** in **red blood cells**, in order to seal off bleeding **blood vessels**. **Photocoagulation** has diverse uses, for example, in **cancer** treatment to destroy **blood vessels** entering a **tumor** and deprive it of nutrients, in the treatment of a detached **retina** to destroy abnormal **blood vessels** in the **retina**, to treat **tumors** in the eye, etc. **NIR light** that is selectively absorbed by slightly intensive **water** and **fat** bands is also used for **tissue coagulation**, for instance, in the treatment of gastric **ulcers**.

photoconductive detector: Photodetector in which an electric potential is applied across the absorbing region and causes a current to flow in proportion to the **irradiance** if the **photon energy** exceeds the **energy** gap between the valence and the conduction band. For the **visible wavelength range**— cadmium sulfide, for **IR**—lead sulfide, silicon doped with arsenide (Si:As), and **mercury-cadmium-telluride (HgCdTe)** are used as photoconductive materials.

photodestruction: Destruction of a **tissue**, a **cell**, or their parts by intensive **light** (**coagulation**, **ablation**) or photochemically by **light** with a moderate **intensity** (**necrosis**). Intensive or focused **laser beams** are usually used.

photodetector: Device that converts optical **energy** to an electric signal. There are numerous optical detectors available on the market that provide a high-sensitive, low-noise, low- and high-optical power detection. They can be relatively slow or extremely fast, with single and multiple detection areas (**pixels**) working in the **UV**, **visible**, and **IR** spectral ranges. Vacuum **photodetectors** such as photocell, **photomultiplier** [**photomultiplier tube (PMT)**], and transmitting television tube (see **dissector**) have been used in **optical imaging**, **microscopy**, and **spectroscopy** from the very beginning. For example, the modern version of the **PMT**, is the **multichannel plate-photomultiplier tube (MCP-PMT)**, which is a highly sensitive and fast image detector. There is a broad class of **photodetectors** and **photodiodes** that are very sensitive, fast, compact, and usually low-cost, such as **PIN photodiode** and **avalanche photodiodes (APDs)**. Solid-state photoconductive detectors are typically used as sensitive **infrared detectors**. **CCDs**, **CMOS** devices, and thermal cameras use solid-state matrix detection and are widely used in biophotonic medical instrumentation. See also **dark noise**, **electronic noise**, **gain**, **quantum detection limit**, **quantum efficiency**, **photon noise**, and **photon shot noise**.

photodiode: Type of **photodetector** capable of converting **light** into either current or voltage, depending upon the mode of operation. **Photodiodes** are **semiconductor** diodes that may be either exposed (to detect vacuum **UV** or **x-rays**) or packaged with a window or **optical fiber** connection ("pig tail") to allow **light** to reach the sensitive part of the device. A **photodiode** is a $p–n$ junction or $p–i–n$ structure. When a **photon** of sufficient **energy** strikes the **photodiode**, it excites an electron, thereby creating a mobile electron and a positively charged electron hole. If the **absorption** occurs in the junction's depletion region, or one **diffusion** length away from it, these carriers are swept from the junction by the built-in field of the depletion region. Thus, holes move toward the anode, electrons move toward the **cathode**, and a photocurrent is produced. For photovoltaic mode at zero bias, the flow of photocurrent out of the device is restricted and a voltage builds up. This is the basis for solar **cells**. In this mode the **photodiode** is often reverse biased, dramatically reducing the response time at the expense of increased noise. This increases the width of the depletion layer, which decreases the junction's capacitance and results in faster response times. The photocurrent is linearly proportional to the **luminance**. The leakage current of a good **PIN photodiode** is so low (<1 nA) that the thermal noise (Johnson–Nyquist noise) of the load resistance in a typical circuit often dominates. **Avalanche photodiodes (APDs)** have a similar structure to regular **photodiodes**, but they are operated with much higher reverse bias, which allows each photo-generated carrier to be multiplied by avalanche breakdown, resulting in internal **gain** within the **photodiode**. The following **photodiodes** provide good sensitivity in their respective **wavelength** ranges: silicon (190–1100 nm), germanium (400–1700 nm), indium gallium arsenide (800–2600 nm), and lead (II) sulfide (<1000–3500 nm). For detection of longer **wavelengths**, **indium antimonide (InSb)** and **mercury cadmium telluride (HgCdTe)** materials are used. Because of their greater **bandgap**, silicon **photodiodes** generate less noise than germanium **photodiodes**. Compared to **photomultipliers**, **photodiodes** have the following advantages: excellent linearity of output current as a function of incident **light**, spectral response from 190–1100 nm (silicon), longer **wavelengths** than other **semiconductor** materials, low noise, high **quantum efficiency** (typically 80%), long lifetime, low cost, compact size and lightweight, and no high voltage requirement. Disadvantages compared to **photomultipliers** are a small area with no or relatively small internal **gain** (for **APD** of 10^2–10^3 compared to up to 10^8 for the **photomultiplier**), and thus much lower overall sensitivity. Only specially designed, usually cooled **photodiodes** with special electronic circuits can be used in **photon**-counting systems. Photodiodes based on **heterostructure** technology are very fast and work in **NIR** range with a high efficiency. For example, **photodiodes** on InGaAs-InGaAlAs-InAlAs **heterostructures** on GaAs substrates provide a low dark current of 500 pA, a responsivity of 0.6 A/W, and a broad **bandwidth** (−3 dB level) of 38 GHz (−5 V reverse bias) for 1.55-μm **radiation**. **Photodiodes** sensitive in the **wavelength** range of 1.1–2.4 μm have been created based on n-GaSb/n-GaInAsSb/p-AlGaAsSb **heterostructures** with a narrow-gap n-GaInAsSb layer.

photodiode array (PDA): Hundreds or thousands (up to 2048) of **photodiodes** of typical sensitive area 0.025 × 1 mm each arranged as a 1D array, which can be used as a position sensor. One advantage of **PDAs** is that they allow for high-speed parallel read out since the driving electronics may not be integrated like a traditional **CMOS** or **CCD** sensor. They are often used in a high-speed **spectroscopy** of biological objects as a detector.

photodisruption: Localized breakdown of semi-transparent biological **tissues** that do not strongly absorb **light** in the **visible** range by an intensive, tightly-focused **femtosecond laser** pulse. The nonlinearity of the process ensures the **absorption**, and therefore material alterations are confined to the extremely small focal volume. Typically, submicrometer-sized photodisrupted regions can be produced inside single **cells**. **Femtosecond** pulses deposit very little **energy** while still causing breakdown, therefore producing surgical **photodisruption** while minimizing collateral damage.

photodynamic diagnoses (PDD): Many **PDT photosensitizers** are also fluorescent, thus **photosensitizer**-based **fluorescence imaging/spectroscopy** is emerging also for guiding surgical resections (not only **PDT**), particularly of **tumor tissue**. The unique feature of **PDD/PDT** technology is that it is allows for easy combination of diagnoses (imaging) and treatment using the same instrumentation by changing the **laser** output **power**. Novel **PDD** technologies include photodynamic **molecular beacons** in which the photoactivation is quenched until the molecules reach specific targets; the use of **nanoparticles**, either as **photosensitizers** or as carriers thereof; and the use of **two-photon fluorescence**.

photodynamic therapy (PDT): Applied to clinical medicine, the use of a compound or drug (**photosensitizer**) that has no or minimal effect alone but that, when activated by **light**, generates one or more reactive chemical species that are able to modify or kill **cells** and **tissues**. As historically defined, the **PDT** reaction should be mediated by **oxygen** through the generation of reactive **oxygen**, most commonly **singlet oxygen** ($^1O_2$). However, there are **photosensitizers** that may use **oxygen**-independent photophysical pathways that may be considered photodynamic agents as well. The clinical status of **PDT** is complex, since there are numerous different **PDT photosensitizers** that have been used in patients to treat a wide variety of diseases, from **cancer** to infection and abnormal **blood vessel proliferation**. Some **photosensitizers** have been approved in different countries for different applications, while others are still in the clinical-trial or pre-clinical evaluation stage. There are also several "hardware" technologies required to apply **PDT** in patients, including different **light** sources (**lasers, LEDs**, and filtered lamps), **light** delivery devices (based particularly on **optical fibers** to reach deep within the body), and "dosimetry" instruments to measure the local **light intensity, photosensitizer** concentration, **oxygen** concentration, or combinations of these. Correspondingly, biophysical and biological models of **PDT** have been developed to systematize the complex interactions of **light, photosensitizer** and **oxygen**, and the resulting effects on **cells** and **tissues**. At the cellular level, there is good understanding of the basic mechanisms of **PDT**-induced damage, with one or more different mechanisms of **cell** death being involved (**necrosis, apoptosis, autophagy**), depending on the **PDT** parameters and cellular characteristics. Likewise, **tissue** may be modified or destroyed by **PDT** either directly by the **cell** death or indirectly by disruption of the **vasculature**, and both local and systemic **immune responses** can be involved in some cases. The multi-component nature of the photophysical, photochemical, and photobiological processes in **PDT** make it a challenging modality to optimize, and much of the clinical progress to date has been largely empirically based. The same complexity provides the opportunity for **PDT** to have many potential applications in biomedicine. Many **PDT photosensitizers** are also fluorescent and thus could be used for **photodynamic diagnoses (PDD)**. Traditional **PDT** is converging with advances from other fields to further exploit the basic concept of **light**-activated drugs.

photodynamic therapy (PDT) photosensitizers: There are numerous **PDT photosensitizers** that have been used on patients to treat a variety of diseases from **cancer** to infection. **Hematoporphyrin derivative (HpD)** was the first **PDT photosensitizer** studied for clinical application in **cancer** detection and treatment in the early 1970s. Photofrin II (Photofrin®), a purified form of **HpD**, was approved for treatment of **bladder cancer** in Canada in 1993. HMME (**hematoporphyrin** monomethyl **ether**), PsD-007 (photocarcinorin), and HiPorfin (second-generation **HpD**) are available. **Foscan**®, approved in Europe in 2001, can have significant clinical benefits. Photogem® was designed and commercialized in Russia. The discovery of **endogenous** photosensitization of **protoporphyrin IX (Pp IX)** induced by **exogenous administration** of prodrug **ALA** (**delta (δ)-aminolevulinic acid**) allowed for the treatment of pre-**malignant** and **malignant skin** lesions at **topical ALA** application. Clinical studies with **ALA-PDD-PDT** drugs Levulan®, Alasens®, and Metvix® (MLA, a methyl ester of **ALA**) showed their efficiency for the treatment of actinic keratoses, **squamous cell** carcinomas, and **basal cell** carcinomas. To treat relatively large solid tumors and to provide extensive **vascular** damage, TOOKAD® (WST09) dye can be used. **Laserphyrin**® is a part of the standard **PDT** protocol for centrally located early-stage **lung cancer** in Japan. **Visudyne**® and **Photosens**® are typically used to eliminate the abnormal **blood** vessels in the eye associated with macular degeneration. **Hypericin**: Naphtodianthrone is a red-colored anthraquinone-derivative which, together with hyperforin, is one of the principal active constituents of hypericum (Saint John's wort). **Hypericin** is under research as a **PDT**-agent, for example, for treatment of transitional **cell carcinoma**. **Antrin**® is used to treat **skin** cancers and in photoangioplasty. **Hexvix**® is approved in Europe for **photodynamic diagnoses (PDDs)** of early **bladder cancer**. Many other PDT dyes commonly used in medicine, such as **toluidine blue O (TBO), methylene blue (MB)**, and **indocyanine green (ICG)**, are used for inflammatory diseases treatment and **bacteria** killing. One such vitamin dye known as **Riboflavin**® was used at extracorporeal **PDT** (photophoresis) of **whole blood** and **blood** components and in a form of Medio-Cross® (**riboflavin/dextran** solution) for cross-linking of the corneal **collagen fibers** induced by **singlet oxygen**.

photoelasticity: Stress-induced **birefringence** and **dichroism** of a medium. This is an experimental method to determine stress distribution in a material. Unlike the analytical methods of stress determination, **photoelasticity** gives a fairly accurate picture of stress distribution even around abrupt discontinuities in a material. The method serves as an important tool for determining the critical stress points in a material and is often used to determine stress concentration factors in irregular geometries, such as **tooth** or **bone**.

photoexcitation: The mechanism of electron excitation by **photon absorption** (see **electronic excitation**, **electronic transition**) when the **energy** of the **photon** is too low to cause **photoionization**. The **absorption** of a **photon** takes place in accordance to the Planck's quantum theory. **Photoexcitation** is exploited in **luminescence**, photochemistry (in particular in **photoisomerization**), dye-sensitized **solar cell**, optically pumped **lasers**, and in some photochromic applications.

Photofrin II (Photofrin®): Effective biological photodynamic dye for red **light** [see **hematoporphyrin derivative (HpD)**]. Its molecular weight is about 500. It has an extinction coefficient of about $5000 \text{ cm}^{-1} \text{ M}^{-1}$ at 626 nm when dissolved in dextrose.

photoionization: Physical process in which an incident **photon** ejects one or more electrons from an atom, ion, or molecule. This is essentially the same process that occurs with the photoelectric effect with metals. In the case of gas and dielectric condensed **media**, such as biological **tissue** components, the term **photoionization** is more common. The ejected electrons, known as photoelectrons, carry information about their pre-ionized states. For example, a single electron can have a kinetic **energy** equal to the **energy** of the incident **photon** minus the electron binding **energy** of the state it left. **Photons** with energies less than the electron binding **energy** may be absorbed or scattered but will not photoionize the atom or ion. For example, to ionize hydrogen or **oxygen**, **photons** need an **energy** greater than 13.6 eV, which corresponds to a **wavelength** of 91.2 nm. For **photons** with greater **energy** than this, the **energy** of the emitted photoelectron is given by $(1/2) \, mv^2 = h\nu - 13.6$ eV, where h is **Planck**

constant and ν is the **frequency** of the **photon**. The **probability** of **photoionization** is related to the **photoionization** cross-section, which depends on the **energy** of the **photon** and the target being considered. For **photon** energies below the ionization threshold, the **photoionization** cross-section is near zero. But with the development of pulsed **lasers**, it has become possible to create extremely intense, **coherent light** where multi-**photon** ionization may occur (see **laser photoionization**).

photoisomerization: Molecular behavior in which structural change between isomers is caused by **photoexcitation**. Both reversible and irreversible **photoisomerization** reactions exist; however, the term usually indicates a reversible process. Photoisomerizable molecules are already put to practical use, for instance, in **pigments** for rewritable CDs, DVDs, and 3D optical-data storage solutions. There is a great interest in the behavior of such molecules to design optically-controlled molecular devices, such as molecular switches, molecular motors, and molecular electronics.

photomechanical effect: When absorbed **light** induces **tissue** stress and may lead to surface **tissue** break-up and ejection.

photomechanical wave: See **laser-generated stress wave**.

photomultiplier: See **photomultiplier tube (PMT)**.

photomultiplier tube (PMT): An extremely sensitive and fast detector of **light** and of other **radiation**, consisting of a vacuum tube in which the electrons released by **radiation** striking a **photocathode** are accelerated to successive dynodes that release several electrons for each incident electron, greatly amplifying the signal obtainable from small quantities of **radiation** (electron multiplier), and then collected by the anode. The internal noise-free **gain** is 10^6 and could be up to 10^8. This makes them ideal for the detection of extremely low **light** or short pulses of **light**. **PMTs** can be used to detect **photons** from 115–1700 nm. Typical applications: detection of **fluorescence**, **chemiluminescence** and **bioluminescence**, **flow cytometry**, environmental **analyzers**, **photon**-counting systems, **gene** chip scanners, particle counters, **spectrophotometry**, **radiation** counters and probes, surface inspection, and **laser** scanning.

photon: Quantum of **electromagnetic radiation (EMR)**, usually considered as an elementary particle that has **energy** $E_{ph} = h\nu$ or $h(c/\lambda)$, where h is the **Planck constant**, ν is the **frequency** of **EMR**, c is the speed of **electromagnetic wave (EMW)**, and λ is the **wavelength** of **EMW**. **Light** can be described as a stream of **photons**. To evaluate the total **energy** of the **light beam**, one must account for each **photon** that was detected or interacted with the target; if the total number of **photons** is N, then $E_{total} = N \times E_{ph} = N \times h\nu$.

photon absorption cross section: Ability of a molecule to absorb a **photon** of a particular **wavelength** and **polarization**. Although the units are given as an area, it does not refer to an actual size area, at least partially because the density or state of the target molecule will affect the **probability** of **absorption**. Quantitatively, the number dN of **photons** absorbed, between the points x and $x + dx$ along the path of a **light beam**, is the product of the number N of **photons** penetrating to depth x times the number ρ of absorbing molecules per unit volume times the **absorption** cross section σ_{abs} : $dN/dx = -\rho\sigma_{abs}N$.

photon diffusion coefficient: General expression for **photon diffusion coefficient**, $D = 3(\mu'_s + \bar{a}\mu_a)^{-1}$, where μ'_s is the **reduced scattering coefficient**, μ_a is the **absorption coefficient**, and $\bar{a}$ is the numerical coefficient depending on the form of the **diffusion** equation (on **scattering anisotropy factor**). Systematic approximation schemes lead to recommendations of $\bar{a} = 0, 1/5, 1/3, 1$. Any of these $\bar{a}$ values gives significantly better agreement with random walk simulations than the **diffusion** equation at $\bar{a} = 0$, with $\bar{a} = 1/3$ being slightly better than the two others. Because values $\bar{a} = 1/5$ and $\bar{a} = 1$ lead to the wrong pulse-front propagation speeds, and only the intermediate value $\bar{a} = 1/3$ gives the correct speed, the **photon diffusion coefficient** should be taken in the form $D \cong (3\mu'_s + \mu_a)^{-1}$. This expression in general gives a better agreement between **diffusion** equation and **RTE**, but in practice it is useful only for relatively high absorbing **tissues** or **tissue** components, when $\mu_a/\mu'_s > 0.01$.

photon diffusion wave (*Synonym*: intensity diffusion wave): See **photon-density wave**.

photon noise: Noise characteristic to **photodetectors** at **light** irradiation. There is **photon shot noise** that causes a fundamental limitation in signal detection and **photon** excess noise, which is determined by **photon** fluctuations originated by a **self-beating** phenomenon or by some imbalance between two outputs of an **OCT** system.

photon scattering cross section: The ability of a particle to scatter a **photon** of a particular **wavelength** and **polarization**. Although the units are given as an area, it does not refer to an actual size area. Quantitatively, the number dN of **photons** scattered, between the points x and $x + dx$ along the path of a **light beam** is the product of the number N of **photons** penetrating to depth x times the number ρ of **scattering** particles per unit volume times the **scattering** cross section σ_{sca} : $dN/dx = -\rho\sigma_{sca}N$.

photon shot noise: Noise caused by the irregularity of photoelectron emission. It induces random errors in a photoelectron measuring system. The mean square of photoelectron current fluctuations is defined by the average photocurrent i and the photodetector's **bandwidth** B_D: $i^2 = 2eiB_D$, where e is the charge of the electron. It is difficult to achieve the **shot noise** limit in practice. The magnitude of this noise increases with the average magnitude of the current or **intensity** of the **light**. However, since the magnitude of the average signal increases more rapidly than that of the **shot noise** (its relative strength decreases with increasing signal), **shot noise** is often only a problem with small currents or **light** intensities. The actual number of detected **photons** is given by a **Poisson**

distribution that approaches a normal distribution for large **photon** numbers with the **standard deviation** of the **photon** noise equal to the square root of the average number of **photons**, then **SNR** $= N/N^{1/2} = N^{1/2}$, where N is the average number of **photons** collected.

photon transport (migration): Process of **photon** travel in a homogeneous or **inhomogeneous medium** with possible macroinhomogeneities. A **photon** changes its direction due to **reflection**, **refraction**, **diffraction**, or **scattering**, and can be absorbed by an appropriate molecule during travel.

photon-correlation spectroscopy: **Noninvasive** method for studying the dynamics of particles on a comparatively large time scale. The implementation of the single-**scattering** regime and the use of **coherent light** sources are of fundamental importance in this case. The spatial scale of testing a **colloid structure** (an ensemble of biological particles) is determined by the inverse of the **wave** vector. **Quasi-elastic light scattering spectroscopy**, **spectroscopy of intensity fluctuations**, and **Doppler spectroscopy** are synonymous terms related to **dynamic light scattering**.

photon-counting system: System that makes use of a specific method of photoelectron signal processing and provides sequential detection of single **photons**. **Photomultipliers (PMTs)** or **avalanche photodetectors (APDs)** are usually used for **photon** counting. The technique is applicable for detecting very weak signals.

photon-density wave: **Wave** of progressively decaying **intensity**. Microscopically, individual **photons** migrate randomly in a **scattering** medium, but collectively they form a **photon-density wave** at a **modulation frequency** that moves away from a **radiation** source.

photonic crystal: Periodic optical (nano)structure that affects the propagation of **electromagnetic waves (EMW)** in the same way that the periodic potential in a **semiconductor** crystal affects the electron motion by defining allowed and forbidden electronic **energy** bands. The absence of allowed propagating **EMW** modes inside the structures, in a range of **wavelengths** called a photonic **bandgap**, gives rise to distinct optical phenomena such as inhibition of spontaneous emission, high-reflecting omnidirectional mirrors, and low-loss waveguiding, among others. Since the basic physical phenomenon is based on **diffraction**, the periodicity of the **photonic crystal** structure has to be in the same length scale as half the **wavelength** of the **EMW**, i.e., ~300 nm for **photonic crystals** operating in the **visible** part of the **spectrum**. **Photonic crystal** structures both in 2D and 3D geometries as well as in microstructured **fibers** (**photonic crystal fibers**) enable the control of the flow and confinement of **light** on the **wavelength** scale. In most cases this confinement in one, two, or all three spatial dimensions is based on the presence of a defect in these structures. Strong modal confinement results, both in large effective nonlinearities and in a control of the **dispersion** characteristics. **Photonic crystals** occur in nature, including in biological **tissues**.

photonic crystal fiber (PCF): This is a microstructured **fiber**, which, in general, is a 2D **photonic crystal** with a regularly repeating 3D structure with a scale on the order of the optical **wavelength**. **Light** in **PCFs** behaves similarly to a **Bragg diffraction** from **crystalline** materials, except that the effect can be seen in the **visible** region. **PCFs** are unique since they can, in theory, make possible extremely low-loss **light** transmission due to the photonic **bandgap** effect. In **PCFs** the waveguiding mechanism is fundamentally different than that of conventional **optical fibers** since it is due to a regular pattern of holes running along the length of the **fiber** rather than variations in the **refractive index** of the **fiber**. This periodic arrangement of normally airfilled holes in the cladding is the main factor in the formation of **waveguide** modes. There are two main types of **PCFs**, those with glass cores and those with hollow cores. A glass-core **PCF** has a high **index of refraction** in the core, and its cladding is a structured 2D **photonic crystal** with a low effective **index of**

refraction. In this type of **PCF**, **light** propagates in the glass core (in analogy with a conventional **optical fiber**) via **total internal reflection**. A **PCF** with a hollow core has a low **index of refraction** compared to the effective **index of refraction** of its cladding. In this type of **fiber**, certain **light** modes propagate through the hollow core due to the photonic **bandgap** mechanism, which localizes and guides **light**. The properties of large, effective nonlinearities and control of the **dispersion** characteristics have been exploited for **supercontinuum** generation. There are a large variety of **PCFs** including **fibers** that employ a 2D-**photonic-crystal** kagome geometry. A kagome lattice consists of a periodic arrangement of three sets of parallel planes, rotated by 60 deg with respect to each other. In the kagome lattice there is no core, and an intersection of the supporting structure alone suffices for guiding **light**, neither requiring a deliberately introduced defect state nor employing photonic **bandgaps**. The guided **light** is effectively confined to a single intersection of the lattice planes, employing **total internal reflection** similar to that in tapered **fibers** or in many other types of **PCFs**. Guided modes in adjacent intersections therefore exhibit only marginal overlap, and the guiding mechanism is broadband. **PCF** manufacturing is based on classical micro- and nanocapillary glass technology containing the following main steps: precision, thin-walled, round glass capillaries are stacked in a bundle, for example, in the shape of a hexagon; the capillaries are then heated to the temperature of glass softening and drawn to create hexagonal polycapillary structures; several of these structures are then assembled in a hexagonal package and drawn again. This procedure is repeated until the desired variable periodicity of air channels is achieved. If one or several capillaries in the center of an initial package are removed or replaced by a glass cylinder, an air or glass core can be created in the final structure. This technology allows one to manufacture micro- and nanostructured **PCFs** from different types of glasses with a great variety of configurations, stacking types (hexagonal, squared, triangular and other), and defect arrangement topologies. **PCFs** allow one to increase the efficiency of nonlinear optical interactions, to control the **dispersion** of **waveguide** modes, and to shift the **wavelength** of a zero **dispersion** in the **visible** range of the **spectrum**. Micro- and nanostructured **PCFs** are used to design **PCF-based capillary biosensors**.

photonic-crystal-fiber (PCF)-based capillary biosensor: Photonic crystal fibers (PCFs) are the basis for biosensors and can be made of glass, silica, polymers, or other materials. Such sensors contain channels and holes that can be filled with samples and reagents, including mixtures of gold or silver **nanoparticles** for effective **SERS**. Hollow-core **PCFs** are viable for molecular sensing because of a rather large interaction length of the probing substance with guided light and a small portion of the probe. **PCF** biosensors can be based on the detection of alterations of **index of refraction**, **absorption**, or **scattering** properties of the probe. **PCF**-based capillary plates also serve for on-line separation of various biological substances and **cells**, such as **DNA** and **blood cells**.

photoplethysmography (PPG): Optically based **plethysmography**. **PPG** is often provided by using a **pulse oximetry** technique in which the **skin** is illuminated, and changes in **light absorption** are measured. The change in volume caused by the **pressure** pulse is detected by illuminating the **skin** with the **light** from a **LED** and then measuring the amount of **light** either transmitted or reflected to a **photodiode**. Each cardiac cycle appears as a peak. Because **blood flow** to the **skin** can be modulated by many other physiological systems, **PPG** can also be used to monitor **breathing**, hypovolemia, and other circulatory conditions. Additionally, the shape of the **PPG** waveform differs from subject to subject, and varies with the location and manner in which the **pulse oximeter** is attached.

photorefractive keratectomy (PRK): Although **PRK** and **LASEK** basically use the same technique, there are minor differences between them. In **PRK**, the **epithelium** is removed and discarded; afterwards, the outermost layer below the **epithelium** is treated with **laser**. See also **LASEK (Laser-Assisted SubEpithelial Keratectomy** or **Laser Epithelial Keratomileusis**).

photorefractive surgery: See **laser refractive surgery**.

photorefractive technique: Detection of **refractive index** gradients above and inside a sample using thermal blooming, thermal lensing, **probe** beam **refraction**, or interferometry and **deflectometry**.

Photosens®:   PDT photosensitizer that contains a mixture of sulfonated aluminium **phtalocyanines** with various degrees of sulfonation. It requires **laser light** of a specific **wavelength** of 675 nm for activation. It has been designed in Russia and tested for various diseases, including treatment of age-related macular degeneration.

photosensitizer: Substance that increases the **absorption** of a **tissue** at a particular **wavelength** band and may significantly accelerate **photothermal** or photochemical reaction. In photomedicine, many diagnostic and treatment technologies use **endogenous** or **exogenous photosensitizers**.

phototherapy: General term accounting for all types of therapy using **light**. See **photochemical therapy**, **photodynamic therapy (PDT)**, **photothermal therapy**, and **low-level laser therapy (LLLT)**.

photothermal (PT):   Related to thermal action of **light**.

photothermal effect: When **laser energy** is absorbed by **tissue**, it results in three photophysical interactions: photomechanical, photochemical, and **photothermal**. **Photothermal** reaction produces **hyperthermia** and **coagulation** of **tissue**. It can be an effective means of **tumor tissue** destruction due to the sensitivity of **tumor cells** to temperature elevation. Among the three interactions, **photothermal** is the most commonly encountered phenomenon in almost all **laser** applications. It causes direct and controllable thermal damage to **tissue**. Because of its effect on **tissue**, thermal damage has been an important factor when a

404

laser is used in clinical treatment. While its enhancement and control are needed when **lesion** removal and **tumor** destruction are concerned, efforts are always required to avoid or to reduce its impact on normal **tissue**.

photothermal flow cytometry: The **flow cytometry** technique that uses **photothermal** detection abilities. Its major advantage is the possibility to provide *in vivo* studies. This method is used for the monitoring and **quantitative measurements** of **cells**, including stem and metastatic **cancer cells**, **nanoparticles**, and other absorbing components within the **blood** and **lymph** streams (see *in vivo* **flow cytometry**).

photothermal immunotherapy: While the **photothermal effect** alone can be used as a basis for **laser** thermotherapy for the large-scale, controlled destruction of **cancer cells**, it has limitations in completely eradicating **cancers**, particularly metastatic **tumors**, either due to the incomplete destruction of target **tumor cells**, or due to metastasis of the **tumor** to other sites. To effectively augment **photothermal therapy**, active immunological stimulation is used. **Photothermal immunotherapy** is a combination of local **selective photothermal treatment** and local immunological stimulation using adjuvant.

photothermal microscopy (PTM): **Microscopy** based on detection of the **photothermal** signal induced by a sharply focused **laser beam**.

photothermal radiometry (PTR): See **optothermal radiometry (OTR)**.

photothermal therapy: General term characterizing all kinds of therapy based on the thermal reaction of a living **tissue** and a **cell** to **light** that is intense enough to produce thermal effects. **Photothermal** effects, **selective photothermolysis**, and **selective photothermal treatments** are behind this therapy. Different lamps and **lasers** are successfully used in **photothermal**

treatments. It includes **laser-induced thermotherapy (LITT)**, **laser-induced hyperthermia (LIHT)**, **laser-induced coagulation (LIC)**, and **laser-induced interstitial thermotherapy (LI-ITT)**.

photovoltaic cell: Semiconductor device (**photodiode**) that generates a voltage when exposed to **light**. When used in zero-bias or photovoltaic mode, the flow of photocurrent out of the device is restricted, and a voltage builds up. The **photodiode** becomes forward biased, and "dark current" begins to flow across the junction in the direction opposite to the photocurrent. This mode is responsible for the photovoltaic effect, which is the basis for solar **cells**—in fact, a solar **cell** is just a large-area **photodiode**.

phthalocyanine: Dye-based **photosensitizer** with an excitation band around 676 nm. It is used in **cancer** diagnostics and **photodynamic therapy**; **Photosens**® is the commercialized product. At **PDT**, the typical **laser power** dose is of 100 J/cm^2.

physiological solution: There are a number of **physiological solutions** that provide safety and normal functioning of **biological cells, tissues**, and organs. They contain electrolytes and organic acids at concentrations that are similar to that in animal or human **serum**. Saline is one **physiological solution** that is a solution of sodium chloride (NaCl) in sterile **water**, used frequently for intravenous **infusion**, rinsing contact **lenses**, and nasal irrigation. Saline solutions are available in various concentrations for different purposes. Normal **saline** is the solution of 0.9% w/v of NaCl. It has a slightly higher degree of osmolality compared to **blood** (hence, although it is referred to as being **isotonic** with **blood** in clinical contexts, this is a technical inaccuracy), about 300 mOsm/L.

pia mater: The fine vascular membrane that closely envelops the **brain** and **spinal cord** under the **arachnoid mater** and the *dura mater*.

picosecond (psec or ps): Unit of time that is equal to 10^{-12} sec (s).

picric acid: The chemical compound formally called 2,4,6-trinitrophenol (TNP). This yellow **crystalline** solid is one of the most acidic **phenols**. In **microscopy**, it is a reagent for staining samples, e.g., **Gram's stain**.

piezoceramics: Piezoelectric materials that are used to make electromechanical sensors and actuators. Lead zirconate titanate (PZT) ceramics is an example. There are several different formulations of the PZT compound, each with different electromechanical properties.

piezodeflector: Device for **light beam** deflection at certain audio or **radio frequencies** using the **acousto-optic effect**. See **acousto-optic (AO) interaction/effect**.

piezodriver: Device that uses the inverse piezoelectric effect in certain asymmetric crystals that is obtained by applying a potential difference to a crystal. An alteration in the size of the crystal takes place.

piezoelectric transducer: Device that uses the piezoelectric effect in certain asymmetric crystals. The effect is obtained by applying an external **pressure** to a crystal. Positive and negative charges are produced on opposite faces of the crystal, giving rise to a potential difference between the faces. The potential difference operates in the opposite direction if tension is applied instead of **pressure**. This potential difference is the signal detected in a crystal **microphone**.

piezo-optical coefficient: Characterizes the efficiency of stress-induced **birefringence** and **dichroism** of a medium (see **photoelasticity**), indicating whether that material is good or not for stress sensors (**piezoelectric transducer**) and **acousto-optic modulators**.

pigment: Any substance whose presence in the **tissues** or **cells colors** them.

pigmentary glaucoma: Form of **glaucoma** that usually appears in young males 20 to 50 years old. In fact, all patients with **pigmentary glaucoma** will necessarily have pigmentary dispersion syndrome prior to the onset of **glaucoma** (i.e., actual optic **nerve** damage and peripheral vision loss). The mechanism of **glaucoma** development in this syndrome is the deposition of **pigment** from the **iris** into the trabecular meshwork (primary site of fluid egress), essentially "plugging" the microscopic spaces through which fluid escapes.

pigmentation: Many **tissues**, such as **skin, iris, sclera,** and **retina**, contain **pigments** (**melanin, bilirubin, myoglobin, hemoglobin**, among others). In **skin**, there are specialized cells called melanocytes that contain melanin. **Red blood cells** (**erothrocytes**) contain **hemoglobin**. Many conditions affect the levels or nature of **pigments** in **cells**. For instance, albinism is a disorder affecting the low level of **melanin** production in animals and humans. Pigment **color** differs from structural **color** in that it is the same for all viewing angles, whereas structural **color** is the result of selective **reflection** or **interference**, usually because of multilayer structures and **light scattering**.

pinhole: See **aperture**.

pink noise (*Synonym*: flicker noise): Also called $1/f$ noise, it is a signal or process with a **frequency spectrum** such that the **power** spectral density is inversely proportional to the **frequency**. In **pink noise**, each octave carries an equal amount of noise **power**. The name arises from being intermediate between **white noise** ($1/f^0$) and red noise ($1/f^2$), more commonly known as Brownian noise. In general it has **power** spectral density of the form $S(f) \propto 1/f^\alpha$, where $0 < \alpha < 2$, with α usually close to 1. These noises occur widely in nature and are a source of considerable interest in many fields. Strictly speaking, the term flicker noise is applied only for

electronic noise. In electronics, **white noise** will be stronger than flicker noise above some corner **frequency**. In biological systems, **pink noise** is present in **heartbeat** rhythms, mental states, and the statistics of **DNA** sequences.

PIN photodiode: Photodiode based on *p–i–n* **semiconductor** structure that has a fast response.

pit: As related to a **tooth**, it is a dental **enamel** hypoplasia in the form of a **pit**.

pixel: Abbreviation for picture element. The smallest element of an image that can be individually displayed. In **optical imaging** technology, a **pixel** is a **focal plane array (FPA)** element—for scanning systems, it is defined by the **IFOV**, and for spot radiometers, by the **FOV**.

plague: An infectious, epidemic disease of high mortality caused by the bacterium *Pasteurella pestis*.

Planck's constant: Denoted *h*, a physical constant that is used to describe the sizes of quanta. It plays a central role in the theory of quantum mechanics, and is named after Max Planck, one of the founders of quantum theory. A closely-related quantity is the reduced **Planck's constant** [also known as Dirac constant ($\hbar = h/2\pi$)]. The Planck constant is also used in measuring **energy** emitted by **light photons**, such as in the equation $E = h\nu$, where *E* is **energy**, *h* is **Planck's constant**, and ν is **frequency**: $h = 6.6262 \times 10^{-34}$ J · sec.

Planck curve (function): Gives the **intensity** radiated by a **blackbody** as a function of **frequency** (or **wavelength**) for a definite body at absolute temperature *T*. This function represents the emitted **power** per unit area of the emitting surface, per unit solid angle, and per unit **frequency** (or **wavelength**). As a function of **wavelength** λ, it is written (for unit solid angle) as $I'\lambda, T = 2hc^2/\lambda^5 \cdot (1/e^{hc/\lambda kT} - 1)$, where *h* is **Planck's constant**, *c*

409

is the **speed of light**, and k is **Boltzmann's constant**. For spectral **radiance** $I'(\lambda, T)$, or **power** per unit surface area, per unit solid angle, per unit **wavelength**, $W \cdot m^{-2} \cdot sr^{-1} \cdot nm^{-1}$, this function peaks for $hc = 4.97\lambda kT$. The peak in the emitted **energy** moves to shorter **wavelengths** as the temperature is increased (**Wien's displacement law**). For normal physiological temperatures, the maximum of **radiation** emitted by a leaving body is in the 10-μm **wavelength** range. The area under the curve increases as the temperature is increased (the **Stefan–Boltzmann law**). See **blackbody curve**.

Planck's law: Describes the spectral **radiance** of **electromagnetic radiation** at all **wavelengths** emitted in the normal direction from a **blackbody** at absolute temperature T. It is written as an expression for emitted **power** per unit area of emitting surface, per unit solid angle, and per unit **frequency** (or **wavelength**) $W \cdot m^{-2} \cdot sr^{-1} \cdot nm^{-1}$. Sometimes, it is written as an expression for emitted **power** integrated over all solid angles $W \cdot m^{-2} \cdot nm^{-1}$. In other cases, it is written as for **energy** per unit volume. See **Planck curve (function)**.

plasma: Clear, waterlike, colorless liquid of **blood** and other body liquids.

plasma-membrane: See **cell membrane**.

plasmid: **DNA** molecule separated from the chromosomal **DNA** and capable of autonomous replication. It is typically circular and double-stranded, and it occurs in **bacteria** and sometimes in eukaryotic organisms.

plasmon: Related to collective excitations of conductive electrons in metals. Depending on the **boundary conditions**, it is commonly accepted to distinguish bulk **plasmons** (3D **plasma**), surface propagating **plasmons** or surface-**plasmon** polaritons (2D films), and surface-localized **plasmons** (**nanoparticles**). A quantum of bulk **plasmons** $h\nu_p$ is about 10 eV for noble metals, as they cannot be excited by **visible light**. The surface **plasmon** polaritons propagate along metal surfaces in a **waveguide**-like fashion. The localized **plasmons** are characterized by the electric component of an external optical field that exerts a force on the conductive electrons and displaces them from their equilibrium positions to create uncompensated charges at the **nanoparticle** surface. As the main effect producing the restoring force is the **polarization** of the particle surface, these oscillations are called "surface **plasmons**" that have a well-defined resonance **frequency** in the **visible** range.

plastic fiber: See **polymer fiber**.

plastic surgery: Surgical techniques to change the appearance and function of a person's body. Some of these operations are called "cosmetic," and others are called "reconstructive."

platelet (*Synonym*: thrombocyte):   Very small, nonnucleated, round or oval disks that are fragments of **cells** from red **bone marrow**. They are found only in mammalian **blood**. There are approximately 200000–400000 per mm^3 in human **blood**. They initiate **blood** clotting by disintegrating and releasing thrombokinase. **Platelets** in the **blood** stream are biconvex, disk-like particles with diameters ranging between 2–4 μm.

pleomorphism: See **polymorphism**.

plethysmography: Measuring changes in volume within an organ usually resulting from fluctuations in the amount of **blood** or air it contains.

pleural effusion: Excess **pleural fluid** that accumulates in the fluid-filled space that surrounds the **lungs**. It is usually diagnosed on the basis of medical history and physical exam, and confirmed by **chest x-ray computed tomography**. Once accumulated fluid is more than 500 ml, there are usually detectable clinical signs in the patient, such as decreased movement of the **chest** on the affected side, dullness to percussion over the fluid, diminished breath sounds on the affected side, decreased vocal resonance, and pleural friction rub.

pleural fluid: This is fluid that fills the space that surrounds the **lungs**. Excessive amounts of such fluid, called **pleural effusion**, can impair **breathing** by limiting the expansion of the **lungs** during inspiration.

P_N **approximation:** The integro-differential of **RTT** is too complicated to be employed for the analysis of **light** propagation in **scattering media**. Therefore, it is frequently simplified by representing the solution in the form of spherical harmonics. Such simplification leads to a system of $(N + 1)^2$ connected differential partial derivative equations known as the P_N **approximation**. This system is reducible to a single differential equation of order $(N+1)$. For example, four connected differential equations reducible to a single **diffusion**-type equation are necessary for $N = 1$ (see **diffusion approximation**).

Pockels cell: Piezoelectric crystal with two plane electrodes for applying an external electric field, placed between two crossed **polarizers**. The basis of its functioning is the linear electro-optical effect, which relates to a change in the **refractive index** of a crystal caused by an external electric field: the phase shift between ordinary and extraordinary rays linearly depends on the electrical field strength. The **Pockels cell** is widely used as an external **laser** or other **light** source **intensity** modulator, as well as an internal **laser** modulator for **giant pulse Q-switching**.

point raster scanning laser Doppler perfusion imaging (LDPI): Raster scan that operates by recording a sequence of point **blood perfusion** measurements along a predetermined raster pathway. This was the first type of **LDPI** system to be developed. Imaging is achieved by using a moveable mirror to scan the **laser beam** over the area in a raster fashion. At each site an individual perfusion measurement is taken. When the scan is complete, the system generates a 2D map from the single point perfusion measurements. The main drawback with this technique is the time required to produce an image. Each individual measurement can be achieved in 4–50 ms. Lowering the **acquisition time** further results in increased noise in the signal.

point spread function (PSF): Describes the response of an imaging system to a point source or point object. Another commonly used term for the **PSF** is a system's impulse response. The degree of spreading (blurring) of the point object is a measure for the quality of an imaging system. In functional terms it is the spatial domain version of the **modulation transfer function (MTF)**. It is a useful concept in Fourier optics, electron **microscopy** and other imaging techniques such as 3D **microscopy** [i.e., **confocal microscopy, fluorescence microscopy**, and **spatial frequency-domain diffuse optical spectroscopy (SFD-DOS)**]. The axial and lateral **PSFs** can be introduced.

point-of-care testing (POCT): Defined as diagnostic testing at or near the site of patient care. The driving notion behind **POCT** is to bring the test conveniently and immediately to the patient. This increases the likelihood that the patient will receive the results in a timely manner. Many biophotonic instruments satisfy this ideology, as **POCT** is accomplished through the use of transportable, portable, and handheld instruments (e.g., pulse oxymeter) and test kits (e.g., lab-on-a-chip). Cheaper, smaller, faster, and smarter **POCT** devices have increased the use of **POCT** approaches by making it cost-effective for many diseases, such as **diabetes**, stroke, **carpal tunnel syndrome (CTS)** and **acute coronary syndrome**.

Poisson distribution: Discrete **probability** distribution function that expresses the **probability** of a number of events occurring in a fixed period of time if these events occur with a known average rate and independently of the time since the last event. It can also be used for the number of events in other specified intervals such as distance, area, or volume. If the expected number of occurrences in a time-interval of given length is λ, then the **probability** that there are exactly n occurrences (n being a nonnegative integer, $n = 0, 1, 2, \ldots$) is equal to $f(n, \lambda) = (\lambda^n e^{-\lambda})/n!$, where e is the base of the natural logarithm ($e = 2.71828$), n is the number of occurrences of an event (the **probability** of which is given by the function), $n!$ is the factorial of n, and λ is a positive real number equal to the expected number of occurrences that occur during the given interval. As a function of n, this is the **probability mass function**. The **Poisson distribution** can be applied to systems with a large number of possible events, each of which is rare. The parameter λ is not only the mean number of occurrences $\langle k \rangle$, but also its **variance** $\sigma_k^2 = \langle k^2 \rangle - \langle k \rangle^2$. Thus, the number of observed occurrences fluctuates about its mean λ with a **standard deviation** $\sigma_k = \sqrt{\lambda}$. These fluctuations are denoted as **Poisson noise** or (particularly in electronics) as **shot noise**. Many other molecular applications of **Poisson noise** have been developed, e.g., estimating the number density of receptor molecules in a **cell membrane**.

Poisson noise: See **Poisson distribution**.

polar aprotic solvent: Solvent that does not contain an O–H or N–H bond. Acetone ($CH_3-C(=O)-CH_3$) is a **polar aprotic solvent**.

polarimetry: Measurement of the **polarization** properties of **light**.

polarizability: The relative tendency of a charge distribution, like the electron cloud of an atom or molecule, to be distorted from its normal shape by an external electric field, which may be caused by the presence of a nearby ion or dipole. The electronic **polarizability** α is defined as the ratio of the induced **dipole moment** P of an atom to the electric field E that produces this **dipole moment** $P = \alpha E$.

polarization: See **light polarization**.

polarization anisotropy: Inequality of **polarization** properties along different axes. Many **tissues** feature **polarization
anisotropy**. Polarization properties of **light** propagating within a
tissue are sensitive to changes in **tissue** morphology. On this basis
a number of **polarization gating** techniques were designed.

polarization gating: Techniques for selection of **diffuse
photon** groups with different pathlengths, in particular **ballistic
photons** or least-**scattering photons**, based on their **polarization**
properties. Because selected groups of **photons** carry information
about **tissue** structure and **absorption** from different depths, these
techniques are used in diffuse **polarization optical tomography**
and **spectroscopy** and in **polarization-sensitive OCT (PS OCT)**.

polarization imaging: By use of simple **polarization** filters,
light from the superficial layers of **tissue** can be differentiated
from **light** backscattered from the **tissue** bulk. For example,
when linearly **polarized light** is incident on the surface of
the **skin**, a small fraction of the **light** (approximately 5%) is
specularly reflected as surface glare (**Fresnel reflection**) from
the **skin** surface due to **refractive index** mismatching between
the two **media**. A further 2% of the original **light** is reflected
from the superficial subsurface layers of the **stratum corneum**.
These two fractions of **light** retain the original **polarization** state
determined by the **polarization** orientation of the incident **light**.
The remaining portion of **light** (approximately 93%) penetrates
through the **epidermis** to be absorbed or backscattered by the
epidermal or dermal matrix. Approximately 46% of this remaining
light is absorbed by the **tissue** and not re-emitted, while the rest is
diffusely backscattered in the dermal **tissue**. This backscattered
portion is exponentially depolarized—more than 10 **scattering**
events are required to sufficiently depolarize **light**—due to
scattering itself and also **tissue birefringence** originating from
dermal fiber structure. The spectral signature of the backscattered
light contains information about the main **chromophores** in the
epidermis (melanin) and **dermis (hemoglobin)**, while the surface
reflections contain information about the surface topography,
such as texture and **wrinkles**. By placing a second **polarization**

filter in front of the detector with **polarization** orientation in parallel (co-polarized, CO) or with perpendicular (cross-polarized, CR) to that of the filter in front of the **light** emitter, it is possible to differentiate between the detection of surface **reflection** and diffusely backscattered **light**. To detect events in the microvascular network, a cross-**polarization** setup is required. There are essentially two different principles employing this setup: **orthogonal polarization spectroscopy (OPS)** and **tissue viability imaging (TiVi)**.

polarized light: See **light polarization**.

polarization optical spectroscopy: Optical **spectroscopy** using polarizied **light** as a **probe** beam and/or detection of transmitted, scattered, or re-emitted **polarized light**. It allows for **polarization** gating of **photons** returning from and carrying spectroscopic information of different compartments of **tissue** under examination.

polarization optical tomography: Optical tomography using polarizied **light** as a **probe** beam and/or detection of transmitted, scattered, or re-emitted **polarized light**.

polarization-maintaining (PM) fiber: Fiber that supports propagation of linearly polarized modes, called LP modes. Indeed, all of the HE_{1n} modes are very much plane polarized, particularly in weakly guiding **fibers** with a small **refractive index** difference between core and cladding. For other modes, many are nearly degenerate, and plane polarized fields can be formed by linear combinations of these nearly degenerate modes—if the weakly guiding approximation is valid. For example, combinations of the following three nearly degenerate modes HE_{21}, TE_{01}, and TM_{01}—result in LP modes. A **single-mode fiber** is actually two-mode, as its fundamental transverse mode has two components with the orthogonal **polarization**. Even for **fibers** with a circular cross section of the core **refractive index** difference for two waves of orthogonal **polarization**, $(n_{\parallel} - n_{\perp}) \sim 10^{-9}$ (for straight **fiber**) and $\sim 5 \cdot 10^{-9}$ (for bent **fiber** with the r = 30 cm). **Fiber birefringence** is characterized usually by the so-called length of **polarization** beats L_p, for which the **phase shift** between orthogonal **light** field **polarization** components is changed by 2π. For the **fiber** with a circular-cross section, L_p = 1–10 m. Transmitted monochromatic **light** can have any **polarization** state—linear, circular, or elliptic— depending on the state of initial **polarization** of the propagating **light** and degree of **fiber** bending or twisting. Transportation of nonmonochromatic **polarized light** via a **fiber** leads to its **depolarization**. The noticeable **birefringence** can be achieved by modification of the core form, **fiber** twisting, and **mechanical stress**. There are many types of commercially available **polarization maintaining (PM) fibers**, one of the most widely spread is PANDA. For **PM fibers**, the length of **polarization** beats is small, L_p = 0.2 − 5.0 cm, which provides disruption of the coupling at mutual **scattering** of the orthogonal components on the inhomogeneities and thus keeps a definite state of **polarization**. **PM fibers** should have $n_{\parallel} - n_{\perp} > 3 \times 10^{-4}$.

polarization-sensitive optical coherence tomography (PS OCT): Specificity of conventional **OCT** can be improved by providing measurements of **polarization** properties of probing **radiation** when it propagates through a **tissue**. This approach was implemented in the **PS OCT**. Advanced **PS OCT** systems provide **tissue** imaging using **Jones matrix** or **Mueller matrix** elements. In the majority of studies using **PS OCT**, the criterion of **pathological** changes in **tissue** is a measured decrease in **tissue** macroscopic **birefringence**. However, it is difficult to provide correct measurements of **birefringence** for depths of more than 300–500 μm. For deeper layers (up to 1.5 mm), a much simpler variant of **PS OCT**, the **cross-polarization OCT (CP OCT)**, can be employed.

polarized reflectance spectroscopy (PRS): Spectroscopy based on detection of backscattered **light** from a **tissue** with **polarization gating** that allows for the selection of **photons** with shorter pathlengths carrying specific information about the **tissue**

417

under study, for instance, about **absorption** of **endogenous** or **exogenous chromophores**.

polarizer: Device, often a crystal or **prism**, that produces **polarized light** from unpolarized **light**. **Laser light** is principally polarized; depending on the **laser** construction, it can provide a high degree of either linear or circular **polarization**.

polydisperse system: Disperse system (medium) with multiple values of characteristic parameters, such as an ensemble of **scatterers** with different sizes and refractive indices. A **cataract** eye **lens** is a good example of a **polydisperse system** because it consists of dielectric particles (aggregated α-crystallins; see $\alpha, \beta,$ **and** γ **crystallins**) with various refractive indices and sizes dispersed in a homogeneous **ground substance**.

polydispersion: Differently sized (and/or with different refractive indices) dispersed particles suspended in a solid, liquid, or gas.

polyethylene glycol (PEG): Any of a series of polymers having the general formula $HOCH_2(CH_2OCH_2)_nCH_2OH$ or $H(OCH_2CH_2)_nOH$ and a molecular weight of about 200 to 20,000. They are obtained by condensation of **ethylene glycol** or ethylene oxide and **water**, and used as an emulsifying agent and lubricant in ointments, creams, etc. **PEGs** with a high molecular weight are used as effective **osmolytes**.

polyglycerylmethacrylate: Substance used in drugs and cosmetic preparations for personal care/use.

polymer fiber (*Synonym*: plastic fiber): **Fiber** made from transparent polymer (plastic) materials (see **fiber**).

polymerized siloxanes: See **silicon oils**.

418

polymorph (*Synonym*: polymorphonuclear leukocyte): Polynucleated, irregularly shaped **white blood cell** exhibiting amoeboid movement. The **nucleus** consists of two or more lobes (up to five in humans) joined by threads. The number of lobes increases with the age of the **cell**. In a healthy person, the distribution of **polymorphs** by the number of lobes remains constant. Any variation indicates a diseased condition. The **cells** are all active **phagocytes**, they are produced continually in **bone marrow**, and they constitute about 70% of all **leukocytes** in humans. The **cytoplasm** of **polymorphs** in humans is granular. Some granulations stain with acid dyes (eosinophils), some with basic dyes (basophils), and some with neutral dyes (neutrophils). All three types increase in number during infection.

polymorphonuclear leukocyte: See **polymorph**.

polymorphism (*Synonym*: pleomorphism): Describes multiple possible states for a single property, for instance, the property of amphiphiles that gives rise to various **aggregations** of **lipids**. It is also defined as the occurrence of two or more structural forms.

polyorganosiloxane (POS) (*Synonym*: silicone): Host **media** for a solid-state **tissue phantom**.

polyp: An abnormal growth of **tissue** (**tumor**) projecting from a **mucous membrane**. If it is attached to the surface by a narrow elongated stalk, it is said to be pedunculated. If no stalk is present, it is said to be sessile. Polyps are commonly found in the **colon**, **stomach**, nose, **urinary bladder**, and **uterus**. They may also occur elsewhere in the body where **mucous membranes** exist, such as the **cervix** and **small intestine**.

polypropylene glycol (PPG): Polymer of **propylene glycol**. Chemically, it is a polyether. The term **polypropylene glycol** or **PPG** is reserved for low-to-medium-range **molar mass** polymers when the nature of the end-group (which is usually a hydroxyl group) still matters.

polysaccharide: A polymeric **carbohydrate** structure consisting of repeating units (either mono- or disaccharides) joined together by glycosidic bonds. These structures are often linear but may contain various degrees of branching. Polysaccharides are often quite heterogeneous, containing slight modifications of the repeating unit. Depending on the structure, these **macromolecules** can have distinct properties from their monosaccharide building blocks. They may be amorphous or even insoluble in **water**. When all the monosaccharides in a **polysaccharide** are the same type, the **polysaccharide** is called a homopolysaccharide, but when more than one type of monosaccharide is present, it is called a heteropolysaccharide. Examples include storage **polysaccharides** such as starch and **glycogen**, and structural **polysaccharides** such as cellulose and chitin. They have a general formula of $C_x(H_2O)_y$ where x is usually a large number between 200 and 2500. Considering that the repeating units in the polymer backbone are often six-carbon monosaccharides, the general formula can also be represented as $(C_6H_{10}O_5)_n$, where $40 \leq n \leq 3000$.

polystyrene microsphere (bead): Used for quality control, **calibration**, and sizing, they are widely seen in clean room certification, filter testing, **light scattering** experiments, **tissue phantoms** design, **cell labeling**, etc. Nanobeads ranging between 40–950 nm, microbeads ranging between 1.00–9.00 μm, and megabeads ranging between 10.0–175.0 μm are available on the market.

polyvinydene fluoride (PVDF): Belongs to piezoelectric materials that are used to make electromechanical sensors and actuators.

pons: Structure located on the **brain** stem. In humans, it is above the medulla, below the midbrain, and anterior to the **cerebellum**.

porosity: Measure of the void spaces in a material, which is measured as a fraction between 0–1 or as a percentage between 0–100%. The term **porosity** is used in multiple fields including biology, for instance, **porosity** of biological **membrane**.

porphyrin: Heterocyclic macrocycle derived from four pyrrole-like subunits interconnected via their α carbon atoms via methyl carbon bridges (=CH–). The macrocycle, therefore, is highly conjugated and consequently deeply colored. The macrocycle has 26π electrons. Many **porphyrins** occur in nature—they are **pigments** found in both animals and plants.

***Porphyromonas gingivalis*:** **Gram-negative bacteria** that are oral anaerobes found in **periodontal lesions** and associated with adult **periodontal** disease.

port wine stain (*Synonym*: cavernous hemangioma): Skin discoloration characterized by a deep red to purple **color** (see **hemangioma**). It is a **vascular** birthmark consisting of superficial and deeply dilated **capillaries** in the **skin**. It is part of the family of disorders known as **vascular** malformations. **Port wine stains** occur most often on the face but can appear anywhere on the body. Many treatments have been tried for **port wine stains** including freezing, surgery, **radiation**, and tattooing. **Lasers** have made the biggest impact on treatment because they are the sole method of destroying the **cutaneous capillaries** without significant damage to the overlying **skin**. The flashlamp-pumped **dye laser** (585 nm) has been the most successful at destroying stains in infants and young children. The **Nd:YAG laser** is used to treat the nodules that may develop in some adult **port wine stains**. Prospective **laser** systems utilize a combination of two different **wavelengths** (595 nm and 1064 nm) used simultaneously with sequential pulses. The advantage of this **laser** system is that it allows for deeper penetration of the **laser beam** and minimizes the post-operative bruising seen in **laser** treatments relative to standard treatments with pulsed **dye lasers**.

positron emission tomography (PET): Medical imaging technique using a radioactive tracer that emits positrons. The positrons react with electrons in the body's molecules to produce gamma rays, which are then detected.

postmenopausal: After **menopause**.

postmortem: Occurring after death. It is a colloquial expression for an examination of the body after death (autopsy).

potassium chromate (K_2CrO_4): Nonscattering, homogeneously absorbing liquid used to construct **tissue phantoms**.

power: Rate of delivery of **energy**. It is normally measured in **watts** (W), that is, **joules** (J) per second (s). The smaller and larger **power** units used in **biomedical optics** and photomedicine to characterize **light** sources and delivery optics include the microwatt (μW), 10^{-6} W; milliwatt (mW), 10^{-3} W; kilowatt (kW), 10^3 W; megawatt (MW), 10^6 W; and gigawatt (GW), 10^9 W.

power density: The **power** of the **light wave** that propagates through a unit area that is perpendicular to the direction of propagation of the **light wave**. **Power density** or **intensity** is measured in W/cm^2 or W/m^2.

preamplifier: An electronic **amplifier** that precedes another **amplifier** to prepare an electronic signal for further amplification or processing.

precancerous: **Tissue lesion** that carries the risk of turning into **cancer**. It is a preliminary stage of **cancer**. These **precancerous lesions** can have several causes: **UV radiation**, **genetics**, and exposure to such **cancer**-causing substances as arsenic, tar, or **x-ray radiation**.

pre-embryo: Performed in the Advanced Reproductive Technologies laboratory after egg (produced in the ovaries each month) aspiration and sperm collection. Oocytes (eggs) are fertilized and form **pre-embryos** (fertilized eggs) or blastocysts (an advanced stage of development of the **pre-embryo**—usually on day 5–6).

premenopausal: Prior to **menopause**.

presbyopia: The eye's diminished ability to focus that occurs with aging. The most widely held theory is that it arises from the loss of elasticity of the **crystalline lens**, although changes in the lens's curvature from continual growth and loss of **power** of the **ciliary muscles** have also been postulated as its cause.

pressure: Force per unit area applied on a surface in a direction perpendicular to that surface. **Pressure** is scalar and has units in pascals, $1 \text{ Pa} = 1 \text{ N/m}^2 = 10^{-5}$ bar (dyn/cm^2) $= 10.197 \times 10^{-6}$ at $= 9.8692 \times 10^{-6}$ atm $= 7.5006 \times 10^{-3}$ Torr (mmHg) $= 145.04 \times 10^{-6}$ psi, where at is the technical atmosphere $= 1 \text{ kgf/cm}^2$, atm is the atmosphere $= 760$ Torr (mmHg), mmHg is an abbreviation for millimeters of mercury, and psi is the pound-force per square inch, $1 \text{ psi} = 6894.76$ Pa. Atmospheric **pressure** at sea level $= 760$ Torr or 14.7 psi. Pressure is transmitted to solid boundaries or across arbitrary sections of fluid normal to these boundaries or sections at every point.

pressure transient: Analysis of **pressure** changes over time.

Prevotella intermedia*:** An obligatory **anaerobic**, black-pigmented, **Gram-negative bacteria** consisting of rods and frequently associated with **periodontal** disease, including adult **periodontitis**, acute necrotizing ulcerative **gingivitis**, and pregnancy **gingivitis**. This organism is also involved in extraoral infections such as nasopharyngeal infection and intra-abdominal infection. It co-aggregates with ***Porphyromonas gingivalis.

Prevotella nigrescens*:** Genospecies that is very close to ***Prevotella intermedia. ***Prevotella intermedia*** is likely to be more associated with **periodontal** sites, whereas ***Prevotella nigrescens*** seems to be more frequently recovered from healthy gingivae.

prickle cells layer: Layer between the ***stratum granulosum*** and ***stratum basale***, characterized by the presence of prickle **cells**— **cells** with delicate, radiating processes connected to similar **cells**, providing a dividing **keratinocyte** of the ***stratum spinosum*** of the **epidermis**.

prism: Transparent optical element with flat, polished surfaces that refract **light**. The exact angles between the surfaces depend on the application. The traditional geometrical shape is that of a triangular **prism** with a triangular base and rectangular sides, and in colloquial use, "**prism**" usually refers to this type. **Prisms** are typically made out of glass but can be made from any material that is transparent to the **light wavelengths** for which they are designed and with **refractive index** different from the surrounding **media**. A **prism** can be used to break **light** up into its constituent spectral **colors**, to reflect **light**, or to split **light** into components with different **polarizations**, such as a **dichroic (dichromatic) prism**, **Wollaston prism**, or **Glan–Taylor polarization prism**. A **prism** is the basic optical element in some **evanescent-wave sensors** and in **attenuated total reflectance Fourier-transform infrared spectroscopy (ATR FTIR)**.

probability: Relative **frequency** with which an event occurs or is likely to occur.

probability density function (PDF): Function that describes the distribution of **probability** over the values of a continuous random variable. The **probability** of a random variable falling within a given set is given by the integral of its density over the set.

probability distribution function: General term when the **probability** distribution is defined as a function over general sets of values. It can be used to denote the **probability density function (PDF)**, the **probability mass function (PMF)**, or a cumulative distribution function.

probability mass function (PMF): Function that gives the **probability** that a discrete random variable is exactly equal to some value.

probe beam: **Light** or **laser beam** used for an object or material probing.

prokaryotes: Organisms without a **cell nucleus** or any other **membrane**-bound organelles. Most are unicellular, but some **prokaryotes** are multicellular. **Bacteria** are **prokaryotes**.

proliferation: **Cell** growth in the context of **cell** development and **cell** division (reproduction). When applied to **cell** division, the term refers to the growth of **cell** populations, where one **cell** (the "mother **cell**") grows and divides to produce two "daughter **cells**."

proliferative disorder: Growth or production of **cells** by multiplication of parts.

propagation constant of electromagnetic wave (EMW): The logarithmic rate of change, with respect to distance in a given direction, of the complex amplitude of any electromagnetic field component. In free space it is $k = \omega/c = 2\pi\nu/c = 2\pi/\lambda$, where ν is the **frequency** of the **EMW** (in particular, an optical **wave**) and λ is its **wavelength**. Because k is proportional to $1/\lambda$, it is also called the **wavenumber**. For the **EMW** propagating in a matter with **refractive index** n, the propagating constant is $k = n\omega/c = 2\pi n\nu/c = 2\pi n/\lambda$.

***Propionibacterium acnes*:** The relatively slow-growing, (typically) aerotolerant anaerobe **Gram-positive bacterium** that is linked to the **skin** condition called acne. This **bacteria** is largely commensal and thus present on most people's **skin**, and it lives on **fatty acids** in the **sebaceous glands** on **sebum** secreted by them. It is named after its ability to generate propionic acid.

propylene glycol (PG): Colorless, viscous, **hygroscopic** liquid, $CH_3CHOHCH_2OH$, used chiefly as a lubricant and as a solvent for **fats**, **oils**, and waxes. It is an **optical clearing agent**.

prostate (prostate gland): Muscular, **glandular** organ that surrounds the urethra of males at the base of the **bladder**.

protein: **Amino acids** joined together in a chain by peptide bonds between their amino and carboxylate groups. An **amino acid** residue is one **amino acid** that is joined to another by a peptide bond. Each **protein** has a unique sequence of **amino acid** residues; this is its primary structure. Just as the letters of the alphabet can be combined to form an almost endless variety of words, **amino acids** can be linked in varying sequences to form a huge variety of **proteins**. The sequence of **amino acids** in a **protein** is defined by the sequence of a **gene**, which is encoded in the genetic code. In general, the genetic code specifies 20 standard **amino acids**. Like other biological **macromolecules**, such as **polysaccharides** and **nucleic acids**, **proteins** are essential parts of organisms and participate in virtually every process within **cells**. Many **proteins** are **enzymes** that catalyze biochemical reactions and are vital to **metabolism**. **Proteins** also have structural or mechanical functions, such as actin and myosin in **muscle** and the **proteins** in the **cytoskeleton**, that form a system of scaffolding that maintains **cell** shape. **Proteins** are also important in **cell** signaling, **immune responses**, **cell adhesion**, and the **cell** cycle. **Proteins** may be purified from other cellular components using a variety of techniques such as ultracentrifugation, precipitation, **electrophoresis**, and chromatography. Methods commonly used to study **protein** structure and function include immunohistochemistry, site-directed mutagenesis, and mass spectrometry. Most **proteins** are linear polymers built from series of up to 20 different L-α-**amino-acids**. Most **proteins** fold into unique 3D structures. The shape into which a **protein** naturally folds is known as its native conformation. Often four distinct aspects of a protein's structure are considered: primary structure (the **amino-acid** sequence), secondary structure (regularly repeating local structures stabilized by hydrogen bonds, such as alpha **helix**, beta sheet, and turns), tertiary structure (the overall shape of a single **protein** molecule providing spatial relationship of the secondary structures to one another; it is generally stabilized by nonlocal interactions, such as the formation of a **hydrophobic** core, salt bridges, hydrogen bonds, disulfide bonds, and post-translational modifications), and quaternary structure (the structure formed by several **protein** molecules, usually called **protein** subunits, that function as a single **protein** complex). **Proteins** may shift between several related structures while they perform their functions— such functional rearrangements involving tertiary or quaternary structures are called conformational changes and are often induced by the binding of a substrate molecule to an enzyme's active site, or the physical region of the **protein** that participates in chemical catalysis, or by the thermal vibrations and the collisions with other molecules in solutions. **Proteins** can be divided into three main classes that correlate with typical tertiary structures: globular **proteins**, **fibrous proteins**, and **membrane proteins**. Almost all globular **proteins** are soluble, and many are **enzymes**. **Fibrous proteins** are often structural, such as **collagen**, the major component of **connective tissue**, or **keratin**, the **protein** component of **hair** and nails. **Membrane proteins** often serve as receptors or provide channels for polar or charged molecules to pass through the **cell membrane**.

proteoglycan: A special class of glycoproteins that are heavily glycosylated. They consist of a core **protein** with one or more covalently attached glycosaminoglycan chain(s). These chains are long, linear **carbohydrate** polymers that are negatively charged under physiological conditions due to the occurrence of sulphate and uronic acid groups.

proteomics: The study of **proteins**, the **gene expression** in health and disease. The identification, profiling, and quantification of **proteins** are characteristic to the structural **proteomics**. Studies of **protein** structure, localization, modification, interactions, activities, and functions belong to functional **proteomics**.

protoporphyrin IX (Pp IX): Pertaining to carbonic acids— its absorbing bands are the same as for other **porphyrins** (see **hemoglobin spectra**), e.g., in diethyl ester solution, **Pp IX** has the following peaks: 403 nm (**Soret band**), 504, 535, 575, and 633 nm (Q bands). **Pp IX** is the immediate heme precursor. **Exogenous administration** of **ALA** (**delta (δ)-aminolevulenic**

acid), an early precursor in heme synthesis, induces accumulation of **endogenous** photoactive **porphyrins**, particularly **Pp IX**. Induced **Pp IX** is used in **cancer** diagnostics and **photodynamic therapy (PDT)**.

psoralene: Pertaining to furocumarins. Its absorbing peaks lie in the UV at 295 and 335 nm. **Psoralene** is used in **photochemical therapy** of **psoriasis** and other **dermatosis (PUVA)**.

psoriasis: Common chronic **skin** disease characterized by scaly patches (**psoriasis** focus or **psoriatic** plaque).

psoriatic: Pertaining to **psoriasis**.

pulp: Soft **connective tissue** at the center for a **tooth** containing **fibroblasts, collagen, blood vessels, nerves**, and **dentin** forming odontoblasts. Apical foramen is an opening at the bottom of the root that connects **pulp** to **periodontal ligament** around the **tooth**; **blood vessels** and **nerves** enter **pulp** here. The **pulp** provides protection due to the presence of odontoblasts that make more **dentin** to protect the **tooth** under conditions of **pulp** assault, e.g., **caries**, and it also provides nutrition due to rich **vascular** supply. **Pulp** shrinks as odontoblasts form more **dentin** during the lifetime of the **tooth**.

pulpal: Related to **pulp**.

pulpitis: Medical condition in which an **inflammation** of the dental **pulp** occurs.

pulse energy: **Energy** of a pulse of pulsed **light**.

pulse laser: **Laser** that generates a single pulse or a set of pulses. A **laser** with **Q-switching** produces so-called **giant pulses**, since a mode-locked **laser** produces ultrashort pulses with a high repetition rate.

pulse oximeter: An instrument for **pulse oximetry**.

pulse oximetry: Technique that measures the quantities of oxy- and **deoxyhemoglobin** in human **blood**-bearing **tissues**. The concept is based on the fact that **light** transmission in human **tissue** varies with arterial pulsations, and comparing the pulsating portion of the red and **infrared** signals should yield **absorption** data for arterial (oxygenated) **blood** alone, as the **absorption** of venous **blood** and other **tissues** are constant or slowly varying. The use of this technique has been firmly established as a "standard of care" in every operating room and intensive care unit. It is used in pulmonary disease studies, in anaesthesiology for monitoring **oxygen saturation** in patients, and in many other applications. The technique has the drawback of being unreliable in conditions of low perfusion (at the site of measurement, normally the finger), subject movement or shivering, and the presence of abnormal **hemoglobins** [**hemoglobin** bound to molecules other than **oxygen**, for instance, **carboxyhemoglobin (COHb)**].

pulse wave: **Wave** of **pressure** sent along the **arteries** by every contraction of the **ventricle**. The increased **pressure** can be felt if the **artery** is pressed against a **bone** (usually in the **wrist**). The **pressure wave** travels much faster than the flow of **blood** through the **artery**. The pulse becomes fainter the farther it is from the **heart**. In the **capillaries**, it completely disappears.

pulsed light: **Light** produced as a single pulse of duration τ_p (**pulsewidth**) measured in seconds (s), or as successive trains of pulses with some repetition rate (**frequency**) f_p measured in **hertz** (1/s). Lamps can generate **light** pulses of duration τ_p in **millisecond** (ms) (10^{-3} s), **microsecond** (µs) (10^{-6} s), or **nanosecond** (ns) (10^{-9} s) ranges, and only **lasers** can generate shorter pulses, i.e., in **picosecond** (ps) (10^{-12} s) and **femtosecond** (fs) (10^{-15} s) ranges with a high repetition rate fp up to 100 MHz. A **laser** with **Q-switching** produces so-called **giant pulses**, as the mode-locked **laser** produces ultrashort pulses with a high repetition rate. Depending on the technology used, the form of

429

the pulses can be different: rectangular, triangle, or Gaussian. To describe energetic properties of pulsed **light**, a few characteristics are introduced, such as pulse **energy** E_p, **peak power** P_p (**power** of the individual pulse), and **average power** for a train of pulses P_{ave}. Peak **power** is calculated as $P_p = E_p/\tau_p$. Thus, for ultrashort pulses, **peak power** can be extremely high even for low or moderate **light** energies, and **tissue** breakdown can be expected; however, the **average power** of **light**, calculated as $P_{ave} = E_p \times f_p$, need not be very high: for example, if a **light** source generates pulses with an **energy** of $E_p = 0.1$ J, at a rate of $f_p = 1$ Hz (one per second) and duration of $\tau_p = 10$ ns, then $P_p = E_p/\tau_p = 107$ W, or 10 MW, as the **average power** is only $P_{ave} = E_p \times f_p = 0.1$ W, or 100 mW.

pulsewidth: Duration of a pulse, τ_p.

pump-beam (pulse): **Laser** (**light**) beam (or pulse) used to pump a nonlinear material or induce an interaction between an optical field and matter to produce lasing or **spectroscopy**.

pupil: Opening of the **iris** of the **eyeball**. Radiating **muscles** dilate the **pupil**, and a ring of **muscle** (a sphincter) around the **pupil** constricts it. The regulation of its size is a reflex action caused by the stimulus of **light** on the optic **nerve**.

purpurin: Photosensitizer of the chloryn family with an excitation band around 660 nm; it is used in **cancer** diagnostics and photodynamic therapy. Purlytin® is the commercialized product. At **PDT**, typical **laser power** dose is 200 J/cm².

PUVA therapy: A form of **photochemical therapy** based on the impregnation of diseased **skin** by a psoralen as a **photosensitizer** and the use of **UVA radiation** to provide the phototoxic effect (reduction of **cell** abnormal **proliferation** due to cross-linking of **DNA** molecules in the **cell** nuclei). It is used to treat **psoriasis** and other **skin** diseases.

pyloric: Pertaining to the region of the **stomach** that connects to the **duodenum**.

pyroelectric detector: Type of thermal **infrared detector** that acts as a current source with output proportional to the rate of change of its temperature.

pyroelectric vidicon (PEV) (*Synonym*: pyrovidicon): Video camera tube with a receiving element fabricated of pyroelectric material and sensitive to **wavelengths** from about 2–20 μm. It is used in **infrared** thermal viewers.

pyrolysis: Irreversible **tissue** damage with carbonization reaching temperatures ~350–450 °C. It is one of the mechanisms of photo-induced **tissue** destruction.

pyrometer: Any instrument used for temperature measurement. A **radiation** or **brightness pyrometer** measures **visible energy** and relates it to **brightness** or **color temperature**. An **infrared pyrometer** measures **infrared radiation** and relates it to target surface temperature.

pyrovidicon: See **pyroelectric vidicon (PEV)**.

pyrrolidonecarboxylic acid (PCA): 2-pyrrolidone-5-carboxylic acid is a cyclic derivative of glutamic acid, which is physiologically present in mammalian **tissues**.

Q-switched laser: Laser operating in **Q-switching** mode.

Q-switching: Sometimes known as **giant pulse** formation, it is a technique by which a **laser** can be made to produce a pulsed output beam. The technique allows the production of **light** pulses with extremely high (gigawatt) **peak power**. Compared to **mode-locking, Q-switching** leads to much lower pulse repetition rates, much higher pulse energies, and much longer pulse durations. Sometimes both techniques are applied at once.

quadrature mixer: An electronic device that mixes signals with different frequencies by the act of squaring.

qualitative measurement: Term describes the classification of themes and interconnections, content analysis, grounded theory and discourse analysis, and reliability and validity, all of which are just as important as they are in **quantitative measurement**. There are computer programs to assist in analysis, and although these might not necessarily save time, they often offer more systematic ways of coding data and identifying connections and themes, for example, the process of obtaining and interpreting **thermal images** based on thermal **contrast** in order to identify anomalies. The purpose is more to determine where a temperature difference exists than what the temperature difference is between the target and its surroundings. On the whole, qualitative research tends to be small scale, simply because it is hugely labor intensive.

quantitative measurement: Quantitative research relies primarily on numbers as the main unit of analysis. It is more commonly used as a primary method in scientific and clinical research, such as drug trials or laboratory experiments where tests may need to be repeated many times, for example, to ensure that a new drug is safe. Another example is the process of obtaining **thermal images** with correct temperature readings. Such measurements are especially useful in situations where the exact temperature or temperature difference of the target determines whether it falls in or out of a determined criteria or range of acceptability. **Quantitative measurement** is also important in R&D and process-control situations.

quantum detection limit: Limit of detection that is defined by the quantum fluctuations of any **light** source, including a **laser**, associated with **spontaneous emission** and defined by the temperature of the medium that emits the **light** being detected. Such fluctuations, as in the case of **photon shot noise**, cause the irregularity of photoelectron emissions that induces random errors in a photoelectron measuring system; mean square of photoelectron current fluctuations is also defined by the average photocurrent i and the photodetector's **bandwidth** B_D: $i^2 = 2eiB_D$, where e is the charge of electron, but the average photocurrent i is proportional to the mean **power** of quantum fluctuations. It is also difficult to achieve the **quantum detection limit** in practice.

quantum dot (QD): **Semiconductor** nanostructure that confines the motion of conduction band electrons, valence band holes, or excitons (bound pairs of conduction band electrons and valence band holes) in all three spatial directions. The confinement can be due to electrostatic potentials (generated by external electrodes, doping, strain, and impurities), the presence of an interface between different **semiconductor** materials (e.g., in core-shell nanocrystal systems), the presence of the **semiconductor** surface (e.g., **semiconductor** nanocrystal), or a combination of these. A **quantum dot** has a discrete quantized **energy spectrum** and contains a small finite number (of the order of 1–100) of conduction band electrons, valence band holes, or excitons, i.e., a finite number of elementary electric charges. These luminescent **nanoparticles** were introduced as biological labels since they were revealed to be rather photostable with variable emission spectra, depending on the size of these particles.

quantum efficiency: Ratio of the number of electrons emitted by a **photodetector** to the number incident at the detector's surface **photons**.

quantum flux: See **intensity**.

quantum yield: For a **radiation**-induced process, it is the number of times that a defined event (usually a chemical reaction step) occurs per **photon** absorbed by the system. This yield is a measure of the efficiency with which absorbed **light** produces some effect. Since not all **photons** are absorbed productively, the typical **quantum yield** is less than 1. **Quantum yields** greater than 1 are possible for photo-induced or **radiation**-induced chain reactions in which a single **photon** may trigger a long chain of transformations. In optical **spectroscopy**, the **quantum yield** is the **probability** that a given quantum state is formed from the system initially prepared in some other quantum state. For example, a singlet-to-triplet transition **quantum yield** is the fraction of molecules that, after being photoexcited into a **singlet state**, cross over to the **triplet state**. The **fluorescence quantum yield** is defined as the ratio of the number of **photons** emitted to the number of **photons** absorbed.

quantum-well laser: **Diode laser** with a quantum-dimension **heterostructure** as a lasing medium. Owing to a high **gain**, it has a high slope of the **watt**/ampere characteristic.

quarter-wave plate: See **lambda (λ)-phase plate**.

quasi-ballistic photons: **Photons** that migrate within a **scattering** medium along trajectories that are close but identical to **ballistic photons**.

quasi-crystalline approximation: First introduced by Melvin Lax to break the infinite heirarchy of equations that results in studies of the coherent field in discrete random **media**, this approximation simply states that the conditional average of a field with the position of one **scatterer** held fixed is equal to the conditional average with two **scatterers** held fixed. It has met with great success for a range of concentrations from sparse to dense and for long and intermediate **wavelengths**.

quasi-elastic light scattering (QELS): See **dynamic light scattering**.

quasi-monochromatic wave (light): **Wave (light)** that has a very narrow but nonzero **frequency** (or **wavelength**) **bandwidth**. It can be presented as a group of monochromatic waves with a slightly different **wavelength**.

quasi-Newton inverse algorithm: **Algorithm** for finding an extreme point. It builds up an approximation of the inverse Hessian of the function and is often regarded as the most sophisticated means of solving unconstrained problems.

quasi-ordered medium: Medium that has a structure very close to being ordered, but is nevertheless not completely ordered due to specific interactions between molecules and molecular structures. Natural media such as **water** and some living **tissues** are examples of **quasi-ordered media**. See also **Ornstein–Zernike equation**, **Percus–Yevick approximation**, and **radial distribution function** *g*(*r*).

quasi-periodic: Almost periodic (process, signal, function, fluctuations, etc.). Almost-periodicity is a property of dynamic systems that appear to retrace their paths through phase space, but not exactly.

radar graph: Similar to line graphs, except that they use a radial grid to display data items. A radial grid displays scale value grid lines circling around a central point, which represents zero. Higher data values are farther from the center point. The **radar graph** type gets its name because it resembles a radar screen. The radial grid is not circular but an equilateral polygon.

radial artery: Main **artery** of the lateral aspect of the **forearm**.

radial distribution function *g*(*r*)**:** Pair distribution function that is a statistical characteristic of the spatial arrangement of the **scatterers**. It is used to describe **light scattering** in a correlated disperse system, such as a **quasi-ordered medium**.

radian: An angular measurement equal to the ratio of the arc length of a circle to its radius. The circumference of a circle is 2π times the radius. Thus, π **radians** = 180 deg, and 1 **radian** = 180 deg/π = 57.29578 deg. A radian is a unit used to express instrument angular **field of view**.

radiance: See **intensity** and **irradiance**.

radiant emittance: Radiometric quantity that characterizes the **power** per unit area of **electromagnetic radiation** at a surface, measured in watts per meter squared (W/m^2). In contrast with **irradiance**, this term is used when the **radiation** is emerging from the surface. For example, all bodies emit **electromagnetic radiation** in the **IR** spectral range and with intensities that correspond to their temperature (see **heat light sources**). This quantity characterizes the total amount of **radiation** present at all frequencies. It is also common to consider each **frequency** in the **spectrum** separately. This is called spectral **radiant emittance** measured in $W/(m^2 \cdot nm)$. If a point source radiates **light** uniformly in all directions and there is no **absorption**, then the **radiant emittance** drops off in proportion to the distance from the object squared, since the total **power** is constant and is spread over an area that increases with the square of the distance from the source. See **radiometry terms**.

radiant exitance: Also called radiosity, it is the total **light energy** (radiant flux) leaving a target surface. This is composed of radiated, reflected, and transmitted components. Only the radiated component is related to target surface temperature. See **radiometry terms** and **radiant emittance**.

radiant (radiation) exposure: Irradiance E integrated over the time of irradiation $H = \int E dt$, the simplified expression of which is $H = E \times t$ when the **irradiance** is constant over the time considered. For a parallel and perpendicularly incident beam not scattered or reflected by the target or its surroundings, **fluence** (F) is an equivalent term.

radiant intensity: Radiometric quantity characterizing solid angular **power density** of **electromagnetic radiation**, measured in **watts** per **steradian** (W/sr).

radiation: **Energy** that travels in the form of waves or high-speed particles. It occurs naturally in sunlight and **sound waves**.

Artificial **radiation** comes from lamps, **lasers, LEDs, ultrasonic transducer, x-rays**, and nuclear sources. See **electromagnetic radiation** and **ionization radiation**.

radiation dosimetry: Measurement or calculation of **radiation** doses. The quantity of **radiation** absorbed by a given mass of material, especially **tissue**, depends upon the strength and distance of the **light** source and the duration of **radiant** exposure.

radiation-transfer equation (RTE): Integro-differential equation (the Boltzmann or linear transport equation) that is a balance equation describing the flow of particles (e.g., **photons**) in a given volume element that takes into account their velocity c, location r, and changes due to collisions (i.e., **scattering** and **absorption**).

radiation-transfer theory (RTT): Basic theory allowing one to calculate **light** distributions in **multiple scattering media** with **absorption**, such as **tissues**. The heart of this theory is the **radiation-transfer equation (RTE)**. The basic parameters are the **scattering coefficient, absorption coefficient, scattering anisotropy factor**, and **reduced scattering coefficient**.

radical: See **free radical**.

radio frequency (RF): Part of the electromagnetic **spectrum** between about 10^6 and 10^9 Hz.

radio-frequency interference (RFI): See **electromagnetic-interference (EMI) noise**.

radiometry terms: Irradiance and **radiant emittance (radiant exitance)** characterize the **power** per unit area of **electromagnetic radiation** at a surface. **Irradiance** is used when the **electromagnetic radiation** is incident on the surface. **Radiant emittance (radiant exitance)** is used when the **radiation** is emerging from the surface. The units for all of these quantities are **watts**

per square meter ($W \cdot m^{-2}$). All of these quantities characterize the total amount of **radiation** present at all frequencies. For consideration of each **frequency** in the **spectrum** separately, spectral **irradiance** and **radiant exitance** (**radiant emittance**) are introduced and measured in $W \cdot m^{-2} \cdot nm^{-1}$.

raffinose: Complex **carbohydrate**; a trisaccharide composed of galactose, fructose, and **glucose**.

raft tissue: Organotypic **tissue** culture (see **cell culture**) systems permitting the growth of differentiated **keratinocytes** *in vitro* or even the creation of a **skin**-equivalent **tissue** model composed of **dermis** with **type I collagen** and **fibroblast cells**, and **epidermis** of differentiated **keratinocytes**.

Raman amplifier: Based on the **stimulated Raman scattering (SRS)** phenomenon, this process, as with other **stimulated emission** processes, allows for all-optical amplification. **Optical fiber** is almost exclusively used as the nonlinear medium for **SRS**, which is therefore characterized by a resonant **frequency** downshift of ~13 THz. The **SRS** amplification process can be readily cascaded, thus accessing essentially any **wavelength** in the **fiber** low-loss guiding window.

Raman laser: **Light** source similar to an ordinary **laser**, but with an **amplifier** medium based on **stimulated Raman scattering (SRS)** rather than on **stimulated emission** from excited atoms or ions. The main attraction of this type of device is that essentially any **Raman laser wavelength** can be achieved with a suitable choice of the pump **wavelength**, provided that both **wavelengths** are within the transparency region of the material and a sufficiently high nonlinearity and/or optical **intensity** are reached.

Raman scattering: Change in **wavelength** of **light** scattered while passing through a transparent medium. The collection of new **wavelengths** is characteristic for the molecular structure of the **scattering** medium and differs from the **fluorescence**

spectrum in being much less intense and unrelated to an **absorption band** of the medium. The frequencies of new lines are combinations of the **frequency** of the incident **light** and the frequencies of the molecular vibrational and rotational transitions. There are a variety of Raman effects such as **resonance Raman scattering (RRS)**, **surface-enhanced Raman scattering (SERS)**, **stimulated Raman scattering (SRS)**, and **coherent anti-Stokes Raman scattering (CARS)**, which can considerably improve typically low signal intensities of spontaneous **Raman scattering** and/or provide lesser **fluorescence** background from most biomolecules.

Raman shifter: Device that is based on **stimulated Raman scattering** phenomenon. Typically, 1st, 2nd, and 3rd Stokes components are induced by a nonlinear medium by pumping a **laser** whose **wavelength** should be shifted. For example, the optimum conversion in the $Ba(NO_3)_2$ crystal at pump with a **Ti: Sapphire laser** (815–900 nm) provides a 1047 cm^{-1} shift and extends the **laser** tuning range to 1300 nm. Gaseous and liquid Raman cells are also available. However, among the most efficient Raman crystals that are suitable for a wide range of pumping pulse duration from **picoseconds** to **nanoseconds**, $Ba(NO_3)_2$, $KGd(WO_4)_2$, and $BaWO_4$ are recommended.

Raman spectroscopy: Spectroscopic technique used in condensed matter (physics, chemistry, and biology) to study vibrational, rotational, and other low-**frequency** modes in a molecular system. It relies on **inelastic scattering** or **Raman scattering** of **monochromatic light**, usually from a **laser** in the **visible**, **NIR**, or near-**UV** range. **Phonons** or other excitations in the system are absorbed or emitted by the **laser light**, resulting in the **energy** of the **laser photons** being shifted up or down. The shift in **energy** gives information about the **phonon** modes in the system. **Infrared spectroscopy** yields similar but complementary information. See **resonance Raman scattering (RRS)**, **surface-enhanced Raman scattering (SERS)**, **stimulated Raman scattering (SRS)**, and **coherent anti-Stokes Raman scattering (CARS)**.

random access second-harmonic-generation (RASH) micro-scope: The major limiting factor of nonlinear microscopes, such as those used in **two-photon fluorescence microscopy** and **second-harmonic generation microscopy**, is their scanning time. The optical measurement of time-dependent processes do not always require the production of full images. Instead, more time should be spent collecting as many **photons** as possible from selective positions where the image plane intersects the biological objects of interest. Using this approach, fast physiological processes, such as neuronal action potentials in the soma of multiple **neurons**, can be recorded at a sampling **frequency** of more than 1 kHz by scanning a set of points within a plane at high speed with two orthogonal **acousto-optic deflectors (AODs)**. On this basis, high-speed, random-access **laser**-scanning systems for **TPF** and **SHG** microscopies were built and applied to record fast physiological signals. **RASH** microscopes are capable of optically recording fast events (~1 ms) in a wide field (150×150 μm^2) and with deep **tissue** penetration in living **brain** slices.

random medium: Specific state of a nonuniform (inhomogeneous) medium characterized by the irregular spatial distribution of its physical properties, including **optical properties**.

random phase screen (RPS) (*Related terms*: deep random phase screen, weakly scattering random phase screen): Specific state of a **random medium** characterized by random spatial variations of the **refractive index** that induce corresponding variations in the **phase shift** of the optical **wave** transmitted through or reflected by the **RPS**.

raw experimental data: Experimental data before processing.

Rayleigh distribution: Probability distribution of a random variable x described by the **probability density function** $p(x) = (x/a^2)\exp(-x^2/2a^2)$, $x \geq 0$. $P(x) = 0, x < 0$. The distribution has a positive asymmetry, and its mode is at the point $x = a$. The mean value and **variance** are, respectively, equal to $\langle x \rangle = (\pi/2a)$ and $\sigma^2 = (4 - \pi)a^2/2$.

Rayleigh (resolution) limit: Resolution of an optical device with a circular **aperture** is limited by the **diffraction** of **light** through that **aperture**. As the **aperture** increases in diameter, the **diffraction** spot gets smaller, increasing the resolution of the instrument. In the case of a circular **aperture**, the **diffraction** pattern has the shape of a disk surrounded by rings; the disk is called the **Airy disk**. If the images of two point sources of **light** overlap such that the centers of the images are closer than the radius of the **Airy disk**, the images are considered to be unresolvable. This definition can be written as $\Delta\theta = 1.22\lambda/D$, where $\Delta\theta$ is the minimum resolvable angular separation of the two objects, λ is the **wavelength** of the **light**, and D is the diameter of the **aperture**.

Rayleigh scattering: Theory that addresses the problem of calculating **scattering** by small particles (with respect to the **wavelength** of the incident **light**) when the individual particle **scattering** can be described as if it is a single dipole, the scattered **irradiance** is proportional to λ^{-4} and increases as a^6, and the angular distribution of the scattered **light** is isotropic. Rayleigh theory is applicable under the condition that $m(2\pi a/\lambda) << 1$, where m is the relative **refractive index** of the **scatterers**, $m = n_s/n_0$, n_s is the **refractive index** of the **scatterers**, n_0 is the **refractive index** of the ground material where **scattering** particles are embedded, $(2\pi a/\lambda)$ is the size parameter, a is the radius of the particle, and λ is the **wavelength** of the incident **light** in a medium.

Rayleigh–Debye theory (approximation): Theory that addresses the problem of calculating the **scattering** by a special class of arbitrarily shaped particles. It requires that the electric field inside the particle be close to that of the incident field and that the particle can be viewed as a collection of independent dipoles that are all exposed to the same incident field.

Rayleigh–Gans theory [approximation (RGA)]: See **Rayleigh –Debye theory (approximation)**.

reactive nitrogen species (RNS): A family of antimicrobial molecules derived from **nitric oxide** (·NO) and **superoxide** ($O_2\cdot-$) produced via the enzymatic activity of inducible nitric oxide synthase 2 (NOS2) and **NADPH oxidase**, respectively. NOS2 is expressed primarily in **macrophages** after induction by cytokines and microbial products. **RNS** act together with **ROS** to damage **cells** and cause nitrosative stress. Therefore, these two species are often collectively referred to as **ROS/RNS**. **RNS** are involved in the signaling pathways from **mitochondria** to nuclei that is considered as one of the mechanisms of **low-level laser therapy (LLLT)**.

reactive oxygen species (ROS): Reactive molecules that contain the **oxygen** atom. They are very small molecules that include **oxygen** ions and peroxides, and can be either inorganic or organic. They are highly reactive due to the presence of unpaired valence shell electrons. **ROSs** form as a natural byproduct of the normal **metabolism** of **oxygen** and have important roles in **cell** signaling. However, during environmental stress (e.g., **UV** or heat exposure), **ROS** levels can increase dramatically and cause **oxidative stress**, which can result in significant damage to **cell** structures. **ROSs** are involved in the signaling pathways from **mitochondria** to **nuclei** which is considered as one of the mechanisms of **low-level laser therapy (LLLT)**.

red blood cell (RBC): See **erythrocyte**.

red/green/blue (RGB): An additive **color** model in which red, green, and blue **light** are added together in various ways to reproduce a broad array of **colors**. The main purpose of the **RGB color** model is for the sensing, representation, and display of images in electronic systems, such as digital cameras, televisions, and computers. The model is based on human perception of **colors**. **RGB** is a device-dependent **color** space. Different devices detect or reproduce a given **RGB** value differently since the **color** elements (such as phosphors or dyes) and their response to the individual R, G, and B levels vary from manufacturer to manufacturer (or even in the same device over time). Thus an **RGB** value does not define the same **color** across devices without some kind of **color** management.

redox: Shorthand for reduction-oxidation reaction, which describes all chemical reactions in which atoms have their oxidation number (oxidation state) changed. This can be either a simple process, such as the oxidation of carbon to yield carbon dioxide or the reduction of carbon by hydrogen to yield methane (CH_4), or it can be a complex process, such as the oxidation of sugar in the human body through a series of very complex electron transfer processes. Oxidation describes the loss of electrons or an increase in oxidation state by a molecule, atom, or ion, while reduction describes the gain of electrons or a decrease in oxidation state by a molecule, atom, or ion.

reduced scattering coefficient: Lumped property incorporating the **scattering** coefficient μ_s and the **scattering anisotropy factor** g: $\mu_s' = \mu_s(1 - g)$ [cm^{-1}]; μ_s' describes the **diffusion** of **photons** in a random walk of step size of $1/\mu_s'$ [cm], where each step involves **isotropic scattering**. This is equivalent to describing **photon** movement using many small steps, $1/\mu_s$, that each involve only a partial (anisotropic) deflection angle if there are many **scattering** events before an **absorption** event, i.e., $\mu_a \ll \mu_s'$ (**diffusion** regime, see **diffusion approximation**); μ_s' is useful in the **diffusion** regime that is commonly encountered when treating how **visible** and **near-infrared light** propagates through **tissues**. For many **tissues**, the **reduced scattering coefficient** obeys a **power** law, $\mu_s' = q\lambda^{-h}$ (cm^{-1}, λ in μm). For example, for a human **forearm** in the **wavelength** range 700–900 nm, constants q and h are determined as 5.50 ± 0.11 and 1.11 ± 0.08, respectively. From Mie theory it follows that the **power** constant h is related to an averaged size of the **scatterers** with the Mie-equivalent radius a_M. Once h is determined, this radius can be derived if the relative **refractive index** between the equivalent spheres and the surrounding medium m is known or determined.

reflectance: See **optical reflectance**.

reflecting (reflection, reflectance) spectroscopy: Spectroscopy that uses for spectral analysis the **light** back-reflected (scattered) by an object.

reflection: See **optical reflection**.

reflection confocal microscopy (RCM): Reflection mode of **confocal microscopy** that is suitable for *in vivo* studies of **tissues**.

refraction: Change in direction of a ray of **light**, **sound**, heat, or the like, while passing obliquely from one medium into another in which its speed is different. The term also describes the ability of the eye to refract **light** that enters it so as to form an image on the **retina**; it is the determination of the refractive condition of the eye.

refractive index: See **index of refraction**.

refractive index mismatch: Difference in the **index of refraction** of two media in contact. A **scattering** medium can be considered as a medium containing **scattering** particles whose **index of refraction** is mismatched relative to the **index of refraction** of the **ground substance** [see **immersion medium (liquid)** and **immersion technique**].

$$\left(\frac{n_{12}^2 - 1}{n_{12}^2 + 2}\right)\frac{1}{\rho_{12}} = \left(\frac{n_1^2 - 1}{n_1^2 + 2}\right)\frac{p_1}{\rho_1} + \left(\frac{n_2^2 - 1}{n_2^2 + 2}\right)\frac{p_2}{\rho_2}$$

refractive index mixture rules: Theoretical mixture rules are based upon the electromagnetic theory of **light** with the implicit restriction that the molecules (or particles) may be considered as dipoles or assemblies of dipoles induced by an external field. The best known mixture rule is that of Lorentz–Lorenz, written for a two-component system, where n_{12}, n_1, and n_2 are the refractive indices of solution, solvent, and solute, respectively, ρ_i and p_i are the density and weight fraction of the i-th component, respectively, and ρ_{ij} is the density of the mixture of the two components.

Dale–Gladstone law formulation is an empirical one: $(n_{12} - 1)/\rho_{12} = [(n_1 - 1)/\rho_1]p_1 + [(n_2 - 1)/\rho_2]p_2$, which is valid for very diluted solutions $(n_{l2} \rightarrow n_l)$ and small differences in **refractive indices** of solute and solvent, $n_2 \rightarrow n_l$. For these limitations, the Dale–Gladstone mixture rule follows from the Lorentz-Lorenz theoretical formula. In its turn, the very widely used **Dale–Gladstone law** is found to be identical with the Arago and Biot equation, $n_{12} = n_1 f_1 + n_2 f_2$, if, in both cases, volume additivity is assumed, $f_1 + f_2 = 1$, where f_1 and f_2 are the **volume fractions** of the respective components in the solution. The **volume fraction** f_i may be obtained from either $f_i = c_i/\rho_i$, where c_i is the concentration in g/cm^3, or from $f_i = p_i \rho_{ij}/\rho_i$. Over an extensive concentration range, the Lorentz–Lorenz equation alone appears to be the reliable equation (W. Heller, "Remarks on refractive index mixture rules," *J. Phys. Chem.* **69**(4), 1123–1129, 1966).

rehydration: The replenishment of **water** and electrolytes lost through **dehydration**.

remineralization: The improvement of the mineral status of mineralized **tissues**. For example, oral **saliva** that is supersaturated with calcium and phosphate provides permanent **remineralization** of teeth that have lost their mineral components (see **demineralization**). **Remineralization** is enhanced by the presence of fluoride.

remittance: Total amount of **light** returned by a surface (**tissue**) whether by **specular reflection**, **diffuse reflection**, or by bulk **scattering**. See **backscattering**.

ren: See **kidney**.

repetition rate (frequency): Number of pulses per second. The **repetition rate** is measured in **hertz**.

reproducibility: One of the main principles of the scientific method, it refers to the ability of a test or experiment to be accurately reproduced or replicated by someone else working independently.

resistor: Two-terminal electrical or electronic component that resists an electric current by producing a voltage drop between its terminals in accordance with Ohm's law.

resonance energy transfer (RET): See **Förster resonance energy transfer (FRET)**.

resonance Raman scattering (RRS): This **Raman scattering** technique allows one to enhance the spontaneous Raman effect and, thus, to overcome the major disadvantage of low signal intensities from most biomolecules. It probes vibrations of **chromophores** and requires careful selection of the excitation **wavelength** to be within the **absorption band** of a **chromophore**. When using **RRS** to boost the Raman signals, single-**photon** excited **fluorescence** must be dealt with. The generally weaker Raman signals can be detected in the presence of intense overlapping **fluorescence** if the Stokes shift of the **fluorescence** emission is large or if the faster **scattering** process is registered before the emission by using time-gating techniques.

respiratory chain: In aerobic respiration, electrons are transferred from **metabolites** to molecular **oxygen** through a series of **redox** reactions mediated by an electron transport chain. The resulting free **energy** is used for the formation of **ATP** and **NAD**. In **anaerobic** respiration, analogous reactions take place with an inorganic compound other than **oxygen** as the ultimate electron acceptor.

retarder: See **optical retarder**.

reticular dermis: See **reticular layer of dermis**.

reticular fiber: Very thin, almost inextensible threads of **reticulin**. They form a network of intercellular **fibers** around and among the **cells** of many **tissues**, e.g., in many large organs such as the **liver** and **kidney**, and also in **tissues** as **nerves** and **muscles**. They especially support and unite **reticular tissue**.

reticular layer of dermis (*Synonym*: reticular dermis): Lower layer of the **dermis**. It is made primarily of coarse **collagen** and elastic **fibers** and is denser than the papillary **dermis**. Reticular **dermis** strengthens the **skin**, providing structure and elasticity. It also supports other **skin** components and appendages such as **sweat glands** and **hair follicles**.

reticular tissue: **Tissue** consisting of a network of reticular **fibers** around and among **cells**, with **lymph** in the intercellular spaces. It occurs in **muscles**, **nerves**, and the larger **glands**.

reticulin: Tough **fibrous protein**, similar to **collagen** but more resistant to higher temperatures and chemical reagents. It occurs in vertebrate **connective tissue** as reticular **fibers**. Reticulin is formed in **embryos** and also in **wounds**. It often changes to **collagen**.

retina: Innermost coat of the posterior part of the **eyeball** that receives the image produced by the eye **cornea** and **crystalline lens**. It is continuous with the optic **nerve** and consists of several layers, one of which contains the rods and cones sensitive to **light**.

retinal: Pertaining to the **retina**.

retinal nerve fiber layer (RNFL): Formed by the expansion of the **fibers** of the optic **nerve**. The **RNFL** comprises bundles of unmyelinated **axons** that run across the surface of the **retina**. The cylindrical organelles of the **RNFL** are axonal **membranes**, **microtubules**, neurofilaments, and **mitochondria**. Axonal **membranes**, like all **cell membranes**, are thin (6–10 nm) **phospholipid bilayers** that form cylindrical shells enclosing the axonal **cytoplasm**. Axonal **microtubules** are long tubular polymers of the **protein** tubulin with an outer diameter of ~25 nm, an inner diameter of ~15 nm, and a length of 10–25 μm. Neurofilaments are stable **protein** polymers with a diameter of ~10 nm. **Mitochondria** are ellipsoidal organelles that contain densely involved **membranes** of **lipid** and **protein**; they are 0.1–0.2 μm thick and 1–2 μm long.

retinol (*Synonym*: vitamin A): **Fat**-soluble, yellow **oil** stored in the **liver**. It is not excreted and can accumulate in the body to produce toxic effects. Retinol is used in the body to produce visual purple, the **pigment** in rods of the **retina**. A deficiency impairs vision and also causes **epithelial cells** to become flattened and heaped up on one another. This leads to xerophthalmia and also to the formation of hard, rough **skin**.

reverberation: The persistence of sound in a particular space after the original sound is removed. When sound is produced in a space, a large number of echos build up and then slowly decay as the sound is absorbed by the walls and air, creating **reverberation** (reverb).

Reynolds number (Re): The ratio of inertial to viscous forces in a gas or liquid flow that quantifies the relative importance of these two types of forces for given flow conditions.

rheumatoid arthritis: Chronic disease marked by **inflammation** of the joints. It is frequently accompanied by marked deformities and is ordinarily associated with manifestations of a general, or systemic, affliction.

rhodamine: Family of related chemical compounds; examples include **Rhodamine** 6G, **Rhodamine** B, and **Rhodamine** 123. They are used as dyes because they fluoresce and can thus be measured easily and inexpensively. **Rhodamines** are generally toxic and are soluble in **water**, methanol, and **ethanol**. Rhodamine B (excitation 510 nm/**fluorescence** 580 nm) is used in biology as a staining fluorescent dye. Rhodamine 123 (excitation 480 nm/**fluorescence** 540 nm) is used in biochemistry to inhibit **mitochondrion** function.

rib: One of a series of curved **bones** that are articulated with the vertebrae and occur in pairs (12 in humans) on each side of the vertebrate body. Certain pairs are connected with the sternum and form the thoracic wall.

Riboflavin® (*Synonym*: vitamin B$_2$): An easily absorbed micronutrient with a key role in maintaining health in humans. It is the central component of the cofactors **FAD** and **FMN** and is therefore required by all flavoproteins. It is required for a wide variety of cellular processes, plays a key role in **energy metabolism**, and is required for the **metabolism** of **fats**, ketone bodies, **carbohydrates**, and **proteins**. Milk, cheese, leafy green vegetables, **liver**, **kidneys**, mature soybeans, **yeast**, and mushrooms are good sources of vitamin B$_2$, but exposure to **light** destroys **riboflavin**. It is used as a **PDT photosensitizer** where, for example, **UVA** (365 nm) **radiation** with concomitant **administration** of Medio-Cross® (**riboflavin/dextran** solution) as a **photosensitizer** generates **singlet oxygen** and **superoxide free radicals**. This process leads to physical cross-linking of the corneal **collagen fibers** and makes it mechanically stronger.

ribonucleic acid (RNA): **Nucleic-acid** polymer consisting of **nucleotide monomers**, which acts as a messenger between **DNA** and **ribosomes** and is also responsible for making **proteins** out of **amino acids**. **RNA** polynucleotides contain ribose sugars and predominantly uracil, unlike **DNA**. It is transcribed (synthesized) from **DNA** by **enzymes** called **RNA** polymerases and further processed by other **enzymes**. **RNA** serves as the template for translating of **genes** into **proteins**, transferring **amino acids** to the **ribosome** to form **proteins**, and also translating the transcript into **proteins**.

ribosomal ribonucleic acid (rRNA): Central component of the **ribosome**, the **protein**-manufacturing machinery of all living

cells. The function of **rRNA** is to decode **mRNA** into **amino acids** and to interact with the **tRNAs** during translation by providing peptidyl transferase activity. The **tRNA** then brings the necessary **amino acids** corresponding to the appropriate **mRNA** codon. See **ribonucleic acid (RNA)**.

ribosome: In the **cytoplasm** of a **cell**, any of the several minute, angular or spherical particles composed of **protein** and **RNA**. It has a **refractive index** that lies within a relatively narrow range (1.38–1.41) and is on the order of 20 nm in diameter.

Riccati–Bessel function: Only slightly different from spherical Bessel function, it applies to cases of **Mie scattering**, where **electromagnetic waves** are scattered by a sphere.

Ringer's solution: An aqueous solution of the chlorides of sodium, potassium, and calcium that is **isotonic** to animal **tissue** and is used topically as a **physiological solution** and, in experiments, to bathe animal **tissues**.

Romanowsky stain: Biological staining technique that uses a mixture of **eosin** Y and modified **methylene blue**, producing a distinctive shade of purple. The demethylation of **methylene blue** in aqueous solution with heat and alkali produces a mixture of **azure** A, **azure** B, methylene violet, and **methylene blue**. **Eosin** Y is then added to produce a "neutral" dye, and the precipitate is dissolved in a mixture of methanol and **glycerol** to form a stable stock solution. This solution is diluted with **water** or an aqueous buffer to form a "working" solution (stable approximately for 3 hours) that is used in the staining of pathology specimens.

root mean square (r.m.s.): Measure of **dispersion** in a **frequency** distribution. It is equal to the square root of the mean of the squares of the deviations from the arithmetic mean of the distribution.

rosaniline hydrochloride: See **fuchsine**.

rotational diffusion: Molecular rotational motion is usually only the rotational rocking near one of the equilibrium orientations. The molecules depend on the interaction with neighbors, and by jumping in time, they are changing their orientation. The activation **energy** is required to change the angle of orientation. Brownian rotational motion can be valid only for comparatively large molecules with slowly changing of orientation angles. In this case, the differential character of rotational motion is valid, and the rotational **diffusion** equation can be written. The interaction of molecules can be considered as the friction foreseen with the moment P proportional to the angle velocity $\Omega, P = \xi\Omega$, where ξ is the rotational coefficient of friction that can be connected with rotational **diffusion coefficient** $D_R = kT/\xi$. In the case of a small macroscopic sphere with radius $a, \xi = 8\pi a 3\eta$, where η is the coefficient of viscosity.

rotational state (level): The particular pattern of **energy** levels (and hence of transitions in the rotational **spectrum**) for a molecule is determined by its symmetry: linear molecules (or linear rotors), symmetric tops (or symmetric rotors) spherical tops (or spherical rotors), and asymmetric tops. Rotational **spectroscopy** (using microwave and/or Raman spectroscopic techniques) studies the **absorption** and emission **electromagnetic radiation** by molecules associated with a corresponding change in the rotational quantum number of the molecule.

rouleaux: Medical term for a condition wherein the **blood cells** clump together, forming what looks like stacks of coins.

ruby laser: The first working **laser** (invented by Theodore Maiman in 1960), it is a **solid-state laser** that uses a synthetic ruby crystal as its **gain** medium, which is pumped by pulse **light** from a spiral or linear xenon lamp. At room temperature, it produces pulses of **visible light** at a **wavelength** of 694.3 nm, which penetrates through **tissues** well. In a free-running mode, **laser** pulses are typically in the **millisecond** range, 1–3 ms, with a pulse **energy** of 1 J in TEM_{00} mode. In contrast to many other **solid-state lasers, ruby lasers** have a low efficiency of 0.1%. They were used extensively in tattoo and **hair** removal but are being replaced by **alexandrite lasers** and **Nd:YAG lasers**. **Ruby lasers** are used in **holography** of big objects and other applications where short pulse and energetic, deep-red **light** is required.

ruthenium red: Inorganic dye ammoniated ruthenium oxychloride, used in **histology** to stain aldehyde-fixed **mucopolysaccharides**. **Ruthenium red** inhibits calcium transport through **membrane** channels and its uptake by isolated **mitochondria**. More often, the term "**ruthenium red**" is used for a ruthenium-containing, red-staining dye that is an organic, polycationic, cell-biology reagent that tightly binds to tubulin dimers and Ryanodine receptors. It is a potent inhibitor of intracellular calcium release by Ryanodine receptors at nanomolar concentrations (~20 nM).

Rytov approximation: First-order approximation that is commonly used to derive a simple expression relating the scattered field to the object in the presence of weak inhomogeneities. In contrast to **Born approximation**, which provides satisfactory description of small-sized weak **scatterers**, the **Rytov approximation** is efficiently used on large, weakly **scattering** objects. This approximation is used to design **algorithms** for **diffraction** medical tomography to determine the structure of large-sized, low **contrast** dielectric objects (related to some kinds of **tissues**).

saccharose (*Synonym: sucrose*): Disaccharide (**glucose** + fructose) with the molecular formula $C_{12}H_{22}O_{11}$. It is best known for its role in human nutrition.

safranin: A biological stain used in **histology** and cytology; other names are **safranin** O, basic red 2, dimethyl **safranin**, or trimethyl **safranin**. It is used as a counterstain in some staining protocols, coloring all **cell** nuclei red. This is the classic counterstain in a **Gram's stain**. It can also be used for the detection of **cartilage**, mucins, and **mast cell** granules, and it is also used as **redox** indicator.

saline: Salt solution that is used for medical treatment. This solution is designed to have the same **osmotic pressure** as **blood**.

saliva: Viscid, colorless, watery fluid secreted into the **mouth** by the **salivary glands**. Its major functions are in tasting, chewing, and swallowing food by keeping the **mouth** moist and starting the digestion of starches. **Saliva** is composed of **water** (99%), **mucin**, bicarbonate, **proteins**, and minerals. Its functions include lubrication (protection of **mucosa**), assistance in the formation of food bolus for effective swallowing, initial enzymatic breakdown of some food components (e.g., amylase), microbial protection (contains **antibodies** and other protective **proteins**, e.g., lysozyme), buffering (contains bicarbonate, phosphate, etc.), **tooth enamel remineralization** (supersaturated with calcium and phosphate), flushing out food debris, and facilitating speech.

salivary gland: There are three major **salivary glands** and hundreds of minor **salivary glands** in the **oral cavity**. Major **salivary glands** are parotid, submandibular, and sublingual **glands**, all of which are paired. Minor **salivary glands** are scattered throughout the oral **mucosa**. **Salivary glands** release their contents (**saliva**) through ducts. Chewing, tasting, or smelling food sends a **nerve** stimulus to the **brain**, which results in secretion of **saliva**. Saliva secretion is low but constant at **baseline**, and it can be stimulated to a high level. Normal salivary levels in the **mouth** are maintained when (1) there is adequate amount of **salivary gland tissue** and (2) the **glands** secrete normal amounts of **saliva**. The amount of **saliva** produced varies widely—in healthy individuals, it ranges from 0.5–1.5 L daily.

sarcoma: **Malignant** growth of abnormal **cells** in **connective tissue**.

saturable absorber: Saturable **absorption** as a physical phenomenon is related to an interband transition where the **energy** of absorbed **photons** is transferred to electrons, which, e.g., for **semiconductor** materials, are brought from the valence band to the conduction band. There is first some fairly rapid thermalization relaxation within the conduction and valence band within, e.g., 50–100 fs, and later (often on a time scale of tens or hundreds of **picoseconds**), the carriers recombine, often with the aid of crystal defects. For low optical intensities, the degree of **electronic excitation** is small, and the **absorption** remains unsaturated. In contrast, at high optical intensities, electrons can accumulate in the conduction band, so that initial states for the absorbing transition are depleted while final states are occupied. Therefore, the **absorption** is reduced. After saturation with a short pulse, the **absorption** recovers, first partially due to intraband thermal relaxation, and later completely via recombination. Saturable absorbers based on this effect are widely used in **laser** technology [see **semiconductor saturable absorber mirror (SESAM)**].

saturation (color): Refers to the perceived **intensity** of a specific **color**. **Saturation** is related to but a distinct concept from **colorfulness** and **chroma**. It is the **colorfulness** of a **color** relative to its own **brightness**.

scalp: Anatomical area bordered by the face anteriorly and the **neck** to the sides and posteriorly.

scanning cytometry: A microscope-based **laser scanning cytometry** that allows one to make **fluorescence** measurements and topographic analysis on individual **cells**. **Laser**-induced **fluorescence** of labeled cellular specimens is detected in multiple discrete **wavelengths**, and the spatially-resolved data are processed to quantify **cell proliferation**, **apoptosis**, **gene expression**, **protein** transport, and other cellular processes. For instance, **confocal microscopy** and two-photon imaging techniques are able to detect fluorescently labeled **cells**, not only *in vitro* but also *in vivo*.

scanning near-field optical microscopy (SNOM) [*Synonym*: near-field scanning optical microscopy (NSOM)]: Principle based on illuminating a sample that is placed within a short distance— much less than the wavelength of the **light**—from the point **light**

source within its near field. The point **light** source is created by irradiating a sub-wavelength diameter **aperture** of 50–100 nm in diameter that defines the **SNOM** resolution. Pulled or etched (tapered) **optical fibers** that are entirely coated with a metal except for an aperture at the fiber's tip are usually employed as point **light** sources. The distance between the point **light** source and the sample surface should be precisely controlled, usually through a feedback mechanism that is unrelated to the **SNOM** signal. At **SNOM** measurement, a point **light** source is scanned over the sample surface with an accuracy of a few **nanometers**, and the optical signal reflected from the surface is collected and detected by the same **optical fiber**.

scanning-probe microscopy (SPM): Includes **atomic-force microscopy (AFM), scanning-tunneling microscopy (STM),** and **near-field scanning optical microscopy (NSOM)**.

scanning-tunneling microscopy (STM): A super-high-resolution microscopy for imaging surfaces at the atomic level. **STM** is based on the concept of quantum tunneling, where a conducting tip is brought very near to the surface to be examined. The resulting tunneling current is a function of tip displacement from the surface, applied voltage between the tip and the surface, and the local density of states of the sample. The scanning of the tip position across the surface allows for gathering information about tunneling current distribution in the form of a surface image. The typical lateral and depth resolution is ~0.1 nm and ~0.01 nm, respectively. **STM** can be used not only in vacuum but also in air and other gases, in water and other liquids, and in a wide temperature range.

scar: Areas of **fibrous tissue** that replace normal **skin** (or other **tissue**) after **injury**. A **scar** results from the biologic process of **wound** repair. Thus, scarring is a natural part of the healing process.

scatterer: An inhomogeneity or a particle of a medium that refracts or diffracts **light** or other **electromagnetic radiation**.

Light is diffused or deflected as a result of collisions between the **wave** and particles of the medium. Sometimes it is a rough surface or a **random phase screen**, also called a **scatterer**.

scattering: Process in which a **wave** or beam of particles is diffused or deflected by collisions with particles of the medium it transverses.

scattering angle: Related to **photon** scattered by a particle so that its trajectory is deflected by a deflection (**scattering**) angle θ in the **scattering** plane and/or by azimuthal angle of **scattering** φ in the plane perpendicular to the **scattering** plane.

scattering anisotropy factor: Measure of the amount of forward direction retained after a **single scattering** event. If a **photon** is scattered by a particle so that its trajectory is deflected by a deflection angle θ, then the component of the new trajectory that is aligned in the forward direction is presented as $\cos\theta$. There is an average deflection angle and the mean value of $\langle\cos\theta\rangle$ is defined as the anisotropy, $g \equiv \langle\cos\theta\rangle$. The value of g varies from -1 to 1: $g = 0$ corresponds to isotropic (**Rayleigh**) **scattering**, $g = 1$ to total forward **scattering** (Mie **scattering** at large particles), and -1 to total backward **scattering**.

scattering coefficient: When a particle with a particular geometrical size redirects incident **photons** into new directions and so prevents the forward on-axis transmission of **photons**, this process constitutes **scattering**. The **scattering** coefficient μ_s [cm^{-1}] describes a medium containing many **scattering** particles at a concentration described as a volume density ρ [cm^3]. The **scattering** coefficient is essentially the cross-sectional area σ_{sca} [cm^{-1}] per unit volume of medium: $\mu_s = \rho\sigma_{sca}$, see **photon scattering cross section**. A **power** law for dependence of the **scattering coefficient** on the **wavelength** is typical for many **tissues**, $\mu_s \propto \lambda^{-h}$; for different **tissue** structures, parameter h ranges between 1–2.

scattering cross section: See **photon-scattering cross section**.

scattering indicatrix: An angular dependence of the scattered **light intensity**. For thin samples, the normalized **scattering indicatrix** is equal to the **scattering phase function**.

scattering medium: Medium in which a **wave** or beam of particles is diffused or deflected by collisions with particles of this medium.

scattering phase function: Function that describes the **scattering** properties of the medium and is in fact the **probability** density function for **scattering** in the direction $\bar{s}'$ of a **photon** traveling in the direction $\bar{s}$. It characterizes an elementary **scattering** act: If **scattering** is symmetric relative to the direction of the incident **wave**, then the **phase function** depends only on the **scattering** angle θ (angle between directions $\bar{s}$ and $\bar{s}'$). Direct measurement of the **scattering phase function** $p(\theta)$ is important for the choice of an adequate model for the **tissue** being examined. It is usually determined from goniophotometric measurements (GPMs) in relatively thin **tissue** samples. Measured-**scattering-intensity** angular dependence is approximated either by the **HGPF** or by a set of **HGPFs**, with each function characterizing the type of **scatterers** and specific contribution to the angular dependence. In the limiting case of a two-component model of a medium containing large and small (compared with the **wavelength**) **scatterers**, the angular dependence is represented in the form of anisotropic and isotropic components. Other approximating functions are equally useful, for example, those obtained from the **Rayleigh–Gans approximation**, ensuing from the Mie theory, or a two-parameter **GKPF**. Some of these types of approximations were used to find the dependence of the **scattering anisotropy factor** g for **dermis** and **epidermis** on **wavelengths** in the range of 300–1300 nm, which proved to coincide fairly well with the empirical formula, $g_e \sim g_d \sim 0.62 + \lambda \times 0.29 \times 10^{-3}$ on the assumption of a 10% contribution of **isotropic scattering** (at least in the spectral range of 300–630 nm); the **wavelength** λ is given in **nanometers**.

scattering plane: Plane defined by positions of a **light** source, a **scattering** particle, and a detector.

scattering spectrum: Spectrum of scattered **light**. It can be differential, measured, or calculated for a certain **scattering** angle or integrated within an angle (field) of view of the measuring **spectrometer**.

Scheimpflug camera: Camera that is based on the Scheimpflug principle. This technique allows for the assessment of the anterior segment of the eye, from the front of the **cornea** to the back of the **lens**, in a sagittal plane. The Scheimpflug principle allows for quantification of the **light** scatter.

Schiff base (*Related term*: azomethine): A functional group that contains a carbon-nitrogen double bond with the nitrogen atom connected to an aryl, alkyl group, a phenyl, or substituted phenyl—but not hydrogen. The general formula is $R_1R_2C=N-R_3$. The **Schiff base** is a stable imine if R_3 is an aryl or alkyl group, and is anil if R_3 is a phenyl or substituted phenyl.

sciatic nerve: Large **nerve** that runs down the lower limb. It is the longest single **nerve** in the body.

sclera: Dense, white, **fibrous membrane** that, with the **cornea**, forms the external covering of the **eyeball**. Scleral regions include the limbal, equatorial, and posterior pole regions.

scleroderma: Disease in which all the layers of the **skin** become hardened and rigid.

sclerotic: Related to dense **fibrous** or tubular **tissue**, i.e., **sclera** or **sclerotic dentin** (**dentin** that has become translucent due to **calcification** of the dentinal tubules as a result of **injury** or normal aging, also called transparent **dentin**). Scleroderma is a **pathological** thickening and hardening of the **skin**. Sclerotic parenchyma applies to **tissue** composed of **cells** with hardened and thickened walls.

sclerotomy: Surgical **incision** of the **sclerotic** coat of the eye.

sea collagen: Used in **cosmetics**. Sea **collagen** is a better choice than bovine **collagen** because of its affinity to the **skin** and its richness in trace elements. Deep **skin moisturizer** prevents and reduces **wrinkles** and lines by redensifying and restructuring the **skin**.

sebaceous gland: Tiny **sebum**-producing **gland** found everywhere except on the palms, **lips**, and soles of the feet. The thicker the density of **hair**, the more **sebaceous glands** are found. They are classified as holocrine **glands**.

sebum: **Sebaceous glands** secrete an oily substance called **sebum** that is made of **fat** (**lipids**) and the debris of dead **fat**-producing **cells**. In the **glands**, **sebum** is produced within specialized **cells** and is released when these **cells** burst. **Sebum** is odorless, but its bacterial breakdown can produce odors.

second-harmonic generation (SHG): Also called **optical frequency doubling**. Nonlinear optical process, in which **photons** interacting with a nonlinear material are effectively "combined" to form new **photons** with twice the **energy**, and therefore twice the **frequency** and half the **wavelength** of the initial **photons**. SHG occurs in materials without a center of symmetry, having a large **hyperpolarizability**. In the past several years, **SHG** has been extended to biological applications, such as imaging molecules that are intrinsically second-harmonic-active in live **cells** [e.g., **collagen** (label-free imaging)] and for studying biological molecules by **labeling** them with second-harmonic-active tags, in particular as a means to detect conformational change at any site and in real time. The major limitation is only noncentrosymmetric biological structures could be imaged.

second-harmonic-generation (SHG) microscopy: An immediate implementation for **TPF microscopy** is represented by **second-harmonic generation microscopy**. SHG has already

459

been largely used for imaging noncentrosymmetric molecules inside **cells**, cellular **membranes**, the **brain**, and other biological **tissues**. In particular, because of its fibrillar structure, **collagen** intrinsically has a high **hyperpolarizability**, providing a strong second-harmonic signal, and it can be imaged inside **skin dermis tissue** using **SHG microscopy**. This technique has been used for investigating **collagen** orientation and its structural changes in healthy **tissues** as human **dermis** or **cornea**, and also for studying its dynamical **modulation** in **tumors**.

sedimentation: Describes the motion of molecules in solutions or particles in suspensions in response to an external force such as gravity, centrifugal force, or electric force. Sedimentation may pertain to objects of various sizes, ranging from suspensions of dust and pollen particles to cellular suspensions to solutions of single molecules such as **proteins** and peptides.

selective laser sintering (SLS):   An additive manufacturing technique that uses a high-**power laser** (for example, a CO_2 **laser**) to fuse small particles of plastic, metal, ceramic, or glass powders into a mass representing a desired 3D object. The **laser** selectively fuses powdered material by scanning cross-sections generated from a 3D digital description of the part on the surface of a powder bed. The physical process can be full melting, partial melting, or liquid-phase **sintering**. Depending on the material, up to 100% density can be achieved with material properties comparable to those from conventional manufacturing methods. This technology has potential for the production of biomaterials and artificial organs. For example, **biocompatible**, microstructured **bone tissue** scaffolds has been designed on the basis of ceramic with axially oriented and random micropores. The industry produces dental **implant** titanium screws using a hybrid structure comprising a fully dense body with a porous surface morphology. It should be noted that this is a highly productive, totally automated process.

selective photothermal treatment: Technique that utilizes a penetrating **laser beam** to enhance **laser–tissue** interaction by *in* *situ* application of **light** absorbers with appropriate **absorption** spectra. While **endogenous light** absorbers can be used for this purpose, it is most common to use **exogenous** absorbers to achieve the selective **light absorption** for appropriate **wavelengths** and appropriate levels of **tissue absorption**. The absorber molecules in the **photothermal** interaction can absorb **light** to reach an excited high-energy state. When the molecules return to their ground states by nonradiative process due to interaction with other molecules, the **energy** is released in the form of heat. If the activation of the absorber molecules continues with a sufficiently high rate, the rate of heat production in the **tissue** can exceed the rate of heat dissipation. As a consequence, the **tissue** temperature increases steadily. The dose of the dye and the **laser fluence** can be adjusted in order to achieve desirable temperature elevation in target **tissue**, resulting in selective **photothermal tissue** destruction. Specifically, an 805-nm **diode laser** and **indocyanine green (ICG)** were first used for thermal treatment of rat **tumors**, both *in vitro* and *in vivo*. As local **laser-light**-induced heaters, plasmonic **nanoparticles** with plasmonic resonance in the **NIR** are now used. Both **CW** and ms-pulse **laser heating** by 808-nm **diode lasers** have similarly short time kinetics (temperature rise up to 46–50 °C over a time of around 40 sec at mean **laser power density** of 1–3 W/cm^2). For example, **gold nanoparticles** (nanoshells) at their local injection mediate **laser** destruction of rat **muscle tissue** *in vivo* (at the depth of 4 mm) without any damage of superficial **tissues**. The use of functionalized **nanoparticles** at **blood** stream injection shows promise for **cancer cell labeling** and follow up **selective photothermal treatment**. This technique is also used for so-called "cold" **tissue laser welding**. The resulting temperature rise induces modifications in the **collagen**, creating intramolecular bridges between the tissue's cut walls. Ultimately, this treatment seals the **wound** with negligible thermal damage to the surroundings and an improved healing process.

selective photothermolysis (SP): **Electromagnetic radiation (EMR)** from **lasers**, lamps, and other sources (including microwave ones) has been used to treat a variety of medical conditions in ophthalmology, dermatology, urology, otolaryngology, and other medical fields. For example, in dermatology, **EMR** sources have been used to perform a wide variety of procedures including treatment of various pigmented **lesions**, removal of **hair**, unwanted veins and tattoos, and **skin** resurfacing. For all of these treatments, **endogenous** (**water**, **melanin**, **hemoglobin**, **proteins**, **lipids**, etc.) or **exogenous** (dyes, ink, carbon particles, metallic **nanoparticles**, etc.) absorbers present in the body are heated by **absorption** of either monochromatic or broadband **EMR**. These cases are well-described by the theory of **selective photothermolysis (SP)**. The aim of **SP** is to provide the permanent thermal damage of targeted **tissue** structures with the surrounding **tissue** held **intact**. The **SP** is based on three general principals: (1) the **wavelength** of **EMR** has to be selected to provide maximum **contrast** of **absorption** of the target versus surrounding **tissue** and other competitive targets, based on **absorption** spectra and location depth of targets. (2) The **pulsewidth** of **EMR** has to be selected to provide maximal **contrast** of heating of the target versus surrounding **tissue**, thus **pulsewidth** τ must be small compared to the thermal relaxation time (TRT) of the whole target, $\approx d^2/Fk$, where d is the size of the target in mm or cm, k is the coefficient of thermal **diffusion** of **tissue** ($k \approx 0.1$ mm^2/s $= 0.001$ cm$^2/s$ for **skin dermis**), and F is the geometrical factor, where $F = 8, 16,$ and 24 for planar, cylindrical, and spherical targets, respectively. Actually, if the condition $\tau \ll$ TRT is met, the heat generated within the target due to **EMR absorption** does not flow out of the structure until it becomes fully damaged (coagulated, injured). This approach provides both selective damage and minimum **light energy** deposition. (3) The **fluence** of the pulse has to be sufficient enough to provide **coagulation** or **ablation** of the target. The new extended theory of **SP** is valid for nonuniformly pigmented structures in **tissue** and postulates the following: (1) the **EMR wavelength** should be chosen to provide sufficient **contrast** between the **absorption coefficient** of the pigmented area and that of the **tissue** surrounding the target and provide **optical density** of pigmented area in the range $1 < \mu_a d < 3$; (2) the **EMR power** should be limited to prevent **absorption** loss in the pigmented area, but it must be sufficient to achieve a heater temperature higher than the target damage temperature; and (3) the **pulsewidth** should be made shorter than or equal to the thermal damage time (TDT), which can be significantly longer than the thermal relaxation time of the target.

selective plane illumination microscopy (SPIM):   By shining a very thin slice of **light** through a relatively large sample (2–3 mm) and then systematically moving (rotation and scanning) the specimen through the **light** sheet, images from each layer can be captured. Because no out-of-focus **light** is created, **SPIM** gives a sharper image of the sample without the usual background blur. **SPIM** minimizes the amount of **light**-induced damage and extends the life of the sample by using thin slices of **light** rather than illuminating the entire sample all at once. The entire procedure is fast enough that detailed 3D images can be acquired in minutes.

self-beating: Signal produced by photomixing the electric components of a scattered field from moveable **cells** or particles.

selfoc lens: See **graded-index (GRIN) lens**.

Sellmeier equation: An empirical relationship between **refractive index** n and **wavelength** λ (in vacuum) for a particular transparent medium. The equation is used to determine the **dispersion** of **light** in the medium (material **dispersion**). This is the development of the **Cauchy equation** to account for anomalous **light dispersion** regions, and to more accurately model a material's **refractive index** across the **UV**, **visible**, and **IR spectrum**. The usual form of the equation is $n^2 = 1 + B_1\lambda^2/(\lambda^2 - C_1) + B_2\lambda^2/(\lambda^2 - C_2) + B_3\lambda^2/(\lambda^2 - C_3)$, where $B_{1,2,3}$ and $C_{1,2,3}$ are experimentally determined Sellmeier coefficients. These coefficients are usually quoted for λ in **micrometers** or **nanometers**.

semen (*Synonym*: **seminal fluid**):   Viscid, whitish fluid produced in the male reproductive organ. It contains spermatozoa.

semiconductor: Material that has an **electrical conductivity** between that of a conductor and an insulator, that is, generally in the range of 10^3 **siemens** per centimeter to 10^{-8} S/cm. **Semiconductor** devices include various types of transistors, photovoltaic **cells** (solar **cells**), many kinds of diodes including **LEDs**, **diode lasers**, silicon controlled rectifiers, digital and analog integrated circuits, and **CCD** and **CMOS** cameras. External external electrical or optical fields may change a semiconductor's resistivity. In a metallic conductor, current is carried by the flow of electrons; in **semiconductors**, current can be carried either by the flow of electrons or by the flow of positively-charged "holes" in the electron structure of the material. Common semiconducting materials are **crystalline** solids, but amorphous and liquid **semiconductors** are also known. Silicon is used to create most **semiconductors** commercially; however, many other materials are used, including germanium, gallium arsenide, and silicon carbide. A pure **semiconductor** is often called an "intrinsic" **semiconductor**. The conductivity of **semiconductor** materials can be drastically changed by adding other elements, called "impurities," to the melted intrinsic material and then allowing the melt to solidify into a new and different crystal. This process is called "doping."

semiconductor optical amplifier (SOA): An **optical amplifier** made with **semiconductor gain** media. Its advantages are (1) a wide range of **gain** center **wavelengths** (750–900 nm for GaAs/Al$_x$Ga$_{1-x}$As and 1100–1600 nm for In$_{1-x}$Ga$_x$As$_{1-y}$P$_y$/InP /Al$_x$Ga$_{1-x}$As), (2) a high **gain** with a broad **bandwidth**, and (3) a fast **gain** response (250 ps).

semiconductor saturable absorber mirror (SESAM): Mirror structure with an incorporated **saturable absorber**, all made with **semiconductor** technology. It is mostly used for the generation of **nanosecond** to **femtosecond** pulses in various types of **lasers** by passive **Q-switching** or **mode-locking**. Typically, a **SESAM** contains a **semiconductor Bragg mirror** and (near the surface) a single quantum-well absorber layer. The materials of the **Bragg mirror** have a larger **bandgap energy** so that essentially no **absorption** occurs in that region. Such **SESAMs** are sometimes called saturable **Bragg reflectors (SBRs)**. For obtaining a large

modulation depth, for example, as required for passive **Q-switching** a thicker absorber layer can be used.

semilogarithmic scale: For example, functions of the kind $y = Be^{-\varphi x}$ are used to describe the **attenuation** of **light intensity** with distance x and may be plotted on a **semilogarithmic scale**. Taking $\log_{10}$ of both sides gives $\log_{10} y = \log_{10} B - \varphi x \log_{10} e = \log_{10} B - 0.434\varphi x$. Plotting $\log_{10} y$ versus x will therefore give a straight line of slope $0.434 \times \varphi$.

seminal fluid (*Synonym*: **semen**): An **Semen**, an organic fluid that usually contains spermatozoa. It is secreted by the sexual **glands** of a male and delivers the spermatozoa to fertilize female ova. In humans, **seminal fluid** also contains several components such as proteolytic and other **enzymes** as well as fructose that promote the survival of spermatozoa and provide a medium through which they can move. During the process of ejaculation (discharge of **semen**), sperm passes through the ejaculatory ducts and mixes with fluids from the seminal vesicles, the **prostate**, and the bulbourethral **glands** to form the **semen**. The seminal vesicles produce a yellowish viscous fluid rich in fructose and other substances that makes up about 70% of human **semen**. The prostatic secretion, influenced by dihydrotestosterone, is a whitish (sometimes clear), thin fluid containing proteolytic **enzymes**, citric acid, acid phosphatase, and **lipids**. The bulbourethral **glands** secrete a clear secretion into the **lumen** of the urethra to lubricate it. The accessory genital ducts, the seminal **vesicle**, **prostate glands**, and the bulbourethral **glands** produce most of the **seminal fluid**.

semi-permeable membrane: See **partially permeable membrane**.

sensory nerve: **Nerves** that receive sensory stimuli such as how something feels and if it is painful. They are made up of **nerve fibers** called sensory **fibers** (mechanoreceptor **fibers** sense body movement and **pressure** placed against the body, and nociceptor **fibers** sense **tissue injury**).

sentinel lymph node: The hypothetical first **lymph node** or group of nodes reached by metastasizing **cancer cells** from a **tumor**. The spread of some forms of **cancer** usually follows an orderly progression, spreading first to regional **lymph nodes**, then the next echelon of **lymph nodes**, and so on, since the flow of **lymph** is directional. The concept of the **sentinel lymph node** is important because of the advent of the **sentinel lymph node biopsy** technique. This technique is used in the staging of certain types of **cancer** to see if they have spread to any **lymph nodes**, since **lymph node** metastasis is one of the most important prognostic signs.

serum: **Blood plasma** with clotting factors removed.

shear rate: Measure of the rate of shear **deformation**. For simple shear cases, the rate is just a gradient of velocity.

shear stress: Stress state where the stress is parallel or tangential to a face of the material, as opposed to normal stress when the stress is perpendicular to the face. For a Newtonian fluid wall, shear stress is proportional to shear rate, where the coefficient of proportionality is the viscosity of the fluid.

sheath: Protective covering **fitting** closely to a structure or a part of an organism, especially an elongated structure or part.

shock wave: In general, this is a type of propagating disturbance. Like an ordinary **wave**, it carries **energy** and can propagate through a solid, liquid, or gas medium, or in the free space if it is **EMR**. **Shock** waves are nonlinear waves characterized by an abrupt, nearly discontinuous change in the characteristics of the medium. Across a **shock** there is always an extremely rapid rise in **pressure**, temperature, and density of the material or flow. A **shock wave** travels through most **media** at a higher speed than an ordinary **wave**. Unlike solitons (another kind of nonlinear **wave**), the **energy** of a **shock wave** dissipates relatively quickly with distance. In **tissues** and biofluids, **shock waves** are generated in **tissues** when a short **laser** pulse with a sufficient **intensity** interacts with a **tissue** due to local **tissue** explosion or thermal **ablation** (for strongly absorbing **tissues** or for transparent **tissues** at **femtosecond laser** excitation caused by optical nonlinear processes, very fast **plasma** heating, and expansion within the **laser** focus).

short-circuit: In electronics, a circuit with a load of an infinitely low resistance or **impedance** through which electric current flows.

short-pass filter: An optical **interference** or **absorptive filter** that attenuates longer **wavelengths** and transmits (passes) shorter **wavelengths** over the active range of the target **spectrum** (usually the **ultraviolet** and **visible** region). In **fluorescence microscopy**, these filters are frequently employed in **dichroic (dichromatic) mirrors (beamsplitters)** and excitation filters (see **epi-fluorescence interference and absorption-filter combinations**).

shot noise: Type of **electronic noise** that occurs when the finite number of particles that carry **energy**, such as electrons in an electronic circuit or **photons** in an optical device, is small enough to give rise to detectable statistical fluctuations in a measurement. It is important in electronics and photoelectronics. The strength of this noise increases with the average magnitude of the current or **intensity** of the **light**. However, because the signal increases more rapidly as the average signal becomes stronger, **shot noise** is often only a problem with small currents and **light** intensities.

Siegert formula: Formula that for **Gaussian statistics** relates the **intensity autocorrelation function** to the first-order **autocorrelation function**.

siemens: The unit of **electrical conductance** that is reciprocal of resistance; hence, one **siemens** (S) is equal to the reciprocal of one ohm.

signal oscillator: This term is used in heterodyne detecting systems for notation of the receiving signal, which can be presented as the **radio-** (or **optical**) **frequency** oscillator and has a slightly different **frequency** than that for the local oscillator [used for converting a high-**frequency** receiving signal to an intermediate **frequency** by mixing the local oscillator signal and receiving signal at an electronic (or photo-) detector].

signal-to-noise ratio (SNR): Ratio of received (detected) signal (an electric impulse) to **noise** (an electric disturbance in a measuring system that interferes with or prevents reception of a signal).

silicon oils (*Synonym*: polymerized siloxanes): Silicon analogues of carbon-based organic compounds that can form (relatively) long and complex molecules based on silicon rather than carbon. Chains are made of alternating silicon-**oxygen** atoms or siloxane, rather than carbon atoms.

silicon waxes: Semi-**crystalline** with a liquid melting point of 53–75 °C, their appearances range from clear and **light**-straw to white and off-white flake. They are semi-occlusive or occlusive formulations, lubricants, emollients, **water** repellents, replacements for **petrolatum**, thickeners, **moisturizers**, and emulsifiers for **water**-in-**oil** and **water**-in-silicone emulsions (up to 80% water content).

silicone: See **polyorganosiloxane**.

silver stain: Substance used to stain histologic sections. This kind of staining is important, especially to show **proteins** (for example type III **collagen**) and **DNA** in both substances inside and outside **cells**. It is also used in temperature-gradient **gel electrophoresis** and in polyacrylamide **gels**.

single scattering: Scattering process that occurs when a **wave** undertakes no more than one collision with particles of the medium in which it propagates.

single scattering approximation: In the case of a **tissue**, it assumes that the **tissue** is sufficiently thin that **single scattering** accurately estimates the **reflection** and transmission for the slab.

single-frequency laser: **Laser** that generates a single **frequency** (one longitudinal mode).

single-integrating-sphere "comparison" technique: This technique uses a single **integrating sphere** containing no baffles but three ports that can be either opened for **light** transmission or closed or covered by a sample or reference standards for the **calibration** (comparison) of **reflectance** or **transmittance** measurements. An additional two ports are used to illuminate samples by a **collimated light beam** and collect the scattered **light** by a **fiber bundle** placed at the "north pole" of the sphere. This technique has an advantage over the conventional double **integrating sphere** technique in that no corrections are required for sphere properties.

single-mode fiber: **Fiber** in which only a single mode can be excited. For a **fiber** with a **numerical aperture** $NA = 0.1$ and **wavelength** 633 nm, the single mode can be excited if the core diameter is less than 4.8 μm (see **fiber-cutoff wavelength**).

single-mode fiber optic Michelson interferometer: **Michelson interferometer** integrated with a **fiber optic single-mode X-coupler**, which optically connects a **light** source, the reference mirror, object, and **photodetector**.

single-mode laser: **Laser** that produces a **light beam** with a Gaussian shape of the transverse **intensity** profile without any spatial oscillations (see **Gaussian light beam**). In general, such **lasers** generate many optical frequencies (so-called longitudinal modes) that have the same transverse Gaussian shape.

single-photon counting mode: See **photon-counting system**.

single-photon emission computed tomography (SPECT): A radiopharmaceutical imaging technique based on detection of the gamma emission produced by a radionuclide [radioisotope, such as gallium (III)] injected into the bloodstream of a patient. To provide more targeted functional imaging of a particular organ or pathology, the radionuclide is often bound to a special radioligand that recognizes a specific type of tissue or cell. As a result, a gamma camera can be used to see radioligand biodistribution in tissues. These data are presented as cross-sectional slices through the patient, providing 3D imaging of blood perfusion, tissue metabolism, and receptor and cellular function. SPECT is applicable to the diagnosis and monitoring of pathologies in the brain, myocardium, skeleton, liver, and in tumors.

singlet oxygen ($^1O_2$): The common name used for the diamagnetic form of molecular **oxygen** (O_2), which is less stable than the normal triplet **oxygen**. Because of its unusual properties, **singlet oxygen** can persist for over an hour at room temperature, depending on the environment. Because of the differences in their electron shells, singlet and triplet **oxygen** differ in their chemical properties. The damaging effects of sunlight on many organic materials (polymers, etc.) are often attributed to the effects of **singlet oxygen**; it is a major species in **PDT cell** damage.

singlet state: In atomic physics, one of the two ways in which the spin of two electrons in an atom or molecule can be combined, the other being a **triplet state**. A single electron has spin $1/2$, and a pair of electron spins can be combined to form a state of total spin 1 (**triplet state**) and a state of spin 0 (**singlet state**). The singlet state is an **excited state** of a molecule that, upon absorbing **light**, can release **energy** as heat or **light** (**fluorescence**) and thus return to the initial (ground) state. It may alternatively assume a slightly more stable, but still **excited state** (**triplet state**), with an electron still dislocated as before, but with reversed spin.

singular eigenfunction method: Method to rigorously solve the **radiation-transfer equation (RTE)**. The **RTE** is solved using

Green's functions in terms of the singular eigenfunctions and their orthogonality relations together with the appropriate **boundary conditions**. The convergence of the numerical results is fast, and the analytical expressions are simple for solving numerically.

sintering: Method for making objects from powder, by heating the material below its melting point (solid state **sintering**) in a **sintering** furnace or by irradiation with **laser light** or microwaves until its particles adhere to each other. Sintering is traditionally used for manufacturing ceramic objects and has also found uses in fields such as powder metallurgy, including biomedical applications. See **selective laser sintering (SLS)**.

sinus: Sack or cavity in any organ or **tissue**, or an abnormal cavity or passage caused by the destruction of **tissue**. In common usage, "sinus" usually refers to the paranasal **sinuses**, which are air cavities in the cranial **bones**, especially those near the nose and connected to it, such as the **maxillary sinus**.

Sjögren's syndrome: An autoimmune disease where **antibodies** against various **tissues** (mainly **glands** in the eyes and **mouth**) cause **gland** destruction, resulting in dry eyes and **dry mouth**.

skeletal muscle: Type of striated **muscle** usually attached to the skeleton. It is mainly composed of **muscle cells (muscle fibers)** containing **myofibrils**, which consist of thin (actin) and thick (myosin) **myofilaments**. **Muscle fibers** are bound together into bundles called fascicles. Skeletal **muscles** are used to create movement, by applying force to **bones** and joints via contraction. They generally contract voluntarily (via somatic **nerve** stimulation), although they can contract involuntarily through reflexes.

skewness: See **asymmetry parameter**.

skin: External protective covering on a body, joined by **connective tissue** to the **muscles**. It generally consists of the inner

subcutaneous fat layer and **dermis**, and an outer **epidermis**, with the upper layer made of *stratum corneum*.

skin appendage: Structures associated with the **skin** such as **hairs**, **sweat glands**, **sebaceous glands**, and nails. They have their roots in the **dermis** or even in the hypodermis.

skin barrier function: Function that protects internal organs from the environment; it resides in the uppermost thin heterogeneous layer, called *stratum corneum*, that is composed of dead **protein**-rich **cells** and intercellular **lipid** domains. This two-compartment structure is renewed continuously, and when the barrier function is damaged, it is repaired immediately. Under low **humidity**, the *stratum corneum* becomes thick, the **lipid** content in it increases, and **water** impermeability is enhanced. The heterogeneous field in the **epidermis** induced by ions such as calcium and potassium regulates the self-referential, self-organizing system to protect the living organism.

skin flap: A tear in the **skin**, away from the body, with one side of the **skin** still attached. It is often used in optically aided *in vivo* studies of **blood microcirculation**, **skin optical clearing**, and drug testing in **animal models** (see **skin flap window**).

skin flap window: Special window surgically made in the **skin** area void of **blood vessels**; an implanted glass plate allows for prolonged *in vivo* studies of **skin vessels**.

skin irritation: Some physical and chemical exposures to the **skin** may cause **dermatitis** with redness, itching, and discomfort.

skin microdermabrasion: Quick, **noninvasive** procedure used to resurface the **skin**. It gently removes only the very top layers of damaged **skin** by "sand blasting" them with tiny crystals. The technique exfoliates and gently resurfaces the **skin**, promoting the formation of new, smoother and clearer **skin**.

skin moisturizer: Often claimed to be either humectants or occlusive agents. Humectants are small **hygroscopic** molecules that penetrate the *stratum corneum*. **Glycerin** is a prime example of this category of **moisturizers**: it is extremely **hygroscopic**, and when left to equilibrate in a moist environment, it will attract **water** until it reaches a level of 55% (w/w), meaning that each molecule of **glycerin** attracts about six molecules of **water**. Glycols and other polyhydroxy molecules like **propylene glycol**, butyleneglycol, **glucose, saccharose**, and sorbitol also work via this mechanism. The other well-accepted mechanism of **skin moisturizers** is that of **occlusion**. This involves predominantly **lipophilic** materials that contain unbranched long-chain alkyl chains without double bonds. More often than not, **moisturizers** that act via this mechanism are mixtures of hydrocarbons, often found in mineral **oil** and other products. For these chemicals, it is critical that they are substantive to the **skin** as well as capable of aligning along their hydrocarbon tails to create an occlusive layer on top of the **skin**. This layer prevents **evaporation** of **water**.

skin reddening: See **erythema**.

skin stripping: Mechanical disruption and reduction of the *stratum corneum* and partially of the living **epidermis**, which are the outermost layers of the **skin**. Medical adhesive tapes and medical glues with such substrates as glass, silica, and metal plates are typically used. The technique is used to study drug delivery and protective filter distribution in the **skin**.

skin type: Due to different content of dark **pigment** (**melanin**), the tone of human **skin** can vary from a dark brown to a nearly colorless pigmentation that may appear reddish due to the **blood** in the **skin**. Europeans generally have lighter **skin, hair**, and eyes than any other group. Africans generally have darker **skin, hair**, and eyes. For practical purposes, such as exposure time for sun tanning or **phototherapy**, six **skin** types are distinguished by Fitzpatrick, listed in order of decreasing **lightness**: I—very light, "nordic," or "celtic" (often **burns**, rarely tans, tends to have **freckles**); II—light, or light-skinned European (usually **burns**, sometimes tans); III—light intermediate, or dark-skinned European (rarely **burns**, usually tans); IV—dark intermediate, "Mediterranean," or "olive **skin**" (rarely **burns**, often tans); V— dark or "brown" (naturally brown **skin**); and VI—very dark or "black" (naturally black-brown **skin**).

skull: Part of the skeleton consisting of the **cranium** and the facial skeleton. The latter includes the sense capsules, the jaws, the hyoid **bone**, and the **cartilage** of the **larynx**. The **skull** may also be divided into the neurocranium and the viscerocranium.

slit-lamp: An optical device consisting of a high-**intensity light** source that can be focused to shine as a slit. It is used in conjunction with a microscope. The lamp facilitates an examination of the anterior segment, or frontal structures, of the human eye, including the eyelid, **sclera**, **conjunctiva**, **iris**, natural **crystalline lens**, and **cornea**. The binocular **slit-lamp** examination provides a stereoscopic magnified view of the eye structures in striking detail, enabling exact anatomical diagnoses to be made for a variety of eye conditions.

slit response function (SRF): A measure of the spatial resolution of an infrared imager, typically plotted as a percent response verses the ratio of the target slit width to the target-to-camera distance.

small angular (angle) approximation: Useful simplification of the laws of trigonometry that is only approximately true for finite angles but correct in the limit as the angle approaches zero. It involves linearization of the trigonometric functions (truncation of their Taylor series). Approximation is useful in many areas of physical science, including optics where it forms the basis of the **paraxial approximation**.

small intestine: The part of the **gastrointestinal tract** (**gut**) following the **stomach** and followed by the large **intestine**, where the vast majority of digestion and **absorption** of food takes place.

In adult humans, it has a diameter approximately 2.5–3 cm in width and is about 5 meters in length, with a normal range of 3–7 m. Due to surface complexity of the inner lining, its inner surface area is approximately 200 m². The small intestine is divided into three structural parts: **duodenum**, **jejunum**, and **ileum**.

S-matrix: See **LSM** [**light-scattering matrix** (**intensity** or **Mueller matrix**)].

smear preparation: Technique used as a precursor in many different staining technologies, it provides distribution, **fixation**, and inactivation of the sampled **cells** on a glass substrate (microscope slide) for further staining and morphology studies. For example, the smear preparation usually calls for the sample bacterium to be placed on a microscope slide (use aseptic technique) with one drop of **deionized water**, then the slide is allowed to air dry for a few minutes followed by heat flaming intended to deactivate **bacteria**. However, for some **bacteria**, such as *M. Tuberculosis*, heat flaming does not deactivate the smear material, whereas 5%-phenol in **ethanol** successfully fixes and deactivates all smears from concentrated sputum samples and from **cell culture** material. See also **blood smears**, **gynecological smears**, and **Pap smears**.

snake photon: Photon that travels in near-forward paths, having undergone few **scattering** events, all of which are in the forward or near-forward direction. Consequently, it retains its image-bearing characteristics to some extent.

Snell's law: Relates the indices of **refraction** n_1 and n_2 of two **media** to the directions of **light** propagation in these **media** in terms of the angles to the normal θ_1 and θ_2 as $n_1 \sin \theta_1 = n_2 \sin \theta_2$. It can be derived from Fermat's Principle or from the **Fresnel equations**. If the incident medium has the larger **index of refraction**, then the angle with the normal is increased by **refraction**. The larger index medium is commonly called the "internal" medium, since air with $n = 1$ is usually the surrounding or "external" medium. The condition for **total internal reflection** can be calculated by setting the refracted angle equal to 90 deg and calculating the incident critical angle θ_c.

sodium fluorescein: Perhaps the most commonly used dye in the biological world, it is a **protein** dye, so some caution is required in its use within the living body. Sodium **fluorescein** has its peak **absorption** at 450 nm and produces a yellow/green emission when stimulated by **light** in the blue region. It is used for **fluorescent angiography**.

sodium lactate: Natural salt that is derived from a natural fermentation product, **lactic acid**, that is produced naturally in foods such as cheese, yogurt, hard salami, pepperoni, sourdough bread, and many others by the action of **lactic-acid** starter cultures (also known as a "good" **bacteria**). **Sodium lactate** can correct the normal acid-base balance in patients whose **blood** has become too acidic. It can also help treat overdoses of certain medications by increasing removal of the drug from the body.

sodium lauryl sulfate: Detergent and surfactant found in many personal care products (soaps, shampoos, toothpaste, etc.). It serves as an enhancer of **skin** permeability for **optical clearing agents**.

soft scattering particles: **Refractive index** of these particles, n_s, is close to the **refractive index** of the ground (**interstitial space**) substance, $n_0 (n_s \geq n_0)$.

soft tissue: A **tissue** composed of closely packed groups of **cells** entrapped in a network of **fibers** through which **water** percolates. At a microscopic scale, the **tissue** components have no pronounced boundaries; they appear to merge into a continuous structure with spatial variations in the **refractive index**. See **adipose tissue, areolar tissue, cervical tissue, connective tissue, episcleral tissue, epithelial tissue, fibrous**

tissue, glandular tissue, lymphoid tissue, malignant tissue, mucosa, muscular tissue, nervous tissue, reticular tissue, scar tissue, tubular tissue, white fibrous tissue, yellow elastic tissue, tissue absorption, tissue birefringence, tissue compartment sizing, tissue optical model, and tissue optics.

solar cell: See photovoltaic cell.

solid-state laser: A laser with an active medium as a matrix of crystal, glass, or ceramic doped by active ions. Different crystal matrices, such as sapphire, yttrium aluminium garnet (YAG), yttrium aluminium perovskite (YAP), alexandrite, yttrium scandium gallium garnet (YSGG), and others are used in lasers. Active ions can be Nd (neodymium), Cr (chromium), Er (erbium), Ho (holmium), Ti (titanium), Tm (thulium), and others. Active ions in different matrices have different laser wavelengths. For example, Cr^{3+} doping sapphire (ruby laser) provides a laser wavelength of 694 nm, but the same ions doping alexandrite crystal (alexandrite laser) give a laser wavelength of 755 nm. Solid-state lasers are pumped by optical radiation from an arc lamp or from another laser, for example, a diode laser. Efficiency of flash lamp pumped laser is about 0.1–5%. Diode laser pumped solid-state lasers have an efficiency in the range of 10–50%. In biomedical applications where femtosecond pulses and a broadband wavelength tuning are critical, lasers based on active media with wide luminescence bands, such as titanium sapphire (Ti:sapphire or Ti:Al_2O_3) laser and Nd:YAP (neodymium: Yttrium aluminum perovskite) laser, are widely used.

somatosensory: Pertaining to the sense of touch that is mediated by the somatosensory system. Touch may simply be considered one of five human senses. However, when a person touches something or somebody, this action gives rise to various feelings: perception of pressure (hence shape, softness, texture, vibration, etc.), relative temperature, and sometimes pain. Thus the term "touch" is actually the combined term for several senses. In medicine, the colloquial term "touch" is usually replaced with "somatic senses" to better reflect the variety of mechanisms involved. The somatosenses include **cutaneous** (**skin**), kinesthesia (movement), and visceral (internal) senses. Visceral senses have to do with sensory information from within the body, such as **stomach** aches.

sonoluminescence (SL): Emission of short bursts of **light** (**luminescence**) from imploding bubbles in a liquid when excited by sound.

sonoluminescence tomography (SLT): Tomography based on **sonoluminescence** signal from **tissues**.

sonophoresis: Process that exponentially increases the **absorption** of **topical** compounds (**transdermal** delivery) into the **epidermis**, **dermis**, and **skin** appendages. It occurs because **ultrasound waves** stimulate micro-vibrations within the **skin epidermis** and increase the overall kinetic **energy** of molecules making up **topical** agents. It is widely used in hospitals to deliver drugs through the **skin**. Pharmacists compound the drugs by mixing them with a coupling agent (**gel**, cream, ointment) that transfers ultrasonic **energy** from the **ultrasound** transducer to the **skin**. The **ultrasound** probably enhances drug transport by **cavitation**, microstreaming, and heating. It is also used in physical therapy. See also **phonophoresis**.

Soret band: Very strong **absorption band** in the blue region of the optical **absorption spectrum** of a haem **protein**.

sound wave: See **acoustic wave**.

spallation: Relaxation of high thermoelastic stress produced by **absorption** of a short **laser** pulse in the irradiated volume at a free (**tissue**–air) surface leads to tensile loading and then mechanical **spallation**. A photomechanical fracture induced by thermoelastic stress waves is an important mechanism of **tissue ablation** by short **laser** pulses. Pulses from **Q-switched**

Nd:YAG lasers (1,064 nm) or **frequency**-doubled (532 nm) with 3–8 **nanoseconds** duration and corresponding **tissue** staining are typically used. **Spallation** is indicated by the formation of **cavitation** bubbles below the irradiated surface and is strongly influenced by impurities serving as nucleation sites. The **cavitation** is caused by the negative part of a bipolar thermoelastic stress **wave**. **Cavitation** and **ablation** are typically observed with various time-resolved methods such as stress detection, video imaging, and an optical pump-probe technique for the detection of individual cavities. Material ejection due to **spallation** is observed in the liquid samples at a **fluence** leading to a temperature below the boiling point. The mechanical action of thermoelastic stress waves is characterized by high stress amplitudes but low energetic efficiency. A model combining **spallation** and **vaporization** is therefore proposed for efficient **tissue ablation**. A **laser**-thin-film **spallation** technique, which was originally developed to measure **adhesion** of thin films, was adopted to determine the interfacial tensile strength of **cells** and mineralized **tissue** to various engineered substrates. Interfacial tensile strengths of living **cells** were successfully measured, and so were its dependence on different surface conditions, including polymer and metal substrates, and the presence or absence of fibronectin treatment and **serum**. The feasibility of the living **cell** isolating-and-placing method using the **laser spallation** technique has been positively demonstrated, suggesting that the method may enhance existing individual living **cell** manipulation techniques for precise placement. It is also possible to convert a longitudinal stress **wave** mode into a shear stress using a pulse shaping **prism** and thus achieve shear **spallation**.

spatial coherence: The ability for two points in space, x_1 and x_2, in the extent of a **wave** to interfere when averaged over time. More precisely, the **spatial coherence** is the cross-**correlation** between two points in a **wave** for all times. The range of separation between the two points over which there is significant **interference** is called the coherence area, A_c. This is the relevant type of coherence for the Young's double-slit **interferometer**. A **single-mode laser beam** with a Gaussian shape (uni-phase beam) for the transverse

intensity profile has a **spatial coherence** close to the ideal one (**correlation coefficient** is close to unity for a whole beam spot). Similarly, a **light beam** on the output of a **superluminescent light diode** and **single-mode fiber** also has a high degree of **spatial coherence**, thus these two spatially **coherent light** sources (**laser** and **SLD**) excite a **single-mode fiber** with a high efficiency due to superior coupling of exciting and propagating modes.

spatial correlation: See **correlation**; valid for spatial variables.

spatial frequency: Spatial harmonic in the **Fourier transform** of a periodic or aperiodic (random) spatial distribution.

spatial frequency-domain diffuse optical imaging (SFD-DOI): A **diffuse optical imaging (DOI)** technique that utilizes structured **light** patterns to form wide-field images of **tissue**. It compares measured data with radiative transport models, based on **radiation-transfer theory (RTT)** solutions, to acquire **NIR** spectra and **absorption** and **scattering** properties of healthy and diseased **tissues**. This technique relies on the concept of the **modulation transfer function (MTF)**. **SFD-DOI** is used to get images of **oxygenated hemoglobin**, **deoxygenated hemoglobin**, **methemoglobin**, **lipids**, and **water** distributions, as well as **tissue** morphology mapping. This technique can be used for **breast tumor** imaging and for dynamical mapping of intrinsic **brain** signals at pre-clinical studies in **animal models**.

spatial frequency-domain diffuse optical spectroscopy (SFD–DOS): A **diffuse optical spectroscopy (DOS)** technique that utilizes structured **light** patterns to form wide-field images of **tissue optical properties**. It compares measured data with radiative transport models, based on **radiation-transfer theory (RTT)** solutions, to acquire **NIR** spectra and **absorption** and **scattering** properties of healthy and diseased **tissues**. This technique relies on the concept of a **modulation transfer function (MTF)**. **SFD-DOS** is used to get spectroscopic information of **oxygenated hemoglobin**, **deoxygenated hemoglobin**, **methemoglobin**, **lipids**, and **water** distributions. Monitoring of **tissue**

morphology changes via the measurement of **scattering** properties is also possible. This technique is sensitive enough to be used for studies of **breast tumor metabolism**, **cancer** detection, and monitoring of therapeutic drug delivery, as well as for detection of intrinsic **brain** signals in **animal models** and evaluation of efficiency of chemotherapeutic drugs.

spatial resolution: Measure of the ability of an **optical imaging** system to reveal the details of an image, i.e., to resolve adjacent elements.

spatial resolution of the instantaneous field of view (IFOV): Smallest target spot size on which an optical imager can produce a measurement, expressed in terms of angular subtense (**mrad** per side). The **slit response function (SRF)** test is used to measure the **spatial resolution of IFOV**.

spatially modulated laser beam (SMLB): **Laser beam** with regular **interference fringes** or irregular **speckle modulation**.

spatially resolved measurements: Related to measurements of **intensity** of scattered **light** from an object, which is typically provided by one or more irradiating plus one or more detecting **optical fibers** separated by distances r_{sd} and oriented either normally or under some angle to the **tissue** surface. **CCD** and **CMOS** cameras can also be used to provide contactless, spatially-resolved measurements by projecting the particular reflecting element of the object to the conjugated **pixel** (or a few **pixels**). The depth profiling of **tissue optical properties** is provided if enough **fibers** or **CCD** detector **pixels** are employed. For many **tissues**, *in vivo* measurements are possible only in the geometry of the **backscattering**. See **spatially resolved reflectance (SRR) technique**.

spatially resolved reflectance (SRR) technique: Technique that uses two or more **optical fibers** to illuminate an object and collect the back-reflected **light**. The positions of the illuminating and

light-collecting **fibers** can be fixed or scanned along the object's surface either perpendicular or at an angle to the object's surface. The depth profiling of **tissue optical properties** is provided if enough **fibers** or **CCD** detector **pixels** are employed. For many **tissues**, *in vivo* measurements are possible only in the geometry of the **backscattering**. The **spatially resolved reflectance (SRR)** $R(r_{sd})$ is defined as the **power** of the backscattered **light** per unit of area detected by a receiver at the surface of the **tissue** at a distance r_{sd} from the source. $R(r_{sd})$ depends on the **optical properties** of the sample, that is, the **absorption coefficient** μ_a, the **scattering** coefficient μ_s, the **phase function** $p(\theta)$, the **refractive index**, and the **numerical aperture (NA)** of the receiving system. The corresponding relation for the **backscattering intensity** as a function of r_{sd} and **optical parameters** for a semi-infinite medium and relatively large r_{sd} can be written on the basis of a **diffusion approximation**. The spatially resolved technique allows one to evaluate the **absorption** and the **scattering** coefficients. When **optical parameters** of **skin** or **mucosa** are under investigation, the small source–detector separations r_{sd} should be used where the **diffusion approximation** is not valid due to proximity to the **tissue** boundary; thus, more sophisticated approximations of the **RTT** solution should be employed. In particular, a numerical solution of the **inverse problem** by the **IMC** method is possible.

specific conductance: See **electrical conductivity**.

specific heat capacity: Also known simply as specific heat, it is an intensive quantity, meaning that it is a property of the material itself and not the size or shape of the sample. Its value is affected by the microscopic structure of the material. Commonly, the amount is specified by mass. For example, **water** has a mass-specific **heat capacity** of about 4186 **joules** per **kelvin** per kilogram. Volume-specific and molar-specific heat capacities are also used. The specific heat of virtually any substance can be measured, including pure elements, compounds, alloys, solutions, and composites.

speckle: Single element of a **speckle** structure (pattern) that is produced as a result of the **interference** of a large number of elementary waves with random phases that arise when **coherent light** is reflected from a rough surface or when **coherent light** passes through a **scattering** medium.

speckle contrast: See **contrast of the intensity fluctuations**.

speckle correlometry: Technique that is based on the measurement of the **intensity autocorrelation function**, characterizing the size and the distribution of **speckle** sizes in a **speckle** pattern caused, for example, by a **scattering** of coherent **light beam** from a rough surface; statistical properties of the **scattering** object's structure can be deduced from such measurements.

speckle interferometry: Technique that uses the **interference** of **speckle** fields.

speckle optical coherence tomography (OCT): An **OCT** technique that does not require transverse scanning and employs subjective **speckles**. A typical experimental setup consists of an **SLD**, mirror **Mach–Zehnder interferometer**, and a **CCD** camera. Radiation produced by the **light** source is focused onto the surface of an object. The incident **light beam** irradiates a surface at an angle of 45 deg. **Light** penetrates into a **tissue** and experiences **scattering** with backscattered **light** emerging at the surface of the object. A fraction of this **light beam** that propagates in the direction perpendicular to the surface of the sample is imaged by the **CCD** camera where this **light beam** is mixed with reference-**wave radiation** reflected from a mirror scanned with a constant rate. Observation of scattered **light** with an **aperture** of finite sizes gives subjective **speckles** in the image plane (the **CCD** camera). In the case where partially **coherent light** is employed, one should consider different groups of **photons** passing through the image plane P_i. Each of these groups consists of **photons** that have traveled a definite pathlength $l_i \pm l_c$. Correspondingly, these **photons** produce their own coherent **speckle** pattern with intensity distribution $S_i(x,y)$. The resulting **speckle** pattern is produced by incoherent superposition $\sum S_i$ of different **speckle** patterns. To locate regions inside an object from which **photons** with a definite pathlength $L = l_i$ come, one should superimpose a reference **wave** with the corresponding pathlength L, then only the **photons** from the chosen group P_i will ensure the required **contrast** V_I, which should be measured. Two sequential exposures are required to measure V_I. After the first one, the phase of the field in the reference beam is shifted by π, and the exposure is repeated. The incoherent component remains unchanged in these two exposures and can be easily subtracted. The pathlength resolution for this system is determined by the **coherence length** l_c of the used **light** source, and using a source with $l_c = 30$ μm, the resulting time resolution is about 100 fs. The main advantage of this scheme is that the generation of a 2D $(x–z)$ tomogram does not require transverse scanning of the beam. Another **speckle OCT** method was shown as an alternative to the **Doppler OCT** in 2D imaging of **blood flow**. Flow information can be extracted using **speckle** fluctuations in conventional amplitude **OCT**. Time-varying **speckle** is manifested as a change in **OCT** image spatial **speckle** frequencies. It was shown that over a range of velocities, the ratio of high-to-low **OCT** image spatial frequencies has a linear relation to flow velocity and that method is sensitive to **blood flow** of all directions without phase information needed. Using **speckle OCT**, 2D images of **blood flow** distributions for *in vivo* hamster **skin** have been produced.

speckle photography: Measuring technique that uses a set of sequential photos of the **speckle** pattern taken at different moments or with different exposures; **full-field technique** can be used to study the dynamic properties of a **scattering** object (see **LASCA**). The updated instruments make use of computer-controlled **CCD** or **CMOS** cameras for averaging and storing the **speckle** patterns.

speckle statistics of the first order: Statistics that define the properties of **speckle** fields at each point.

speckle statistics of the second order: Statistics that show how fast the **intensity** changes from point to point in a **speckle** pattern, i.e., they characterize the size and the distribution of **speckle** sizes in the pattern.

speckle structure: See **speckle**.

spectral OCT: See **frequency-domain OCT**.

spectral radar: See **frequency-domain OCT**.

Spectrolon®: Very white reflective plastic used as the "white reference" in spectral measurements and in **integrating sphere spectrometers**.

spectrometer: General term characterizing any kind of spectrally sensitive measuring instrument, such as a spectrophotometer, spectroscope, or spectrograph, used in **spectroscopy** to measure properties of **electromagnetic radiation (EMR)** over a specific **wavelength** or **wavenumber** range. The variable measured is most often the **EMR intensity** but could also be, for instance, the **intensity modulation** depth or **phase shift**, the **intensity** fluctuations, the **polarization** state, or thermal or acoustic signals. "Spectrometer" is a term that is applied to instruments that operate over a very wide range of **wavelengths**, from gamma rays and **x-rays** into the **far-infrared**, **terahertz**, and microwaves. A large number of different **spectrometers** are used in **biophotonics** to analyze biological object structure, and they function from the atomic/molecular level to **cell/tissue** structural-compound level. Biophotonic **spectrometers** can perform the following techniques: **absorption spectroscopy**, **near-infrared spectroscopy (NIRS)**, **differential optical absorption spectroscopy (DOAS)**, **diffuse optical spectroscopy (DOS)** (**integrating sphere spectrometers**), **reflecting (reflection, reflectance) spectroscopy**, **time-resolved spectroscopy (TRS)**, **frequency-domain diffuse reflectance spectroscopy (FD-spectrometer)**, **spatial frequency-domain diffuse optical spectroscopy (SFD-DOS)**, **terahertz time-domain**

spectroscopy (THz-TDS), light scattering spectroscopy (LSS), infrared spectroscopy, attenuated total reflectance Fourier-transform infrared spectroscopy (ATR FTIR), fluorescence spectroscopy, laser-induced fluorescence (LIF) spectroscopy, luminescence lifetime spectroscopy, polarization optical spectroscopy, polarization gating spectroscopy, orthogonal polarization spectroscopy (OPS), polarized reflectance spectroscopy (PRS), Raman spectroscopy, Doppler spectroscopy, quasielastic light-scattering spectroscopy, spectroscopy of intensity fluctuations, photon-correlation spectroscopy, diffusion wave spectroscopy (DWS), optoacoustic (OA) spectroscopy, photothermal spectroscopy, thermal gradient spectroscopy (TGS), emission spectroscopy, and laser-induced breakdown spectroscopy (LIBS). Many modern microscopy systems are actually spectrometers.

spectrophotometry: Spectroscopic method and instrument for making photometric comparisons between parts of spectra.

spectroscopy: Science that deals with the use of the **spectrometer** and with **spectrum** analysis. The following spectroscopic techniques are widely used in **biophotonics** to analyze biological object structure and functioning on the atomic/molecular level to **cell/tissue** structural compound level: **absorption spectroscopy, near-infrared spectroscopy (NIRS), differential optical absorption spectroscopy (DOAS), diffuse optical spectroscopy (DOS) (integrating sphere spectrometers), reflecting (reflection, reflectance) spectroscopy, time-resolved spectroscopy (TRS), frequency-domain diffuse reflectance spectroscopy (FD-spectrometer), spatial frequency-domain diffuse optical spectroscopy (SFD-DOS), terahertz time-domain spectroscopy (THz-TDS), light scattering spectroscopy (LSS), infrared spectroscopy, attenuated total reflectance Fourier-transform infrared spectroscopy (ATR FTIR), fluorescence spectroscopy, laser-induced fluorescence (LIF) spectroscopy, luminescence lifetime spectroscopy, polarization optical spectroscopy, polarization gating spectroscopy, orthogonal polarization spectroscopy (OPS), polarized reflectance spectroscopy**

(PRS), **Raman spectroscopy**, **Doppler spectroscopy**, **quasielastic light-scattering spectroscopy**, **spectroscopy of intensity fluctuations**, **photon-correlation spectroscopy**, **diffusion wave spectroscopy (DWS)**, **optoacoustic (OA) spectroscopy**, **photothermal spectroscopy**, **thermal gradient spectroscopy (TGS)**, **emission spectroscopy**, and **laser-induced breakdown spectroscopy (LIBS)**.

spectroscopy of intensity fluctuations: See **photon-correlation spectroscopy**.

spectrum: Range of frequencies or **wavelengths**.

spectrum analysis: Ascertaining the number and character of the constituents combining to produce a signal spectrogram.

spectrum analyzer: An instrument for conducting **spectrum** analysis of a signal.

specular: Pertaining to or having the properties of a mirror.

speed of light: In free space, **speed of light** $c = 299,792,458$ m/s or approximately 3×10^8 m/s. The speed at which **light** propagates through transparent materials, such as glass or **tissues** (eye **cornea**), is less than c. The ratio between c and the speed v at which **light** travels through a material is called the **refractive index** n of the material ($n = c/v$). For example, for **visible light**, the **refractive index** of glass is typically around 1.5, meaning that **light** in glass travels at $v = c/1.5 \approx 2 \times 10^8$ m/s. For the human eye **cornea**, $n \approx 1.38$, and thus **light** in the **cornea** travels at $v = c/1.38 \approx 2.17 \times 10^8$ m/s.

spherocyte: Sphere-shaped **erythrocyte**; an auto-hemolytic anemia (a disease of the **blood**) characterized by the production of **spherocytes**. It is caused by a molecular defect in one or more of the **proteins** of the **erythrocyte cytoskeleton** (usually ankyrin, sometimes spectrin). Because the **cell** skeleton has a defect, the

blood cell contracts to its most surface-tension efficient and least flexible configuration (a sphere) rather than the more flexible donut shape.

spin: The angular momentum intrinsic to a body. In classical mechanics, the spin angular momentum of a body is associated with the rotation of the body around its own center of mass. In quantum mechanics, spin is particularly important for systems at atomic length scales, such as individual atoms, protons, or electrons. Such particles and the spin of quantum mechanical systems ("particle spin") possess several nonclassical features, and for such systems, spin angular momentum cannot be associated with rotation but instead refers only to the presence of angular momentum.

spinal cord: Long, thin, tubular bundle of **nervous tissue** and support **cells** that extends from the **brain** (the medulla, specifically). The **brain** and **spinal cord** together make up the **central nervous system**. The **spinal cord** extends down to the space between the first and second lumbar vertebrae. It is around 45 cm long in men and around 43 cm long in women. The enclosing bony vertebral column protects the relatively shorter **spinal cord**. The **spinal cord** functions primarily in the transmission of neural signals between the **brain** and the rest of the body but also contains neural circuits that can independently control numerous reflexes and central pattern generators. The **spinal cord** is protected by three layers of **tissue**, called spinal meninges, that surround the cord. The *dura mater* is the outermost layer, and it forms a tough protective coating. Between the *dura mater* and the surrounding **bone** of the vertebrae is a space, called the epidural space, that is filled with **adipose tissue**, and it contains a network of **blood vessels**. The arachnoid is the middle protective layer, the space between the arachnoid and the underlying *pia mater* contains **cerebrospinal fluid (CSF)**, and it is called subarachnoid space. The medical procedure known as a "spinal tap" involves using a needle to withdraw **CSF** from the subarachnoid space, usually from the lumbar region of the spine.

The *pia mater* is the innermost protective layer, which is very delicate and tightly associated with the surface of the **spinal cord**.

spirits: See **alcohol**.

spleen: Highly **vascular**, **glandular**, ductless organ situated in humans at the cardiac end of the **stomach**. It serves chiefly in the formation of **lymphocytes**, in the destruction of worn-out **erythrocytes**, and as a reservoir for **red corpuscles** and **platelets**.

spontaneous emission: **Light** is emitted by atoms (molecules) of the **light** source material that can be a gas, a liquid, or a solid. Atoms can be in the different **excited states** when electrons possess **energy** according to their position in relation to the **nucleus** of an atom. Excitation of atoms (molecules) can be provided in different ways: by heating, by electrical discharge, or by optical pumping. An excited atom (molecule) is able to relax during the so-called lifetime of the **excited state** by emitting a **photon** spontaneously (**spontaneous emission**) or lose **energy** nonradiatively following collisions with other atoms (molecules). The rate of **spontaneous emission** for fluorescent compounds commonly used in **biomedical optics** is within the range of 0.5–20 ns. Atomic optical transition is typically an **electronic transition**, where **energy** is given out as **electromagnetic radiation** in the optical range. At **vibrational transitions**, the emittance of **infrared light** is possible. **Spontaneous** and **stimulated emission** by atoms are also the basis for the **Planck curve** (function). Direction of spontaneously emitted **photons** is random, and the **frequency** (**wavelength**) is also random in the limits of the **bandwidth** of **luminescence** of the excited transition. As a result, most spontaneous emitting **light** sources have an isotropic direction of emission and a wide range of frequencies (polychromatic).

spore: Reproductive structure adapted for **dispersion** and surviving for extended periods of time in unfavorable conditions. Spores form part of the life cycles of many plants, algae, **fungi cells**, and some protozoans.

Sprague Dawley rat: Strain of albino rat used extensively in medical research. Its main advantage is its calmness and ease of handling. This strain was first produced by the Sprague Dawley farms in Madison, Wisconsin. The adult body weight is 250–300 g for females and 450–520 g for males. The typical life span is 2.5–3.5 years. These rats typically have an increased tail-to-body-length ratio compared to **Wistar rats**.

sputum: Matter that is expelled from the respiratory tract, such as **mucus** or phlegm, mixed with **saliva**, which can then be spat from the **mouth**. It is usually associated with air passages in diseased **lungs**, bronchi, or upper respiratory tract and also a case of pneumonia. It can be found to contain **blood** if in a chronic cough possibly caused by severe cases of tuberculosis. It is usually used for microbiological investigations of respiratory infections. The best sputum samples contain very little **saliva**, as this contaminates the sample with oral **bacteria**.

squames: Flat, keratinised, dead **cells** shed from the outermost layer of a stratified **squamous epithelium**.

squamous cell: Flat, scale-like **epithelial cells** belonging to the most superficial layer of **epithelial tissue**.

squamous cell carcinomas: Form of **cancer** of the **carcinoma** type that may occur in many different organs, including the **skin**, **mouth**, **esophagus**, **prostate**, **lungs**, and **cervix**. It is a **malignant tumor** of **epithelium** that shows **squamous cell** differentiation.

squamous epithelium: An **epithelium** characterized by containing **squamous cells**. It may possess only one layer of these **cells**, in which case it is referred to as simple **squamous epithelium**, or it may possess multiple layers, referred to as stratified **squamous epithelium**. Both types perform differing functions, ranging from nutrient exchange to protection.

standard deviation: See **root mean square**.

standard error: Related to a method of measurement or estimation when the **standard deviation** of the sampling distribution is associated with the estimation method. The term may also be used to refer to an estimate of that **standard deviation** derived from a particular sample used to compute the estimate. The **standard deviation** of the error (the difference between the estimate and the true value) is the same as the **standard deviation** of the estimates themselves.

standard error of the mean (SEM): The **standard deviation** of the selected sample mean over all possible samples (of a given size) drawn from the measurements. The **SEM** can refer to an estimate of that **standard deviation**, computed from the sample of data being analyzed at the time.

***Staphylococcus*:** Any of several spherical **bacteria** of the genus *Staphylococcus*, occurring in pairs, tetrads, and irregular clusters, certain species of which, such as *S. Aureus*, can be pathogenic for man.

***Staphylococcus* toxin (ST):** Some *Staphylococcus* produce a **toxin** that is responsible for food poisoning. This **toxin** is heat stable. **Bacteria** can be killed during processing, but the **toxin** may remain behind.

stasis: Stopping of **blood flow** or flows of other biological fluids in the organism.

statistical approach: Approach based on statistics as a mathematical science.

statistically significant: A result that is unlikely to have occurred by chance, i.e., there is statistical evidence that there is a difference. The amount of evidence required to accept that an event is unlikely to have arisen by chance is known as the significance level or critical *p*-value: in traditional Fisherian statistical hypothesis testing, the *p*-value is the **probability**

conditional on the null hypothesis of the observed data or more extreme data. In general, a 5% or lower p-value is considered to be **statistically significant**. Popular levels of significance, usually denoted as α, are 5% (0.05), 1% (0.01), and 0.1% (0.001).

statistics: Mathematical science pertaining to the collection, analysis, interpretation or explanation, and presentation of data. It is applicable to a wide variety of academic disciplines.

Stefan–Boltzmann law: It states that the total **energy** radiated per unit surface area of a **blackbody** in unit time, known as **radiant emittance** j and measured in W/m^2, is directly proportional to the fourth **power** of the blackbody's absolute temperature T: $j = \sigma T^4$. For a more general case of a **graybody**, which radiates a portion of **energy density** characterized by its **emissivity** $\varepsilon(\lambda)$, $j = \varepsilon(\lambda)\sigma T^4$. The total **power** of the object **radiation** $P = Aj$, where A is the object surface area in m^2. The constant of proportionality σ, called the **Stefan–Boltzmann constant**, is nonfundamental in the sense that it derives from other known constants of nature, $\sigma = (2\pi^5 k^4)/(15c^2 h^3) = 5.670400 \times 10^{-8}$ J s^{-1} m^{-2} K^{-4}, where k is **Boltzmann's constant**, h is **Planck's constant**, and c is the **speed of light** in vacuum. Thus, at $T = 100$ K, the **energy flux** density $j = 5.67$ W/m^2, and at $T = 1000$ K, $j = 56,700$ W/m^2.

stem cell: **Cells** found in all multi-cellular organisms. They are characterized by the ability to renew themselves through mitotic **cell** division and differentiate into a diverse range of specialized **cell** types. There are two broad types of mammalian **stem cells**: embryonic **stem cells** that are isolated from the inner **cell** mass of blastocysts, and adult **stem cells** that are found in adult **tissues**. In a developing **embryo**, **stem cells** can differentiate into all of the specialized embryonic **tissues**. In adult organisms, **stem cells** and progenitor **cells** act as a repair system for the body, replenishing specialized **cells** but also maintaining the normal turnover of regenerative organs, such as **blood**, **skin**, or intestinal **tissues**. **Stem cells** can now be grown and transformed into specialized **cells** with characteristics consistent with **cells** of various **tissues** such as **muscles** or **nerves** through **cell culture**. Highly plastic adult **stem cells** from a variety of sources, including umbilical-cord **blood** and **bone marrow**, are routinely used in medical therapies. Embryonic **cell** lines and autologous embryonic **stem cells** generated through therapeutic cloning have also been proposed as promising candidates for future therapies.

stenosis: Narrowing of a canal (as in the walls of **arteries** or a cardiac **valve**).

step-index fiber: A **fiber** with a step-transverse profile of **refractive index** of core to cladding.

stepper motor: Machine that converts electrical **energy** into mechanical **energy** by steps. It is used as the computer-controlled mechanical drivers of optical stages.

steroid: Terpenoid **lipid** characterized by a carbon skeleton with four fused rings. Different **steroids** vary in the functional groups attached to these rings. Hundreds of distinct **steroids** are found in plants, animals, and **fungi cells**. All **steroids** are derived either from the sterol lanosterol (animals and **fungi cells**) or the sterol cycloartenol (plants). Both sterols are derived from the cyclization of the triterpene squalene.

stimulated Brillouin–Mandelshtam scattering (SBMS): For intense beams (e.g., **laser light**) traveling in a medium such as an **optical fiber**, the variations in the electric field of the beam itself may produce acoustic vibrations in the medium via the electrostriction effect. The beam may undergo **Brillouin–Mandelshtam scattering (BMS)** from these vibrations, usually in the opposite direction of the incoming beam—this is a phenomenon known as **stimulated Brillouin–Mandelshtam scattering (SBMS)**. For liquids and gases, typical **frequency** shifts are on the order of 1–10 GHz (**wavelength** shifts of ~1–10 pm for **visible light**). **SBMS** is one effect by which optical phase conjugation can take place.

stimulated emission: The generation of **electromagnetic radiation** that is characterized by the creation of a new **photon** identical to the excitation **photon** that initially interacted with the atom. As a result, instead of one **photon**, two **photons** with the same **wavelength**, phase, **polarization**, and direction of propagation are generated. Intensive **stimulated emission** of **light** by a group of atoms (molecules) is possible when the higher **energy** levels of these atoms are populated more intensively than the lower ones (inverse population). **Stimulation emission** is the basic concept for lasing. Population inversion can be provided by different methods including single- or multi-component gas-discharge systems (gas **lasers**), optical pumping (gas, liquid and **solid-state lasers**), or quantum **heterostructures** with confined discrete **energy** levels (**diode lasers**). **Spontaneous** and **stimulated emission** by atoms are also the basis for the **Planck curve** (function).

stimulated emission depletion microscopy (STED microscopy): Technique that uses the nonlinear de-excitation of fluorescent dyes to overcome the resolution limit imposed by **diffraction** with standard **confocal laser scanning microscopes** and conventional far-field **optical microscopes**. **STED-microscopy** reduces the size of the excited region by using a very short excitation pulse that is immediately followed by a "depletion" pulse tuned to an emission line of the fluorescent dye. This depletion pulse causes **stimulated emission**, moving electrons from the **excited state** (from which **fluorescence** occurs) to a lower **energy** state. The wavefront of the depletion beam is altered in such a way that it is focused to a ring instead of a spot, featuring a dark spot of zero **laser intensity** in the center. While this dark spot is itself **diffraction**-limited, the **intensity** distribution is continuous and is zero only at the center. Therefore, using a bright depletion pulse causes almost all of the electrons excited by the excitation pulse to return to the ground state, leaving only the region of the sample very close to the axis of the depletion beam excited. After both pulses have been sent, **fluorescence** from the remaining excited dye molecules is detected by the microscope. Resolution improvements over confocal **laser scanning microscopy (LSM)** of up to 12-fold have been reported.

stimulated Raman scattering (SRS): Phenomenon where a lower-**frequency** "signal" **photon** induces the **inelastic scattering** of a higher-**frequency** "pump" **photon** in a nonlinear optical medium. As a result of this, another "signal" **photon** is produced, with the surplus **energy** resonantly passed to the vibrational states of the nonlinear medium. This process is the basis for **Raman amplifiers**.

stochastic optical reconstruction microscopy (STORM): See **photo-activated localization microscopy (PALM)**.

Stokes parameters: Four numbers, I, Q, U, and V, representing an arbitrary **polarization** of **light**. I refers to the **irradiance** or **intensity** of the **light**. The parameters Q, U, and V represent the extent of horizontal linear, 45-deg linear, and circular **polarization**, respectively.

Stokes shift: The difference (in **wavelength** or **frequency** units) between positions of the band maxima of the **absorption** and **luminescence** (**fluorescence**) spectra of the same **electronic transition**. When a molecule or atom absorbs **light**, it enters an excited electronic state. The **Stokes shift** occurs because the molecule loses a small amount of the absorbed **energy** before re-releasing the rest of the **energy** as **fluorescence**, depending on the time between the **absorption** and the re-emission. This **energy** is often lost as thermal **energy**.

Stokes vector: Vector that is formed by the four **Stokes parameters**.

Stokes wave: Induced (scattered) **wave** that has a **frequency** less than the **frequency** of the incident **radiation**.

Stokes–Raman scattering: **Energy** of the Raman-scattered **photons** is lower than the **energy** of the incident **photons**.

stomach: Saclike enlargement of the alimentary canal that forms an organ for storing, diluting, and digesting food. It is situated between the **esophagus** and **duodenum**, and divided into a **fundus**, cardiac portion, **pyloric** portion, and pylorus.

stratum basale: See **epidermis**.

stratum corneum (**SC**): See **epidermis**.

stratum granulosum: See **epidermis**.

stratum spinosum: See **epidermis**.

streak camera (*Synonym*: synchroscan streak camera): An instrument for recording the temporal profile of **light intensity** with a high time resolution (of about 10 ps), displayed as a spatial profile. Synchronous scanning controlled by a reference (**trigger** beam) **light** pulse is provided.

stress: Internal distribution of force per unit area that balances and reacts to external loads applied to a body. **Stress** is a second-order tensor with nine components, but it can be fully described with six components due to symmetry in the absence of body moments. **Stress** is often broken down into its shear and normal components as these have unique physical significance. Stress can be applied to solids, liquids, and gases. Static fluids support normal **stress** (**hydrostatic pressure**) but will flow under **shear stress**. Moving viscous fluids can support **shear stress** (dynamic **pressure**). Solids can support both shear and normal stress, with ductile materials failing under shear, and brittle materials failing under normal **stress**. All materials have temperature-dependent variations in stress-related properties, and non-Newtonian materials have rate-dependent variations.

stress amplitude: Value of a **stress**.

stress distribution: **Stress** is a second-order tensor with nine components.

stroke: Classified into two major categories: ischemic and hemorrhagic. The most common cause of ischemic **stroke** is the blockage of an **artery** in the **brain** by a clot, thrombosis, embolism, or stenosis. Hemorrhagic **strokes** are the result of the rupture of a cerebral **artery**, which can lead to spasm of the **artery** and various degrees of bleeding. Ischemic **stroke** is a complex entity with multiple etiologies and variable clinical manifestations. When an ischemic **stroke** occurs, the **blood** supply to the **brain** is interrupted, and **brain cells** are deprived of the **glucose** and **oxygen** they need to function. **Stroke** causes physical disruption of neuronal **tissue** that sets into motion secondary damage resulting in the death of additional **tissue**. Hypoperfusion and **ischemia**-induced increases in the formation of **superoxide** and **nitric oxide (NO)** have been reported after **stroke**, predicting a role for **oxidative stress** during damage.

stromal layer (stroma): Supporting framework, usually of **connective tissue**, of an organ as distinguished from the parenchyma, e.g., the main layer of the eye **sclera** and **cornea**.

structure function: Function that describes the second-order statistics of a random process and is proportional to the difference between values of the **autocorrelation function** for zero and arbitrary values of the argument. The structure function is more sensitive to small-scale fluctuations.

structured illumination microscopy (SIM): Wide-field **microscopy** (no scanning beam) at structured illumination (SI) used to break the **diffraction limit** of **light**. The SI (or patterned illumination) relies on the specific **microscopy** protocols and extensive post-exposure software analysis. The main concept of SI is to illuminate a sample with patterned **light** and increase the resolution by measuring the fringes in the Moiré pattern (from the **interference** of the illumination pattern and the sample). By taking several frames with the illumination shifted by some phase, it is possible to computationally separate and reconstruct the **Fourier transform (FT)** image, which has much more resolution information. The reverse FT returns the reconstructed image to a super-resolution image; this process enhances the resolution by a factor of 2 (because the SI pattern cannot be focused to anything smaller than half the **wavelength** of the excitation **light**). To further increase the resolution, one can introduce nonlinearities that show up as higher-order harmonics in the FT. Each higher-order harmonic in the FT allows for another set of images that can be used to reconstruct a larger area in reciprocal space, and thus a higher resolution. Less than 50-nm resolving power is achievable, more than five times that of the microscope in its normal configuration. The main problems with SI are that saturating excitation **powers** cause more photodamage and lower **fluorophore** photostability, and sample drift must be kept to below the resolving distance. The principle of wide-field **microscopy** combined with structured **laser** illumination [spatially modulated illumination (SMI)] allows for a size resolution of 30–40 nm (approximately 1/16–1/13 of the **wavelength** used). It is now possible to undertake 3D analyses of whole **cells** within short observation times (a few seconds). By combining spectral precision distance/position determination **microscopy** (SPDM) and SMI, known as Vertico-SMI **microscopy**, a resolution of ~10 nm in 2D and 40 nm in 3D in wide-field images of whole living **cells** has been achieved. Wide-field 3D "nanoimages" of whole living **cells** currently still take about two minutes.

student's t-test: See **t-test**.

subcutaneous: See **hypodermic**.

subdermis (subdermal): Skin layer that primarily consists of globular **fat cells**.

subepidermal: Situated immediately below the **epidermis**.

subject arm of an interferometer: Arm on which an object under study is placed.

subjective speckle: Speckles produced in the image space of an optical system (including an eye).

submucosa: Tissue layer under the **mucous membrane**.

sucrose: See **saccharose**.

sugar: White, **crystalline carbohydrate**, soluble in **water** and sweet to the taste. Sugars are classified as reducing or nonreducing, according to their reaction with Fehling's solution, and also as monosaccharides or disaccharides, according to their structure. **Glucose**, fructose, galactose, and mannose are monosaccharides, and **sucrose** is a disaccharide.

sulci: Superficial **fissures** that increase the surface area of the cerebral **cortex**. The *pia mater* dips down into the **fissures**.

sulfonated tetraphenyl porphines (TPPS$_n$): Photosensitizing dyes that localize in **cell lysosomes**. The extralysosomal location of hydrophylic TPPS$_3$ and TPPS$_4$ in close proximity to the **plasma membrane** can also be found. The **Soret band** of the dye is 400–440 nm, with the emission maxima at 655 nm (dye) and 610 nm (photoproduct).

sum frequency generation (SFG): In optics, a nonlinear optical process that is more generally applied to high-intensity (**laser**) **light** interaction with matter than **second-harmonic generation (SHG)**. **SFG** requires two simultaneous **light beams** (**lasers**) with different frequencies. It is a so-called "parametric process," where the photons satisfy energy conservation with no changes to the matter. In addition, a condition of momentum conservation must be fulfilled, i.e., phase-matching of the three waves (two incident waves and one generated) as they travel through the medium. More accurate fulfillment of this condition produces more-efficient **SFG**. If the interaction length becomes longer, the phase matching should be more precise. As with **SHG**, biomedical applications of **SFG** include **tissue** and **cell optical spectroscopy** and **imaging**.

sunscreen: Substance that protects the **skin** from sunlight, especially from **UVC** and **UVB radiation**. Typically, this is a lotion, spray, **gel**, or other **topical** product that absorbs or reflects some of the **UV radiation** on the **skin** exposed to **light**, and thus helps protect against sunburn and prevent the development of **squamous cell carcinomas** and **basal cell carcinomas**. **Sunscreens** contain one or more **UV** filters—organic chemical compounds that absorb **UV light** (for example, oxybenzone), inorganic **nanoparticles** that reflect, scatter, and absorb **UV light** (titanium dioxide, zinc oxide, or a combination of both), and organic particles that mostly absorb **light** (such as organic chemical compounds that contain multiple **chromophores**) but may also reflect and scatter a fraction of **light** like inorganic particles.

supercontinuum: There are a variety of nonlinear optical effects that allow for the generation of a very broadband **EMR** at a short pulse **laser** excitation. **Photonic crystal** structures in both 2D and 3D geometries, as well as in microstructured **fibers** (**photonic crystal fibers**), enable the control of the flow and confinement of **light** on the **wavelength** scale. In most cases, this confinement in one, two, or all three spatial dimensions is based on the presence of a defect in these structures. The strong modal confinement results in large effective nonlinearities and in a control of the **dispersion** characteristics. These properties have been exploited for **supercontinuum** generation in microstructured **fibers** with impressive spectral broadening at an **intensity** level accessible with **mode-locked laser** systems. Continua of remarkable width were first reported for regular microstructured **fibers** where **light** is guided by **total internal reflection** inside the defect of a photonic **crystal fiber** with extension from 350 to 2200 nm, i.e., over 2.6 optical octaves. Tapered **fibers** provide a similar spectral width. In kagome structure, the guided **light** is effectively confined to a single intersection of the lattice planes, employing **total internal reflection** similar to that in tapered **fibers** or in many other types of microstructured **fibers**. Guided modes in adjacent intersections therefore exhibit only marginal overlap, and the guiding mechanism is broadband with the **supercontinuum**

extended from 200 to 1750 nm. **PCF** at **femtosecond laser** excitation creates a broadband (low-coherent) **light** source suitable for a superresolution **OCT**.

superior sagittal sinus: Also known as the superior longitudinal sinus, it occupies the attached or convex margin of the falx cerebri; also known as the cerebral falx, so named for its sickle-like form, it is a strong, arched fold of *dura mater* that descends vertically in the longitudinal **fissure** between the cerebral hemispheres.

superluminescent light diode (SLD): Very bright diode **light** source with a broad **bandwidth**. It is usually manufactured using a **laser diode** technology (**heterostructure**, **waveguide**, etc.), but without reflecting mirrors (either there is an antireflection coating on the diode faces or their out-of-parallelism is provided). The main difference from a **LED** is that an **SLD** has a uniform wavefront of the output **radiation**, which allows one to couple its **radiation** into a single-mode **fiber**. **SLDs** are used in different medical **OCT** systems.

superoxide: An anion with the chemical formula O_2^-. It is important as the product of the one-electron reduction of dioxygen O_2, which occurs widely in living systems. With one unpaired electron, the **superoxide** ion is a **free radical**. It is biologically toxic and is deployed by the immune system to kill invading microorganisms. In **phagocytes**, **superoxide** is produced in large quantities by the **enzyme NADPH oxidase** and several other **enzymes**, as well as a byproduct of mitochondrial respiration. Because **superoxide** is toxic, nearly all organisms living in the presence of **oxygen** contain isoforms of the **superoxide** scavenging **enzyme, superoxide dismutase (SOD)**. **Superoxide** may contribute to the pathogenesis of many diseases, and also to aging via the **oxidative stress** that it inflicts on **cells**. The most widely accepted view is that **cell** damage caused by **oxidative stress** is one of several factors limiting lifespan.

superoxide dismutase (SOD): Extremely efficient **enzyme**. It catalyzes the neutralization of **superoxide** nearly as fast as the two substances can diffuse together spontaneously in solution. Other **proteins**, which can be both oxidized and reduced by **superoxide**, have weak **SOD**-like activity (e.g., **hemoglobin**). Genetic deactivation of **SOD** produces deleterious **phenotypes** in organisms ranging from **bacteria** to mice and have provided valuable information about possible mechanisms of toxicity of **superoxide** *in vivo*.

surface-enhanced Raman scattering (SERS) [*Related term*: **surface-enhanced Raman spectroscopy (SERS)**]: Strong increase in Raman signals from molecules if those molecules are attached to submicron metallic structures. For a rough surface due to excitation of **electromagnetic resonances** by the incident **radiation**, such enhancement may be of a few orders. Both the excitation and Raman scattered fields contribute to this enhancement. Thus, the **SERS** signal is proportional to the fourth power of the field enhancement factor.

surface-enhanced Raman spectroscopy (SERS): A high-resolution and sensitive spectroscopic technique based on the **surface-enhanced Raman scattering (SERS)** phenomenon.

surface-plasmon resonance: Also known as surface **plasmon** polaritons, surface **electromagnetic waves** propagate parallel to a metal/dielectric interface. For electronic surface **plasmons** to exist, the real part of the dielectric constant of the metal must be negative and its magnitude must be greater than that of the dielectric. This condition is met in the **visible-IR wavelength** region for air/metal and **water**/metal interfaces (where the real dielectric constant of a metal is negative and that of air or **water** is positive). The excitation of surface **plasmons** by **light** is denoted for planar surfaces, as for **nanometer**-sized metallic structures, it is called localized **surface plasmon resonance**. Typical metals that support surface **plasmons** are silver and gold, but metals such as copper, titanium, or chromium can also support surface-**plasmon** generation. Surface **plasmons** have been used to enhance the surface sensitivity of several spectroscopic methods including

fluorescence, **Raman scattering** (see **surface-enhanced Raman scattering**), and **second harmonic generation**.

surfactant: Wetting agents that lower the surface tension of a liquid, allowing easier spreading, and lower the interfacial tension between two liquids.

sweat gland: In humans, there are two kinds of **sweat glands**, that differ greatly in both the composition of the sweat and its purpose. Eccrine **sweat glands** are distributed over the entire body surface but are particularly abundant on the **palms** of **hands**, soles of feet, and on the forehead. These **glands** produce sweat that is composed chiefly of **water** with various salts and is used for body temperature regulation. Apocrine **sweat glands** develop during the early- to mid-puberty ages (approximately around the age of 15) and release more than normal amounts of sweat for approximately a month; they subsequently regulate and release normal amounts of sweat. They are located wherever there is body **hair**.

swelling: Enlargement of organs caused by accumulation of excess fluid in **tissues** called **edema**. It can occur throughout the body (generalized), or only some part or organ is affected (localized). It is considered one of the five characteristics of **inflammation**.

swept-laser source: Single-wavelength **laser** that is rapidly tuned (swept) over a broad spectral range. This is an alternative **light** source for **OCT** systems, which usually use **light** sources that provide a wide range of **wavelengths** simultaneously, such as **SLDs** and **femtosecond titanium–sapphire lasers**. **Swept-laser sources** allow for the measurement of **interference** signals at individual **wavelengths** sequentially with high spectral resolution, which is especially critical for a high-speed and high-resolution **frequency-domain OCT**. **Semiconductor optical amplifiers (SOAs)** are one of the most widely used **gain media** for rapidly swept **lasers** because of (1) their wide range of **gain** center **wavelengths**; (2) high **gain** with a broad **bandwidth**, which provides great flexibility in choosing a tunable filter and cavity configuration for wide range and fast tuning; and (3) the **gain** response time (250 ps), which is much shorter than the micro- or **millisecond** time response of other **gain media** such as titanium–sapphire and rare-earth doped **fibers**. Rapidly scanned intracavity filters provide high **wavelength**-sweep speeds exceeding 1,000 nm/ms. For example, Thorlabs' **swept-laser source** SL1325-P16 has output **power** P = 12 mW at central **wavelength** λ_0 = 1325 nm and spectral width $\Delta\lambda$ = 110 nm with scanning rate over the full operating **wavelength** range of 16 kHz. Santec's **swept-laser source** has $P \geq 20$ mW at central **wavelengths** λ_0 = 1070, 1330, and 1550 and spectral width $\Delta\lambda \geq$ 170 nm with scan speed from 1 to 50 kHz.

symmetric molecule: Refers to molecular geometry. Molecules have fixed equilibrium geometries—bond lengths and angles—about which they continuously oscillate through vibrational and rotational motions. A **symmetric molecule** contains identical bonds. For example, trigonal-planar, tetrahedral, and linear bonding arrangements often lead to symmetrical, nonpolar molecules that contain polar bonds.

symmetric vibrational mode: For example, a linear triatomic molecule moving when each atom that oscillates—or vibrates—along a line connecting them may be in symmetric or anti-symmetric vibrational mode relative to the central atom.

synchroscan streak camera: See **streak camera**.

synergetic (synergistic): Refers to the phenomenon in which two or more discrete influences or agents acting together create an effect greater than that predicted by knowing only the separate effects of the individual agents.

synovial fluid: Viscous fluid found in the cavities of synovial joints. The principal role of **synovial fluid** is to reduce friction between the articular **cartilage** of synovial joints during movement. The inner **membrane** of synovial joints is called the synovial **membrane**, and it secretes synovial fluid into the joint cavity. This fluid forms a thin layer (roughly 50 μm) at the surface of **cartilage** and also seeps into microcavities and irregularities in the articular **cartilage** surface, filling all empty space. Synovial **tissue** is sterile and composed of vascularized **connective tissue** that lacks a **basement membrane**. Synovial **fluid** is made of hyaluronic acid and lubricin, proteinases, and collagenases. It exhibits non-Newtonian flow characteristics. The viscosity coefficient is not a constant, and the fluid is not linearly viscous—viscosity decreases and the fluid thins over a period of continued **stress**. It also contains phagocytic **cells** that remove microbes and the debris that results from normal wear and tear in the joint.

systematic errors: In **tissue** optical and spectroscopic studies, the errors caused by finite **tissue** volume, curved surfaces, **tissue** inhomogeneity while scanning, finite source and detection size, uncertainty in their relative positions, etc. They can be much larger than random errors induced by **shot noise**.

Système International d'Unités (International System of Units) (SI): The modern form of the metric system that is generally a system of measurement devised around seven base units and the convenience of the number ten. It is the world's most widely used system of measurement, both in everyday commerce and in science. Base units: meter (m)—length (l), kilogram (kg)—mass (m), second (s)—time (t), ampere (A)—electric current (I), kelvin (K)—thermodynamic temperature (T), **candela** (cd)—luminous **intensity** (I_v), **mole** (mol)—amount of substance (n). Standard prefixes for the **SI** units of measure: multiples—deca- (da) $\times 10^1$, hecto- (h) $\times 10^2$, kilo- (k) $\times 10^3$, mega- (M) $\times 10^6$, giga- (G) $\times 10^9$, tera- (T) $\times 10^{12}$, peta- (P) $\times 10^{15}$, exa- (E) $\times 10^{18}$, zetta- (Z) $\times 10^{21}$, yotta- (Y) $\times 10^{24}$; subdivisions—deci- (d) $\times 10^{-1}$, centi- (c) $\times 10^{-2}$, milli- (m) $\times 10^{-3}$, micro- (μ) $\times 10^{-6}$, nano- (n) $\times 10^{-9}$, pico- (p) $\times 10^{-12}$, femto- (f) $\times 10^{-15}$, atto- (a) $\times 10^{-18}$, zepto- (z) $\times 10^{-21}$, yocto- (y) $\times 10^{-24}$.

T84: Carcinoma cell line.

target background temperature: Apparent **ambient temperature** of the scene behind and surrounding the target, as viewed from the instrument. When the **field of view** of a point-sensing instrument is larger than the target, the target **background temperature** will affect the instrument reading. It is also called the surroundings temperature and **foreground temperature**.

temoporfin (mTHPC): A **photosensitizer** of the chloryn family with an excitation band around 655 nm. It is used in **cancer** diagnostics and **photodynamic therapy (PDT)**. **Foscan**® is the commercialized product. At **PDT**, typical **laser** dose is of 20 J/cm².

temporal coherence: Measure of the average **correlation** between the value of a **wave** at any pair of times, separated by delay τ. It states how monochromatic a **light** source is, or, in other words, how well a **wave** can interfere with itself at a different time delay. The delay over which the phase or amplitude of a **wave** wanders by a significant amount (and hence the **correlation** decreases by significant amount) is defined as the **coherence time** τ_c. At τ = 0, the degree of coherence is perfect, whereas it drops significantly by delay τ_c. The **coherence length** l_c is defined as the distance the **wave** travels in time τ_c.

tendon: Cord of **white fibrous tissue**, it usually attaches **muscle** to **bones**. It consists mostly of parallel, densely packed **collagen fibers** arranged in parallel bundles interspersed with long, elliptical **fibroblasts**. In general, **tendon fibers** are cylindrical in shape with diameters ranging from 20 to 400 nm. The ordered structure of **collagen fibers** running parallel to a single axis makes **tendon** a highly **birefringent tissue**.

Tenon's capsule: Adherent to episcleral **tissue**.

tensor: Term with slightly different meanings in mathematics and physics. In the mathematical fields of multilinear algebra and differential geometry, a tensor is a multilinear function. In physics and engineering, the same term usually means what a mathematician would call a tensor field: an association of a different (mathematical) tensor with each point of a geometric space, varying continuously with position. In the field of **diffusion** tensor imaging, for instance, a tensor quantity that expresses the differential permeability of organs to **water** in varying directions is used to produce scans of the **brain**. Perhaps the most important engineering examples are the stress tensor and strain tensor, which are both second-rank tensors and are related in a general linear material by a fourth-rank elasticity tensor. The rank of a particular tensor is the number of array indices required to describe such a quantity.

terabit per second (Tb/s): A unit of data transfer rate equal to 10^{12} b/s (see **bit**).

terahertz (THz): Unit for expression of **frequency** of **electromagnetic wave**; 1 THz = 10^{12} Hz. **IR radiation** with a **wavelength** of 10 μm in the free space oscillates with a **frequency** of 30 THz.

terahertz time-domain spectroscopy (THz-TDS): Implies coherent generation and detection of THz pulses using **visible femtosecond laser** pulses. The **terahertz frequency** range is located between the **IR** and microwave ranges (1 THz → 300 μm → 33 cm^{-1} → 4.1 meV → 47.6 °K). **Terahertz radiation** is a prospective tool for biomedical **spectroscopy** and imaging. A big advantage for medicine is the fact that THz **photons** are nonionizing. Many vibration transitions of small biomolecules correspond to THz frequencies. Inhomogeneities less than 100 μm in diameter, which cause strong **scattering** of **visible** and **IR light**, do not cause strong **scattering** in THz range. The use of THz **spectroscopy** to study systems of biological significance seems reasonable due to its high sensitivity to **water** properties, hydrogen bonds, and molecule conformation. There is a rather good **contrast** between **muscle** and **fat tissue** layers and between regions of healthy **skin** and **basal cell carcinoma**, including *in vivo* studies. **Tissue** response to THz frequencies is very sensitive to the presence of free and bounded **water**. This potentially allows one to differentiate benign and **malignant tumors** in **cancer** diagnostics because the **water** state is different in those **tumor** types. Determination of **absorption bands** and transparency windows for certain **tissues** and substances participating in **metabolic processes** is necessary for the development of THz tomography. The knowledge of **tissue** properties in the **terahertz** range will allow one to detect and monitor substances with characteristic complex **refraction** spectra, which could be important for precise marking of the margins of pathologic focus. However, it is not easy to provide **terahertz spectroscopy** in **tissues** because **absorption** by the **amino acids** and the most other biomolecules is masked by much stronger **water absorption** in the 1–3 THz spectral region.

texaphyrins: **Photosensitizers** of **porphyrin** family with an excitation band around 730 nm, they are used in **cancer** diagnostics and **photodynamic therapy** (**PDT**). Lu-tex®, Lutrin®, Optrin®, and **Antrin**® are the commercialized products. At **PDT**, the typical **laser** dose is 150 J/cm².

thalamus: Pair and symmetric part of the **brain**. It constitutes the main part of the diencephalons. In the caudal (tail) to oral (**mouth**) sequence of neuromeres, the diencephalons is located between the mesencephalon (cerebral peduncule, belonging to the **brain** stem) and the telencephalon.

theranostics: Term composed from two words, therapy and diagnostics, and can be used to describe that in the framework of a technology in which diagnostics and therapy are provided. For biophotonic technologies, two important examples are the **photodynamic diagnoses (PDD)** and the **photodynamic therapy (PDT)**, as well as **optical imaging** enhanced by the **gold**

nanoparticles (by using their unique **scattering** properties) of a **tumor** and its treatment by **laser-induced hyperthermia (LIHT)** mediated by these particles (using their strong **absorption** properties) with the same **laser** but of increased **power** density at therapy.

therapeutic window (*Synonym*: diagnostic window): Generally, the spectral range from 600 to 1900 nm within which the **penetration depth** of **light beams** for most living **tissues** and **blood** is the highest. Certain phototherapeutic and diagnostic modalities take advantage of this range for **visible** and **NIR light**. Within this general optical window, heterogeneous multicomponent **tissues** exhibit the **absorption bands** of **hemoglobin**, **fat**, and **water** within a wider window between 600 and 1400 nm, and the narrower one between 1550 and 1900 nm, where the lowest percentage of **light** is attenuated. The narrow spectral range from 1400 to 1550 nm is blocked for penetration by a high **absorption** of **water**. For longer **wavelengths**, there is another narrow, barely transparent window between two **water** bands from 2100 to 2400 nm (see **water absorption bands**).

thermal blooming: Major effect in high-**power laser beams** transmitting through a gaseous medium as well as the atmosphere. Due to this nonlinear heating effect, the beam pattern is deformed through the propagation path.

thermal capacitance: This term is used to describe **heat capacity** in terms of an electrical analog, where loss of heat in analogous to loss of charge on a capacitor. Structures with high **thermal capacitance** lose heat more slowly than those structures with low thermal capacitance.

thermal conductance: See **heat conductance**.

thermal conduction: See **heat conduction**.

thermal conductivity: See **heat conductivity**.

thermal damage (*Related terms*: ablation and coagulation): Damage to a **tissue** occurs when it is exposed to a high temperature for a long time period.

$$\Omega(\tau) = \ln\left(\frac{C(0)}{C(\tau)}\right) = A \int_0^\tau e^{-\frac{E_a}{RT(t)}} dt$$

The damage function is expressed in terms of an Arrhenius integral, where τ is the total heating time (s), $C(0)$ is the original concentration of undamaged **tissue**, $C(\tau)$ is the remaining concentration of undamaged **tissue** after time τ, A is an empirically determined constant (s^{-1}), E_a is an empirically determined activation **energy** barrier (J/mole), R is the universal gas constant (8.32 J/mole · K), and T is the absolute temperature (K). With **noninvasive** optical diagnostics and some photochemical applications of **light**, one must keep **tissue** below the damaging temperature, called the critical temperature T_{crit}. This temperature is defined as the temperature where the damage accumulation rate, $d\Omega/dt$, is equal to 1.0: $T_{crit} = E_a/R \ln(A)$. The constants A and E_a can be calculated on the basis of experimental data when **tissue** is exposed to a constant temperature. For example, for pig **skin**, $A = 3.1 \times 10^{98}$ and $E_a = 6.28 \times 10^5$ J/mole, which gives $T_{crit} = 59.7$ °C. With **CW light** sources, due to increases in the temperature difference between the irradiation and the surrounding **tissue**, conduction of heat away from the **light absorption** region into surrounding **tissue** increases. Depending on the **light energy**, large **tissue** volumes may be damaged. For pulsed **light**, little heat is usually lost during the pulse duration since **light absorption** is a fast process, whereas heat conduction is relatively slow, and, therefore, more precise **tissue** damage is possible.

thermal diffusivity: In **heat-transfer** analysis, the ratio of **heat conductivity** to volumetric **heat capacity**, i.e., the ratio of thermal conductivity (k_T) to the product of density (ρ) and specific **heat capacity** (c_p), $a_T = k_T/\rho c_p$, is expressed in units of m^2 s^{-1} or cm^2 s^{-1}. **Thermal diffusivity** shows the ability of a material to distribute thermal **energy** after a change in heat input. A body with a high diffusivity will reach a uniform temperature distribution faster than a body with lower diffusivity. For many **soft tissues**, these values lie within the rather narrow range defined by the thermal diffusivity of **tissue** components, such as type I **hydrated collagen** (50% **water**), 1.03×10^{-7} m^2/s, and pure **water**, 1.46×10^{-7} m^2/s. Therefore, the characteristic thermal time response of a bio-object, defined by its dimension R_o (the radius for a cylinder form) as $\tau_T \sim (R_o)^2/a_T$, can be estimated as 10^{-3} s for a **cell**, 3×10^{-2} s for a small **blood vessel**, 10^2 s for a finger, and more than 10^4 s for a whole **arm**.

thermal display resolution: Precision with which an instrument displays its assigned measurement parameter (temperature), usually expressed in degrees, tenths of degrees, hundredths of degrees, etc.

thermal effusivity: Measure of the resistance of a material to temperature change $e = (k_T \rho c_p)^{1/2}$, where k_T is the **heat conductivity**, ρ is the bulk density, and c_p is the volumetric specific **heat capacity**. It is a measure of material's ability to exchange thermal **energy** with its surroundings. If two semi-infinite bodies, initially at temperatures T_1 and T_2, are brought in perfect thermal contact, the temperature at the contact surface T_m will be given by their relative effusivities, $T_m = T_1 + (T_2 - T_1)[e_2/(e_2 + e_1)]$.

thermal expansion coefficient: During **heat transfer**, the **energy** that is stored in the intermolecular bonds between atoms changes. When the stored **energy** increases, so does the length of the molecular bond. As a result, solids typically expand in response to heating and contract on cooling. This response to temperature change is expressed as its **thermal expansion coefficient**. The coefficient of thermal expansion is used in two ways: as a volumetric **thermal expansion coefficient** (liquids and solids) and as a linear **thermal expansion coefficient** (solid state).

thermal gradient spectroscopy (TGS): As it applies to *in vivo* **glucose** sensing, it is based on measuring the fundamental

absorption bands of **glucose** at 9.1–10.5 μm using the body's naturally emitted **IR radiation** as an internal source of **radiation**. The cooling-induced **skin** transparency allows for monitoring the **IR** emission from the **interstitial fluid** and **cutaneous** layers. A linear response between *in vivo* **TGS**-detected **glucose** and reference **blood glucose** values has been reported at clinical studies for several individuals with Type 1 **diabetes**. Different modifications of this method and corresponding instrumentation for more precise quantifying of **glucose** in a human body have been defined. The simplicity of this method makes it quite appealing. However, the overlap between the effect of **glucose** on the signal and temperature variations due to circadian periodicity, as well as temperature and **blood flow** response to **glucose** change, should be eliminated or accounted for.

thermal image: Received by a **thermal imager** that creates pictures of heat rather than **light**. It measures radiated **IR energy** and converts the data to corresponding maps of temperatures. Today, instruments provide temperature data at each image **pixel**. Images may be digitized, stored, manipulated, processed, and printed out.

thermal image processing: Analysis of **thermal images**, usually by computer, and their enhancement for computer or visual analysis. In the case of an **infrared** image or thermogram, this could include temperature scaling, spot temperature measurements, thermal profiles, image manipulation, subtraction, and storage.

thermal imaging: Procedure for taking **thermal images** of a target.

thermal length: The **length of thermal diffusivity** that characterizes the distance in a medium where heat diffuses during the heating **laser** pulse.

thermal lensing: Virtual **lens** that is induced in a transparent material by its local heating, particularly by **laser beam**

absorption. The local changes in the **refractive index** of a sample induce such a **lens** for some period. Such an effect can be used to estimate **tissue** optical and thermal properties if a probing **laser beam** is applied.

thermal noise (*Related term*: Johnson–Nyquist noise): Noise that is generated by the random thermal motion of charge carriers (usually electrons) inside an electrical conductor, which happens regardless of any applied voltage. It is approximately **white noise**. The amplitude of the signal has very nearly a Gaussian **probability density function**. The **r.m.s.** voltage due to thermal noise V_n, generated in a **electrical resistance** R (ohms) over **bandwidth** Δf (**hertz**) is given by $V_n = \{4k_B T R \Delta f\}^{1/2}$, where k_B is Boltzmann's constant (joules per kelvin) and T is the resistor's absolute temperature (kelvin). As the amount of thermal noise generated depends upon the temperature of the circuit, very sensitive circuits such as **OMA** are often cooled in liquid nitrogen to reduce the noise level.

thermal radiation: Mode of heat flow that occurs by emission and **absorption** of **electromagnetic radiation**, propagating at the **speed of light**. Unlike conductive and convective heat flow, it is capable of propagating across a vacuum. The form of **heat transfer** that allows **infrared** thermography to work since **infrared energy** travels from the target to the detector by **radiation**.

thermal relaxation time (TRT): Time to dissipate the heat absorbed during a **laser** pulse.

thermal resolution: See **minimum resolvable temperature (difference) [MRT(D)]**.

thermal sensitivity: See **minimum resolvable temperature (difference) [MRT(D)]**.

thermodynamic activity: Ions in solution are in constant motion. This movement is temperature dependent, i.e., as **water** becomes hotter, the particles within it move faster and, conversely, as it becomes cooler, they slow down.

thermodynamic temperature: See **absolute (Kelvin) temperature scale**

thermoelastic effect: Generation of **mechanical stress (acoustic) waves** via the time-dependent thermal expansion of a sample.

thermography: Hardware and software for target thermal imaging and **thermal image** processing.

thigh: In humans, the thigh is the area between the pelvis and buttocks, and the **knee**. Anatomically, it is part of the lower limb. The single **bone** in the thigh is called the femur. This **bone** is very thick and strong (due to the high proportion of cortical **bone**); it forms a ball and socket joint at the hip, and a condylar joint at the **knee**.

thin lens: The approximation that ignores optical effects due to the thickness of **lenses** and simplifies ray-tracing calculations. It is often combined with the **paraxial approximation** in techniques such as ray transfer matrix analysis. The **focal length** f of a thin **lens** is given by the equation $1/f \approx (n-1)[(1/R_1)-(1/R_2)]$, where n is the **index of refraction** of the **lens** material, and R_1 and R_2 are the radii of curvature of the two **lens** surfaces. Here, R_1 is taken to be positive if the first surface is convex, and negative if the surface is concave. The signs are reversed for the back surface of the **lens**: R_2 is positive if the surface is concave, and negative if it is convex. In air, the **focal length** is the distance from the center of the **lens** to the principal foci (or **focal points**) of the **lens**. For a converging **lens** (for example, a convex **lens**), the **focal length** is positive and is the distance at which a beam of **collimated light** will be focused to a single spot. For a diverging **lens** (for example, a concave **lens**), the **focal length** is negative and is the distance to the point from which a **collimated** beam appears to be diverging after passing through the **lens**. For a thin **lens** in the paraxial ray approximation, the object (s) and image (s') distances are related by the equation $(1/s) + (1/s') = 1/f$.

thionine (*Synonyms*: thionine acetate, Lauth's violet): A strongly staining metachromatic dye that is widely used for biological staining. It can also be used as a **Schiff base** reagent in quantitative staining of **DNA**.

third-harmonic generation (THG): If a narrow-band optical **wave** pulse at a **frequency** ω propagates through a nonlinear medium with a nonzero Kerr **nonlinear susceptibility** $\chi^{(3)}$ due to nonlinearity, the result will be a signal at **frequency** 3ω (see **second harmonic generation**).

thorax: See **chest**.

three-photon fluorescence microscopy: **Microscopy** that employs both **ballistic photons** and scattered **photons** at the **wavelength** of the third harmonic of incident **radiation**. It possesses the same advantages as **two-photon fluorescence microscopy**, but it ensures a somewhat higher **spatial resolution** and provides an opportunity to excite **chromophores** with shorter **wavelengths**.

throat: The anterior part of the **neck** in front of the vertebral column. It consists of the **pharynx** and **larynx**. An important feature of the **throat** is the epiglottis, a flap that separates the **esophagus** from the **trachea** and prevents inhalation of food or drink. The **throat** contains various **blood vessels**, various pharyngeal **muscles**, the **trachea** (windpipe), and the **esophagus**.

thrombocyte: See **platelet**.

thymus: An organ located in the upper anterior portion of the **chest** cavity just behind the sternum. The main function of the

thymus is to provide an area for T-**lymphocyte** maturation, which is vital in protecting against autoimmunity.

thyroid: One of the larger endocrine **glands** in the body, this **gland** is found in the **neck** just below the Adam's apple. The **thyroid** controls how quickly the body burns **energy**, makes **proteins**, and regulates how sensitive the body should be to other **hormones**.

Tikhonov regularization: The most *commonly* used regularization method of ill-posed **inverse problems**. In statistics, the method is also known as ridge regression. It is related to the Levenberg–Marquardt **algorithm** for nonlinear **least-squares** problems. To solve an overdetermined system of linear equations, given as $Ax_\lambda = b$, with the preference to a particular solution with desirable properties, the regularization term is included in the minimization: $\|Ax_\lambda - b\|^2 + \lambda \|x_\lambda\|^2$, where $\|Ax_\lambda - b\|^2$ is the least square or residual norm, $\|x_\lambda\|^2$ is the regularized norm, and λ is the regularization parameter.

time-correlated single-photon counting (TCSPC) technique: Time-resolved single-**photon** counting method and instrument (see **photon-counting system**) used to receive low-**intensity** short **light** pulses.

time-dependent radiation-transfer theory (RTT): Theory that is based on the time-dependent integro-differential, **radiation-transfer equation (RTE)** (the Boltzmann or linear transport equation), which is a balance equation describing the time-dependent flow of particles (e.g., **photons**) in a given volume element that takes into account their velocity c, location $\bar{r}$, and changes due to collisions (i.e., **scattering** and **absorption**).

time-division multiplexing (TDM): Multiplexing technique in which each signal is separated into many segments, each one very short in duration.

time-domain technique: Spectroscopic or imaging technique that uses **ultrashort laser pulses**. See **time-gating**, **time-resolved imaging**, **time-resolved measurements**, **time-resolved optical absorption and scattering tomography** (**TOAST**), and **time-resolved spectroscopy** (**TRS**).

time-gating: Method for selecting **photon** groups with different arriving times to a detector within a selected and moveable time window. It is used in **diffuse optical tomography** and **spectroscopy**. Time-gating may be purely electronic, optical, or a combination of the two.

time-of-flight (**TOF**): Describes a variety of methods that measure the time that it takes for an object (for instance, molecule), particle (for instance, **nanoparticle**), or acoustic, electromagnetic, or other **wave** to travel a distance through a medium. In **biomedical optics**, this is the mean time of **photon** travel between two points that accounts for the **refractive index** and **scattering** properties of the medium (see **time-domain technique**). This method is used to measure the **tissue**-dependent optical pathlength over a range of optical **wavelengths** from which composition and properties of the **tissue** can be analyzed and **tissue** abnormalities can be imaged. In optical interferometry, the pathlength difference between sample and reference arms can be measured by **TOF** methods, such as **frequency modulation** followed by **phase shift** measurement or cross-**correlation** of signals (see **cross-correlation measurement device**). Such methods are used in LIDAR and **laser** tracker systems. In ultrasonic flow-meter measurement, **TOF** is used to measure the speed of signal propagation in a collinear direction with the flow—upstream and downstream of flow of a medium—in order to estimate total flow velocity. In optical flow velocimetry, **TOF** measurements are made perpendicular to the flow by timing when individual particles cross two or more locations along the flow. In **time-of-flight** mass spectrometry, ions are accelerated by an electrical field to the same kinetic **energy** with the velocity of the ion depending on the mass-to-charge ratio. This technique is used to determine mass-to-charge ratio; see **laser microprobe mass analysis (LAMMA)**.

time-resolved imaging: Method based on **time-resolved measurements** where **ballistic photons** can be used to produce precise **tissue** images similar to **x-ray computed tomography**; however, in many **tissues**, because of strong **scattering**, this group of **photons** is typically negligibly small. **Zigzag photons** or **snake photons**, having undergone a few **scattering** events (all of which are in the forward or near-forward direction), retain the image-bearing characteristics to some extent, but these **photons** are detectable. Due to a high **intensity**-of-**diffusion** component, it is much more practical to use **diffuse photons** to evaluate **optical properties** of **tissues**, although **spatial resolution** may not be very high in that case. To improve the **spatial resolution** of **diffusion** methods, various approaches for selective detection of informative **photons** are suggested, such as **spatially resolved**, angle-resolved, and **polarization gating**.

time-resolved measurements: Measurements that use pulsed or modulated **laser beams** for irradiating **tissues** under study and separating (**time-gating**) different groups of scattered **photons** at their detection in the forward (transillumination) or the backward (**backscattering**) directions. These groups of **photons** are so-called **ballistic photons** (coherent), **quasi-ballistic photons** (zigzag or snake), and **diffuse photons** that are typically the largest group of **photons** that migrated for a longer time in a **tissue** along multi-step random trajectories. Each of these groups carries information about optical (morphological) properties of a **tissue**.

time-resolved optical absorption and scattering tomography (TOAST): An image reconstruction package developed at University College London that employs a finite-element method forward model and an iterative reconstruction **algorithm**.

time-resolved spectroscopy (TRS): This is related to **time-resolved measurements** with the aim of producing spectroscopic information.

518

time-share control: Regime that ensures that at one time an optical signal of only a given **wavelength** passes through the whole system.

tip-enhanced Raman spectroscopy (TERS): A combination of **surface-enhanced Raman spectroscopy (SERS)** with **scanning-probe microscopy (SPM)**, providing spatial resolution down to the nanometer scale. **TERS** uses a metallic (usually silver- or gold-coated **AFM** or **STM**) tip to enhance the Raman signals of molecules placed in its vicinity. The spatial resolution is approximately the size of the tip apex (20–30 nm). **TERS** has a sensitivity down to the single-molecule level.

tissue: Aggregate of similar **cells** and **cell** products forming a definite kind of structural material. See **adipose tissue, areolar tissue, cervical tissue, connective tissue, episcleral tissue, epithelial tissue, fibrous tissue, glandular tissue, hard tissue, hard oral tissue, lymphoid tissue, malignant tissue, mucosa, muscular tissue, nervous tissue, reticular tissue, scar tissue, soft tissue, tubular tissue, white fibrous tissue,** and **yellow elastic tissue.**

tissue absorption: Absorbed **light** is converted to heat or radiated in the form of **fluorescence**; it is also consumed in photobiochemical reactions. The **absorption spectrum** depends on the type of predominant **absorption centers** and **water** content (**chromophores**) of **tissues**. Absolute values of **absorption coefficients** for typical **tissues** lie in the range of $10^{-2} - 10^4$ cm^{-1}. In the **ultraviolet (UV)** and **infrared (IR)** ($\lambda \geq 2000$ nm) spectral regions, **light** is readily absorbed, which accounts for the small contribution of **scattering** and the inability of **radiation** to penetrate deep into **tissues** (see **tissue penetration depth**). The **absorption spectrum** of biological **tissue** is usually expressed in terms of the **wavelength** dependence of the **absorption coefficient**. Since **water** is the major component of any **soft tissue**, an **absorption coefficient** of 75% **water** only slightly differs from experimental values for real **tissues**. The **absorption** of diffuse **light** by **skin pigments** is a measure of **bilirubin** content, **hemoglobin** concentration and its **saturation** with **oxygen**, and the concentration of pharmaceutical products in **blood** and **tissues**. These characteristics are widely used in the diagnostics and monitoring of various diseases.

tissue birefringence: Phenomenon that results primarily from the linear anisotropy of **fibrous** structures that form **connective tissues**. The **refractive index** of a medium is higher along the length of a **fiber** than along the cross section. A specific **tissue** structure is a system composed of parallel cylinders that creates a uniaxial **birefringent** medium with the **optic axis** parallel to the cylinder axes. This is called form **birefringence**. A large variety of **tissues** such as eye **cornea**, **tendon**, **cartilage**, eye **sclera**, *dura mater*, testis, **muscle**, **nerve**, **retina**, **bone**, **tooth**, **myelin**, etc., exhibit form **birefringence**. All of these **tissues** contain uniaxial and/or biaxial **birefringent** structures. For instance, in **bone** and **tooth**, these are mineralized structures originating from **hydroxyapatite** crystals that play an important role in **hard tissue birefringence**. In particular, dental **enamel** is an ordered array of such crystals surrounded by a **protein/lipid/water** matrix. **Tendon** consists mostly of densely packed **collagen fibers** arranged in parallel bundles cylindrical in shape with diameters ranging from 20 to 400 nm; the ordered structure of **collagen fibers** running parallel to a single axis makes **tendon** a highly **birefringent tissue**. Arteries have a more complex structure than **tendons**; however, as with **tendon**, the cylindrical **collagen** and **elastin fibers** are ordered mainly along one axis, thus causing the **tissue** to be **birefringent**. **Myocardium**, on the other **hand**, contains **fibers** oriented along two different axes; it consists mostly of cardiac **muscle fibers** arranged in sheets that wind around the ventricles and atria, and it is typically **birefringent** since the **refractive index** along the axis of the **muscle fiber** is different from that in the transverse direction. Reported **birefringence** values for **tendon**, **muscle**, **coronary artery**, **myocardium**, **sclera**, **cartilage**, and **skin** are on the order of 10^{-3}. **PS OCT** allows for the measurement of linear **birefringence** in turbid **tissue** with a high precision: for rodent **muscle**, 1.4×10^{-3}, for normal porcine **tendon**, $(4.2 \pm 0.3) \times 10^{-3}$, and when thermally treated (90 °C, 20 s), $(2.24 \pm 0.07) \times 10^{-3}$, for porcine **skin**, $(1.5–3.5) \times 10^{-3}$, for bovine **cartilage** 3.0×10^{-3}, and for bovine **tendon**, $(3.7 \pm 0.4) \times 10^{-3}$. Such **birefringence** provides 90%-phase retardation at a depth on the order of several hundred **micrometers**. The magnitude of **birefringence** is related to the density and other properties of the **collagen fibers**, whereas the orientation of the fast axis indicates the orientation of the **collagen fibers**. The amplitude and orientation of **birefringence** of the **skin** and **cartilage** are not as uniformly distributed as in **tendon**. The densities of **collagen fibers** in **skin** and **cartilage** are not as uniform as in **tendon**, and the orientation of the **collagen fibers** is not distributed in as orderly a fashion.

tissue compartment sizing: **Cells** and **tissue** structure elements vary in size from a few tenths of **nanometers** to hundreds of **micrometers**; **blood cells** (**erythrocytes**, **leukocytes**, and **platelets**) exhibit the following parameters: normal **erythrocyte** in **plasma** has the shape of a concave–concave disc with a diameter varying from 7.1 to 9.2 μm, a thickness of 0.9–1.2 μm in the center, 1.7–2.4 μm on the periphery, and a volume of ~90 μm³. **Leukocytes** are formed like spheres with a diameter of 8–22 μm. **Platelets** in the **blood** stream are biconvex disc-like particles with diameters ranging from 2 to 4 μm. Normally, **blood** has about 10 times as many **erythrocytes** as **platelets** and about 30 times as many **platelets** as **leukocytes**. Most other mammalian **cells** have diameters in the range of 5–75 μm. In the epidermal layer, the **cells** are large (with an average cross-sectional area of about 80 μm²) and quite uniform in size. **Fat cells**, each containing a single **lipid** droplet that nearly fills the entire **cell** and therefore results in eccentric placement of the **cytoplasm** and **nucleus**, have a wide range of diameters from a few microns to 50–75 μm. **Fat cells** may reach a diameter of 100–200 μm in **pathological** cases. There are a wide variety of structures within **cells** that determine **tissue light scattering**. **Cell** nuclei are on the order of 5–10 μm in diameter. **Mitochondria**, **lysosomes**, and **peroxisomes** have dimensions of 1–2 μm. **Ribosomes** are on the order of 20 nm in diameter, and structures within various organelles can have dimensions up to a few hundred **nanometers**. Usually, the **scatterers** in **cells** are not spherical. The models of prolate ellipsoids with a ratio of the ellipsoid axes between 2 and 10 are more typical. The hollow organs of the body are lined with a thin, highly cellular surface layer of **epithelial tissue** that is supported by underlying, relatively acellular **connective tissue**. In healthy **tissues**, the **epithelium** often consists of a single, well-organized layer of **cells** with en-face diameter of 10–20 μm and height of 25 μm. In **dysplastic epithelium**, **cells** proliferate, and their nuclei enlarge and appear darker (hyperchromatic) when stained. Enlarged nuclei are primary indicators of **cancer**, **dysplasia**, and **cell** regeneration in most human **tissues**. In **fibrous tissues** or **tissues** containing fiber layers (**cornea**, **sclera**, *dura mater*, **muscle**, **myocardium**, **tendon**, **cartilage**, **vessel** wall, **retinal nerve fiber layer**, etc.) composed mostly of **microfibrils** and/or **microtubules**, typical diameters of the cylindrical structural elements are 10–400 nm. Their length varies from 10–25 μm to a few millimeters. For some **tissues**, the size distribution of the **scattering** particles may be essentially monodispersive, and for others it may be quite broad. Examples for the two are transparent **eye cornea stroma**, which has a sharply monodispersive distribution, and turbid eye **sclera**, which has a rather broad distribution of **collagen fiber** diameters.

tissue dehydration: See **dehydration**.

tissue demineralization: See **demineralization**.

tissue laser welding: **Laser** welding is a technique used to produce immediate closure of **wounds**. A variety of **lasers** are used for sealing many **tissue** types, including **blood vessels**, urethra, **nerves**, *dura mater*, **skin**, **stomach**, and **colon**. **Tissue laser welding** enables a reduction in foreign-body reaction, bleeding, suture and needle **trauma**, as well as in surgical times and skill requirements. Although the precise molecular mechanism of **tissue laser welding** is still unknown, it is widely considered to be a thermal phenomenon. **Laser** irradiation induces thermal changes in connective-**tissue proteins** within cut **tissues**, resulting in a bond between the two adjoining edges. The dosimetry of the **laser** irradiation and of the induced temperature rise are crucial in order to minimize the risk of heat damage to the **tissue**. To overcome this problem and to improve the localization of **laser light absorption** into **tissue**, the application of photo-enhancing **chromophores** or metallic **nanoparticles** has been proposed as a safer technique (see **selective photothermal treatment**). The use of **wavelength**-specific **chromophores** or plasmonic **nanoparticles** makes a differential **absorption** possible between the stained (labeled) region and the surrounding **tissue**. The advantage is primarily the selective **absorption** of **laser radiation** by the target without needing precise focusing of the **laser beam**. Lower **laser** irradiances can be used because of the increased **absorption** of stained **tissue**. **Indocyanine green (ICG)**, **fluorescein**, basic **fuchsine**, and fen 6 are often-used dyes. On the **tissue**, **laser-welding** natural adhesives, such as **blood**, **plasma**, fibrinogen, and **albumin** are applied. Following **laser**-induced **coagulation**, these materials act as glues that form an inter-digitated matrix among the **collagen fibers**. **Water** is also used as an **endogenous chromophore** for absorbing near- and **far-infrared laser light**. For example, the welding of a corneal **wound** is achieved after staining the cut walls with a **water** solution of **ICG** and irradiating with a **diode laser** emitting at 810 nm that operates at low **power** (12–17 W/cm^2 at the corneal surface). The result is a localized heating of the cut that induces a mild and controlled welding of the **stromal collagen**, thereby minimizing the risk of thermal **injury**.

tissue optical index (TOI): Developed as a **contrast** function by combining **diffuse optical spectroscopy (DOS)** measurements: **TOI** = ctHHb × ctH_2O / (%lipid), where ctHHb is the **deoxyhemoglobin** concentration, ctH_2O is the **water** concentration, and %lipid is the **lipid** concentration. Spatial variations in **TOI** allow one to rapidly locate the maximum **cancer lesion** optical **contrast**.

tissue optical model: Biological **tissues** are optically inhomogeneous and absorbing **media**. Their average **refractive index** is higher than that of air, thus partial **reflection** of the **radiation** at the **tissue**/air interface (**Fresnel reflection**) takes place while the remaining part of **radiation** penetrates the **tissue**. **Multiple scattering** and **absorption** are responsible for **light beams** broadening and eventually decaying as they travel through a **tissue**. The bulk **scattering** causes a large portion of **radiation** to be scattered in the backward direction. **Light** propagation within a **tissue** depends on the **scattering** and **absorption** properties of its compartments: **cells, cell** organelles, and various **fiber** structures. The size, shape, and density of these structures, and their refractive indices play important roles in the propagation of **light** in **tissues** (see **tissue compartment sizing**). The great diversity and structural complexity of **tissues** require the development of adequate optical models accounting for the **optical properties** of **tissues**. Two major approaches are currently used: (1) **tissue** modeled as a medium with a continuous random spatial distribution of **optical parameters**, and (2) **tissue** considered as a discrete ensemble of **scatterers**. The choice of approach is determined by both the structural specificity of the **tissue** under study and the kind of **light-scattering** characteristics that are to be described. Many **tissues** can be represented as a random continuum of the inhomogeneities of the **refractive index** with a varying spatial scale. This approach is applicable for **tissues** with no pronounced boundaries between elements that feature significant heterogeneity. The process of **scattering** by these structures may be described under certain conditions using the model of a **phase screen**. In accordance with the second approach, biological **media** are often modeled as ensembles of particles since many **cells** and micro-organisms are close in shape to spheres, ellipsoids, or rods. A system of noninteracting, homogeneous, spherical particles is the simplest **tissue** model. Mie theory rigorously describes the **diffraction** of **light** by a spherical particle. The further development of this model involves accounting for more complex structure of the spherical particles, namely, the multilayered spheres and the spheres with radial nonhomogeneity, anisotropy, and **optical activity**. Since a **connective tissue** consists of **fiber** structures, a system of long cylinders is the most appropriate model for it. **Muscular tissue**, **skin dermis**, cerebral **membrane** (*dura mater*), **eye cornea**, and

sclera belong to this type of **tissue** formed essentially by **collagen fibrils**. **Light diffraction** by a single homogeneous or multilayered cylinder has also been well described. Attempts to describe **light scattering** by a system of interacting particles as a more realistic **tissue** model (quasi-ordered spherical particles or cylinders) have been made.

tissue optical properties control: Any kind of physical or chemical action, such as **mechanical stress** or changes in **osmolarity** that induces reversible or irreversible changes in the **optical properties** of a tissue [see **controlling of tissue optical properties**, **immersion medium (liquid)**, **immersion technique**, **matching substance**, **mechanical stress**, and **optical clearing**].

tissue optics: Field of R&D describing how **light** propagates in **scattering** and absorbing **media** such as biological **tissue**, and applying optical methods for medical imaging, diagnosis, and therapy. It encompasses modeling of the **light** transport in **tissues**, measurement of **tissue** optical transport parameters, and development of models that can explain the **optical properties** of **tissue** and their dependence on the number, size, and arrangement of the **tissue** compartments, as well as **light-tissue** interaction phenomena including **photothermal**, photomechanical, and photochemical effects [see **ablation**, **hyperthermia**, **coagulation**, **laser heating**, **laser-induced interstitial thermotherapy (LITT)**, **photochemical therapy**, **photodynamic therapy**, **photothermal therapy**], and **optoacoustic** and **acousto-optic interactions**. Nonlinear optics of **tissues**, as a part of **tissue** optics, is a new field of research and biomedical applications. See also **tissue absorption**, **tissue birefringence, tissue optical models, tissue optical properties control, tissue penetration depth, tissue refractive index, tissue refractive index measurement**, and **tissue scattering**.

tissue penetration depth: See also **penetration depth of light**. In the **ultraviolet (UV)** and **infrared (IR)** ($\lambda \geq 2000$ nm) spectral regions, **light** is readily absorbed, which accounts for the inability of **radiation** to penetrate deep into **tissues** (only through one or two **cell** layers). Short-**wave visible light** penetrates typical **tissues** as deep as 0.5–2.5 mm, where upon it undergoes an *e*-fold decrease of **intensity**. In this case, both **scattering** and **absorption** occur. In the **wavelength** range of 600–1600 nm, **scattering** prevails over **absorption**, and **light** penetrates to a depth of 8–10 mm within a more narrow optical window from 700 to 1100 nm (see **therapeutic/diagnostic window**).

tissue phantom: An artificial model of actual **tissue** that mimics its optical, structural, and functional properties. Various **tissue phantoms** used for **calibration** and dosimetry of optical diagnostic, imaging, and therapeutic techniques and instruments have been developed. Available **tissue phantoms** provide **calibration** and **light** dosimetry of **CW**, time-domain, and **frequency-domain diffuse reflectance** and **fluorescence spectroscopy** and **tomography**; **polarization-gating spectroscopy** and **tomography**; **optoacoustic** and pulsed **photothermal spectroscopy** and **tomography**; **OCT** and **confocal microscopy**; **noninvasive glucose** monitoring, **oxymetry**, and Doppler-**flowmetry**; and **laser ablation** and **PDT** (see **phantom**). Liquid, **gel**-like, and solid-state **phantoms** are typically used. Liquid **phantoms** consist of a **scattering** medium, an **absorbing medium**, a diluent, and, in some cases, **fluorophores**. Some common **scattering media** are **Intralipid**, Nutralipid, or Liposyn. Other common **scatterers** are milk or **micron**-sized **latex** (polystyrene) spheres. Polystyrene microspheres exhibit low **fluorescence**. Absorbing **media** include some biological dyes, such as **trypan blue**, **Evans blue**, **indocyanine green**, **methylene blue**, and **Photofrin II**, as well as black **India ink** and natural **pigments**, such as **melanin** and **hemoglobin**. The resulting suspension has the desired intrinsic **optical properties** of the simulated **tissue** in norm, pathology, or at experimental conditions. These **optical properties** include the **absorption coefficient** μ_a, the **scattering coefficient** μ_s, and the **scattering anisotropy factor** *g*. For **soft tissues**, typical **optical properties** are $\mu_a \approx$ 0.5 to 5.0 cm^{-1}, $\mu_s \approx$ 0.2 to 400 cm^{-1}, and $g \approx$ 0.6 to 0.9 for **visible** and **NIR wavelengths**. The typical mixtures approximately close to 10%-**Intralipid** (**scatterers**) and $\sim$ 0.01%-**India ink** (absorbers) are used to model **tissue optical properties** in the far red/**NIR** range. A liquid **phantom** system is very easy to prepare; however, it cannot be used to make samples of realistic complexity and stability. **Gelatin** in combination with **scattering** nano- and **micrometer**-sized particles as **scatterers** and **melanin** and **hemoglobin** as absorbing fractions are used in **gel**-like **phantoms**. Solid-state **phantom** samples have been made using either transparent hosts, like polymers, epoxy resin, silicone, or **gelatin**, or using inherently **light-scattering** materials, such as wax. Optical epoxy resins are used to build solid-state **phantoms** with titanium dioxide or other particles as **scatterers** and **Indian ink** as absorber. Steps toward realistic complex geometries have been layered samples, inserted inhomogeneities, and **phantoms** mimicking whole organs. Multilayered **phantoms** have been developed in the past to mimic, for example, the **skin**, the human **head**, and the **cervix**.

tissue refractive index: Mean **refractive index (RI)** $\bar{n}$ of a **tissue** is defined by the **RIs** of its **scattering** particle material n_s and ground (surrounding) matter n_0. The **RIs** of **tissue** structure elements and the **tissue** itself can be derived using the **Gladstone and Dale law**, as $\bar{n} = \sum_{i=1}^{N} n_i f_i, \sum_i f_i = 1$, where n_i and f_i are the **refractive index** and **volume fraction** of the individual components, respectively, and N is the number of components. At a microscopic scale, the **soft-tissue** components have no pronounced boundaries. They appear to merge into a continuous structure with spatial variations in the **RI**. To model such a complicated structure as a collection of particles, it is necessary to resort to a statistical approach. The **tissue** components that contribute most to the local **RI** variations are the **connective tissue fibers** (bundles of **elastin** and **collagen**), cytoplasmic organelles (**mitochondria**, **lysosomes**, and **peroxisomes**), **cell** nuclei, and **melanin** granules. The average background index is defined as the weighted average of **RIs** of the **cytoplasm** and the **interstitial fluid**, n_{cp} and n_{is}, as $\bar{n}_0 = f_{cp} n_{cp} + (1 - f_{cp}) n_{is}$, where f_{cp} is the **volume fraction** of the fluid in the **tissue** contained inside the **cells**, $\bar{n}_0 = 1.362$ for $n_{cp} = 1.367$ and $n_{is} = 1.355$, and $f_{cp} = 0.6$. The **RI** of **scattering** particle material, $\bar{n}_s = \bar{n}_0 + f_f(n_f - n_{is}) + f_{nc}(n_{nc} - n_{cp}) + f_{or}(n_{or} - n_{cp})$, where the subscripts f, is, nc, cp, and or refer to the **fibers**, **interstitial fluid**, nuclei, **cytoplasm**, and organelles. The multiplying factors f are the **volume fractions** of the elements in the solid portion of the **tissue**. The **RI** of the connective-**tissue fibers** is about 1.47, which corresponds to about 55% **hydration** of **collagen**, its main component; $n_{nc} = n_{or} = 1.40$, thus, $\bar{n}_s = \bar{n}_0 + f_f(n_f - n_{is}) + (1 - f_f)(n_{nc} - n_{cp})$. **Collagen** and **elastin fibers** consist of approximately 70% of the **fat**-free dry weight of the **dermis**, 45% of the **heart**, and 2–3% of the nonmuscular internal organs. Therefore, depending on **tissue** type, f_f may be as small as about 0.02 or as large as 0.7, and the mean **refractive index** variations that correspond to these two extremes are $n_s = 1.397$ and 1.452. For some **hard tissues** or **melanin** granules in **skin** or eye **iris**, **refractive index** of **scatterers** can be as high as 1.5–1.7. **RI** determines **light reflection** and **refraction** at the interfaces between air and **tissue**, **optical fiber** and **tissue**, and **tissue** layers. It also strongly influences **light** propagation and distribution within **tissues**, defines **speed of light** in **tissue**, and governs how the **photons** migrate. It is worth noting that *in vitro* and *in vivo* measures may differ significantly—this difference can be accounted for by the decreased refractivity of ground matter, $\bar{n}_0$, due to impaired **hydration**. **Tissue** is modeled as a mixture of **water** and a bio-organic compound of a **tissue**. For instance, the **RI** of human **skin** can be approximated by a 70/30 mixture of **water** and **proteins**, assuming that **proteins** in the **visible** and **NIR** have a constant **RI** value of 1.5, $n_{skin}(\lambda) = 0.7n_W(\lambda) + 0.3 \times 1.5$.

tissue refractive index measurement: Refractivity measurements in a number of strongly **scattering tissues** and **blood** can be performed using various techniques. One of the techniques is a **fiber optic refractometer** based on the simple concept that the cone of **light** issuing from an **optical fiber** is dependent on the indices of the cladding material (**tissue**); using this simple and sensitive technique, it was found that at 633 nm, **fatty tissue** has the largest **refractive index (RI)** (1.455), followed by **kidney tissue** (1.418), **muscular tissue** (1.410), and then **blood** and **spleen** tissues (1.400). The lowest **RIs** were found in **lungs** and **liver** (1.380 and 1.368, respectively). There is a tendency for **RIs** to decrease with increasing **light wavelength** from 390 to 700 nm.

The principle of **total internal reflection** at **laser beam** irradiation is also used for **tissue** and **blood refraction** measurements, and the results are typically presented in the form of a Cauchy **dispersion** equation as $n = A + B\lambda^{-2} + C\lambda^{-4} + D\lambda^{-6}$, for human **blood plasma** in the range from 400 to 1000 nm $n_{bp}(\lambda) = 1.3254 + 8.4052 \times 10^3\lambda^{-2} - 3.9572 \times 10^8\lambda^{-4} - 2.3617 \times 10^{13}\lambda^{-6}$. For modeling of the behavior of **RI** of **tissues**, **blood**, and their components, one may use a remarkable property of **proteins** that equal concentrations of aqueous solutions of different **proteins** all have approximately the same **RI**, n_{pw}, and it varies almost linearly with concentration, $C_p, n_{pw}(\lambda) = n_w(\lambda) + \beta_p(\lambda) \times C_p$, where n_w is the **RI** of **water** and β_p is the specific refractive increment, and C_p is measured in grams per 100 ml (grams per deciliter). For example, the **RI** of human **erythrocyte cytoplasm**, defined by the **cell**-bounded **hemoglobin** solution, can be found from this equation at $\beta_p = 0.001942$, valid for a **wavelength** of 589 nm. That is, for normal **hemoglobin** concentration in **RBC cytoplasm** of 300–360 g/l, the **RBC RI**, $n_{RBC} = 1.393$–1.406. Other materials of specific biological interest are the **carbohydrates**, lipoids, and **nucleic acid** compounds. The first two usually have low values of β, in the region of 0.0014–0.0015, and **nucleic acids** have higher values, 0.0016–0.0020. Some other techniques of **RI** measurements of biological liquids are also available. A short-pulse time delay technique was also successfully applied for **RI** estimation of normal and **malignant breast tissue**; for the known thickness of the sample and the measured shift Δt of the transmitted pulse peak relative to the delay time measured through a layer of air of the same thickness, the mean phase **RI**, n, of a **tissue** sample can be evaluated. Very short pulses should be used in such measurements, thus, the **group refractive index** [$n_g = n - \lambda(dn/d\lambda)$] should be used and determined. The time delay in the pulse arrival for a **tissue** sample of thickness d is $\Delta t = (d/c_0)(n_{g1} - n_{g2})$, where c_0 is the **light** velocity in free space, n_{g1} is the effective (mean) group **RI** of a **tissue**, and n_{g2} is the group **RI** of the homogeneous reference medium (air). The effective group **RI** of a **tissue** is $n_{g1} = f_s n_{gs} + (1 - f_s)n_{g0}$, where f_s is the **volume fraction** of the **scatterers** composing a **tissue**, n_{gs} is the group **RI** of the **scatterers**, and n_{g0} is the group **RI** of the ground material of a **tissue**; $n = 1.403$ was found for normal and 1.431 for **malignant breast tissue**. **OCT** provides simple and straightforward measurements of the **RI** both *in vitro* and *in vivo*. The in-depth scale of **OCT** images is determined by the optical pathlength z_{opt} between two points along the depth direction. Because a broadband **light** source is used, the optical pathlength is proportional to the group **RI** n_g and geometrical pathlength z as $z_{opt} = n_g z$, and usually $n_g \cong n$.

tissue scattering: Mixture of Rayleigh (isotropic) and Mie (anisotropic) **scattering** is characteristic for many **tissues** as a **tissue optical model**. The input of each kind of **scattering** depends on **tissue compartment sizing** and **refractive index**. As a result, a **power** law for dependence of the **scattering** coefficient on the **wavelength** is typical. However, because of strong **tissue absorption** in the **ultraviolet (UV)** and **infrared (IR)** ($\lambda \geq 2000$ nm) spectral regions, **light** is more absorbed than scattered, and **radiation** does not penetrate deep into **tissues** (see **tissue penetration depth**). For short-**wave visible light**, both **scattering** and **absorption** occur with 15–40% of the incident **radiation** being reflected (backscattered). In the **wavelength** range of 600–1600 nm, **scattering** prevails over **absorption**, **light** penetrates deeply, and the **intensity** of the reflected **radiation** increases to 35–70%.

tissue shrinkage: Loss of volume and weight caused, for instance, by **tissue dehydration**.

tissue viability imaging (TiVi):   Based on analysis of the **RBC** concentration in any **skin** site of arbitrary size by way of single image or video acquisition by low-cost cameras utilizing **cross-polarization imaging** technology. For single image acquisition, the flash of a consumer-end **RGB** digital camera is used as a broadband **light** source, and the camera **CCD** acquires an instantaneous image in three 8-**bit** primary **color** planes. **Color** filtering is performed on-camera by three 100 nm **bandwidth color** filters: blue ($\approx$400–500 nm), green ($\approx$500–600 nm), and red ($\approx$600–700 nm). Using **polarization** imaging and the

Kubelka–Munk model (KKM), a spectroscopic **algorithm** was developed that is not dependent on incident **light intensity**, taking advantage of the physiological fact that green **light** is absorbed more by **RBCs** than red **light**. TiVi represents the first low-cost technique designed to image **tissue hematocrit** in real time.

titanium dioxide (TiO$_2$): **Semiconductor** material. Its electronic **energy** structure is represented by two bands, namely, a conduction band and valence band with an **energy** gap (**bandgap**) between them. Being excited by a **photon**, an electron from the valence band goes to the conduction band, generating a positive-charged hole in the valence band. Only **photons** with energies larger than the **bandgap** can be absorbed. The formed charged carriers can recombine either radiatively (by emitting a **photon**) or nonradiatively (releasing **energy** as heat). Electrons and holes can recombine on a particle surface, reducing or oxidizing surrounding molecules, and thus producing **radicals**. TiO$_2$ is a wide-**bandgap semiconductor** with a **bandgap** that varies for different material structures: 3.11 eV for brookite, 3.00 eV for rutile, and 3.20 eV for anatase at room temperature. The interband transition is symmetry-forbidden (indirect), and the **absorption** efficiency is shifted to the **UVB wavelengths** (290–320 nm). Anatase is thermodynamically stable for diameters smaller than 11 nm, and rutile is stable for sizes larger than 35 nm.

titanium dioxide (TiO$_2$) particles: An insoluble white powder that is used extensively in many commercial products, including paint, **cosmetics**, plastics, paper, and food as an anti-caking or whitening agent and **UV-light**-protection substance. It is produced and used in the workplace in varying particle-size fractions, including fine and ultrafine sizes (monodisperse nanosized, ~100 nm). Uncoated particles can damage **tissue** and **cells** at irradiation by **UV** or blue **light** due to a strong **photocatalytic effect**. These **nanoparticles** are used for **light**-mediated **bacteria** killing and for bleaching plant **cell** mass (**pulp**). **Nanoparticles** tend to form aggregates and agglomerates of 100–200 nm in size, resulting in worsening their protecting properties as **sunscreens** in the **UVB** range and shifting the pronounced attenuation to the longer-**wavelength UVA** and **visible** regions of the solar **spectrum**. Novel manufacturing technologies, e.g., mechanochemical processing, enable the production of nano-powders without such disadvantages and with a narrow size distribution (25 ± 4 nm) that can be successfully used in **sunscreens**. Usually, size distribution of TiO$_2$ particles is 15–20% around the mean value. The protective efficiency of nano-sized particles of TiO$_2$ in **sunscreens** depends on their size. They absorb and scatter **UV radiation** most efficiently at sizes of 60–120 nm. Because particles scatter **UV** and not **visible light**, the **sunscreen** made on the basis of these particles appears to be transparent. TiO$_2$ **nanoparticles** are commonly used with a surface covered by inert coating materials, such as SiO$_2$ or Al$_2$O$_3$, to improve their **dispersion** in **sunscreen** formulations and prevent radical generation at **light-tissue** interaction mediated by **nanoparticles** via the **photocatalytic effect**.

titanium sapphire (Ti:sapphire or Ti:Al$_2$O$_3$) laser: Titanium sapphire crystal as pumped by an **argon laser** provides **laser radiation** tunable in the **wavelength** range from 700 to 960 nm with a few **watts** in **CW** mode, and in mode-locked regime—the pulse duration is on the order of 100–150 fs with a pulse repetition rate of 76–82 MHz, a mean **power** around 10 mW, and maximal **energy** of 10 nJ. Coherent Model 890 is a **CW** system tunable in the range 690–1100 nm with a **power** of no less than 3.5 W (with maximum near 7 W) upon pumping by a **CW argon laser** of 20 W **power**, and in the range 700–1020 nm with a **power** of no less than 1.1 W (with maximum higher than 2 W) upon pumping by an **argon laser** of 8 W of **power**. The **laser** operates in the single-mode regime, and its **radiation** is linearly polarized and well stabilized. A low-cost **CW titanium sapphire laser** tunable within the range 700–1100 nm is typically pumped by a standard, industrial, **frequency**-doubled **Nd-YAG laser** (532 nm).

toluidine blue O (TBO): Common name is **toluidine blue**, also known as tolonium chloride. It is a blue thiazin **cationic** (basic) dye used in **histology**, *in vivo* **lesions** demarcation, and **PDT** of microbial **cells**. The empirical formula of the dye is C$_{15}$H$_{16}$N$_3$SCl, the formula weight is 305.8, the aqueous solubility is 3.82%, and the **ethanol** solubility is 0.57%. Depending on the producer, the **absorption** maximum can be at any of the following **wavelengths**: 620–622, 632, 640.4, or 626 nm. It is often used to identify **mast cells** by virtue of the heparin in their cytoplasmic granules. It is also used to stain **proteoglycans** and **glycosaminoglycans** in **tissues** such as **cartilage**. The strongly acidic macromolecular **carbohydrates** of **mast cells** and **cartilage** are colored red by the blue dye, a phenomenon called **metachromasia**. Alkaline solutions of **TBO** are commonly used for staining semi-thin (0.5–1 μm) sections of resin-embedded **tissue**. At high **pH** (about 10), the dye binds to **nucleic acids** and all **proteins**.

tomographic reconstruction: Mathematical procedure of obtaining 3D images by which the size, shape, and position of a hidden object can be determined.

tomography: Imaging by sections or sectioning (the Greek word *tomos* conveys the meaning of "a section" or "a cutting"). A device used in **tomography** is called a tomograph, while the image produced is a tomogram. The method is used in medicine, biology, and other sciences. In most cases it is based on the mathematical procedure called **tomographic reconstruction**. There are many different types of tomography, including **x-ray computed tomography**, **magnetic resonance imaging (MRI)**, **functional MRI (fMRI)**, **positron-emission tomography (PET)**, **single-photon-emission computed tomography (SPECT)**, **diffuse optical tomography**, **optical coherence tomography (OCT)**, **optical-projection tomography (OPT)**, **acousto-optic tomography (AOT)**, and **optoacoustic tomography (OAT)**.

tongue: Muscular organ covered by oral **mucosa**. Numerous tiny projections on the surface are called papillae. Taste buds lie in many of these papillae; they are also in soft **palate** and back of the **throat**. There are regional sensitivities on the **tongue** to different tastes. There are also small **salivary glands** in the **tongue**. **Tonsils** and adenoids at the back of the **tongue** are immune **tissue**.

tonometer: An instrument for determining **pressure** or tension, particularly that for measuring the tension within the **eyeball**.

tonsils: Areas of **lymphoid tissue** on either side of the **throat**. An infection of the **tonsils** is called tonsillitis. Most commonly, the term "**tonsils**" refers to the palatine **tonsils** that can be seen in the back of the **throat**. Like other organs of the **lymphatic system**, the **tonsils** act as part of the immune system to help protect against infection. In particular, they are believed to help fight off pharyngeal and upper-respiratory-tract infections.

TOOKAD® (**WST09**): **PDT photosensitizer** that contains palladium bacteriopheophorbide. It requires **laser light** of a specific **wavelength** of 763 nm with **fluence** in the range 50–200 J/cm^2 at 150 mW/cm^2 for activation. **TOOKAD®** can be used to treat relatively large, solid **tumors**, such as localized **prostate cancer**. For *in vivo* applications, the most prominent feature of **TOOKAD®** is its fast clearance while staying exclusively within the **vascular** network. Because of these properties, a **TOOKAD®**-mediated **PDT** procedure causes extensive **vascular** damage and thus is also referred to as **vascular-targeted PDT (VT-PDT)**.

tooth: Hard body composed of **dentin** surrounding a sensitive **pulp** and covered on the crown with **enamel**. The crown is a portion of the natural **tooth** visible in **mouth** above the gumline, and it also refers to artificial replacement for crown. The layers from outside in are **enamel**, **dentin**, and **pulp**. The root is a portion of the **tooth** under the gumline that anchors the **tooth** in **bone** (layers from outside in: **cementum**, **dentin**, and **pulp**).

tooth plaque: See **dental plaque**.

topical: Means that medication is applied to body surfaces such as the **skin** or **mucous membranes**. Some **hydrophobic** chemicals such as steroid **hormones** can be absorbed into the body after being applied to the **skin** in the form of a cream, **gel**, or lotion. **Transdermal** patches have become a popular means of administering some drugs for birth control, **hormone** replacement therapy, and prevention of motion sickness. In dentistry, a **topical** medication may also mean one that is applied to the surface of teeth.

total hemoglobin (THb): Sum concentration of **oxy-** and **deoxyhemoglobin**; total **tissue hemoglobin** concentration $ctTHb = ctO_2Hb + ctHHb$.

total internal reflection (TIR): Reflection of **light** at the interface between **media** of different **refractive indices** when the angle of incidence is larger than the critical angle (defined by the relative **refractive index** of the interfaced **media**). When **light** is incident upon a medium of lesser **index of refraction**, the ray is bent away from the normal so that the exit angle is greater than the incident angle. Such **reflection** is commonly called "**internal reflection**." The exit angle will then approach 90 deg for some critical incident angle θ_c, and for incident angles greater than the critical angle there will be **total internal reflection**. The critical angle can be calculated from **Snell's law** by setting the **refraction** angle equal to 90 deg. **Total internal reflection** is important in **fiber optics** and is employed in polarizing **prisms**. For example, $\theta_c = 48.6$ deg for a **water** and air interface. Measurement of the critical angle can be used to determine the **index of refraction** of a medium.

total internal reflection fluorescence (TIRF) microscope: **Microscope** based on the **total internal reflection** phenomenon (see **evanescent wave**) and designed to observe **fluorescence** in a thin surface layer of a specimen, thus avoiding being flooded by **light** from deeper layers.

total radiant energy fluence rate: See **fluence rate**.

total transmittance: Optical **transmittance** of a turbid sample T_t measured using the **integrating sphere** that collects all transmitted **light**, unscattered and scattered, in the forward direction.

toxin: Any of a group of poisonous, usually unstable compounds generated by micro-organisms or plants, or of animal origin. Certain toxins are produced by specific pathogenic micro-organisms and are the causative agents in various diseases. Some are capable of inducing the production of **antibodies** in certain animals.

trabeculae: Rodlike **cells** or a row of **cells** forming supporting structures lying across spaces or lumina, e.g., outgrowths of the **cell** wall across the **lumen** of tracheids, the supporting meshwork in spongy **bone**.

trachea: Common biological term for an airway through which respiratory air transport takes place in organisms.

transdermal: Through **skin**.

transepidermal water loss (TEWL): Describes the total amount of **water** lost through the **skin**, a loss that occurs constantly by passive **diffusion** through the **epidermis**. Although **TEWL** is a normal physiological phenomenon, if it rises too high, the **skin** can become dehydrated, disrupting form and function, and potentially leading to infection or transepidermal passage of deleterious agents.

transfer matrix method: Assumes that **light** consists of various plane waves traveling with oblique angles through the sample. The latent bulk image is obtained by first calculating the vertical amplitude dependence of the field resulting from the excitation with one plane **wave** of definite amplitude. It is applicable to the analysis of a stratified medium. Using the vector version of the transfer matrix **algorithm**, arbitrarily **polarized light** can be simulated.

transfer ribonucleic acid (tRNA): A small **RNA** molecule (usually about 74–95 **nucleotides**) that transfers a specific active **amino acid** to a growing polypeptide chain at the ribosomal site of **protein** synthesis during translation. It has a 3′ terminal site for **amino acid** attachment. This covalent linkage is catalyzed by an aminoacyl **tRNA** synthetase. It also contains a three-base region called the anticodon that can base pair to the corresponding three-base codon region on **mRNA**. Each type of **tRNA** molecule can be attached to only one type of **amino acid**, but because the genetic code contains multiple codons that specify the same **amino acid**, **tRNA** molecules bearing different anticodons may also carry the same **amino acid**.

transillumination digital microscopy (TDM): Light transillumination **microscopy** based on the usage of fast and high-resolution **CCD** and **CMOS** cameras and corresponding software (see **digital microscopy**). It is applicable for *in vivo* **flow cytometry**, monitoring of **blood** and **lymph vessel** dynamics, and **cell** imaging within **lymph nodes**. For example, **TDM** of rat **mesentery** is a promising model for studying some microlymphatic functions in norm, its response to drugs, and for experimental modeling of pathologies. In parallel with routine imaging (whole lymphangion, neighboring **blood** microvessels, lymphatic walls, leaflets of **valve**, and flowing single **cells**) and obtaining quantitative data (**lymph** and **blood** microvessel diameters, amplitude, and rate of lymphatic phasic contractions), **TDM** allows one to obtain more detailed parameters of phasic contractions (velocity of wall movement, duration of contraction and its periodicity), **valve** function (duration of **valve** cycle and its periodicity, **correlation** between **valve** function and phasic contractions), and **lymph** flow parameters (mean **cell** velocity, relation of forward and backward **cell** velocity, and **cell** concentration). It works well with other optical measuring techniques such as **laser speckle imaging, photothermal** or **optoacoustic flow cytometry**, and **fluorescence imaging**. *In vivo*, label-free, high-speed (up to 40,000 frames per second), high-resolution (up to 300 nm), real-time imaging of circulating individual **erythrocytes, leukocytes**, and **platelets** in fast **blood flows** is possible.

transition matrix (T-matrix) approach: This approach is similar to the Mie theory used for nonspherical objects such as spheroids. The T-matrix for the spherical particles is diagonal.

transmittance: See **optical transmittance**.

transport albedo: Introduced as **albedo** with the **scattering coefficient** replaced by the **reduced scattering coefficient**, i.e., $\Lambda' = \mu'_s/(\mu_a + \mu'_s)$.

transport coefficient: The coefficient related to transport of a **photon** in a **multiple scattering medium** with the anisotropic character of **single scattering**, $\mu'_t = \mu_a + \mu'_s$, where μ_a is the **absorption coefficient** and μ'_s is the **reduced scattering coefficient**.

transport mean free path (TMFP): Pathlength of a **photon** (cm) defined as $l_t = (1/\mu'_t) = (\mu_a + \mu'_s)^{-1}$, where $\mu'_t = \mu_a + \mu'_s$ is the **transport coefficient**. The **TMFP** in a medium with anisotropic **single scattering** significantly exceeds the **MFP**, $l_t \gg l_{ph}$. The l_t is the distance over which the **photon** loses its initial direction.

transpupillary: Through the eye **pupil**.

transscleral: Through the eye **sclera**.

transverse excited atmospheric pressure (TEA) CO$_2$ laser: Gas **CO$_2$ laser** in which a glow discharge is maintained without arc formation at atmospheric **pressure** by using a discharge that is transverse rather than parallel to the **optic axis**. Mode-locked, tunable, and minuture **lasers** of that type are available.

trauma: An often-serious and body-altering physical **injury**, such as the removal of a limb.

trazograph: Derivative of 2, 4, 6-triiodobenzene acid, molecular weight of about 500. **Water**-soluble colorless liquid usually used at concentrations of 60 or 76% as an intravenous **x-ray** contrasting agent. Very good agent for **optical clearing** of **fibrous tissue** owing to its high **osmolarity** and high **index of refraction**.

tremor: An unintentional, somewhat rhythmic **muscle** movement involving to-and-fro movements (oscillations) of one or more parts of the body. It is the most common of all involuntary movements and can affect the **hands**, arms, **head**, face, vocal cords, trunk, and legs. Most tremors occur in the **hands**. In some people, **tremor** is a symptom of another neurological disorder.

trigger beam: Part of a **laser beam** used to synchronize the measuring system (for example, the **streak camera**).

triphenylmethane: Biological dye (stain)

triplet state: See **singlet state**.

trypan blue: Vital stain that is used to **color** dead **tissues** or **cells** blue. It is a diazo dye. Live **cells** or **tissues** with **intact cell membranes** will not be colored. Since **cells** are very selective in the compounds that pass through the **membrane**, in a viable **cell** **trypan blue** is not absorbed. However, it traverses the **membrane** in a dead **cell**. Hence, dead **cells** are shown as a distinctive blue **color** under a microscope.

tryptophan: Colorless, **crystalline**, aromatic essential **amino acid** that occurs in the seeds of some leguminous plants. It is released from **proteins** by tryptic digestion and is important in the nutrition of animals.

T-scan: A transversal scanner producing fast lines in an image. This can be produced by controlling either the transverse scanner along the x-coordinate, along the y-coordinate, or along the polar angle θ, with the two other scanners fixed. A T-scan is used in **OCT** systems.

T-scan-based B-scan: Where the x-scanner produces the **T-scans** and the axial scanner advances slower in depth along the z-coordinate. This type of scan has a net advantage in comparison with the **A-scan**-based **B-scan** procedure as it allows for the production of **OCT** transverse (or en-face) images for a fixed reference path, images called **C-scans**. 3D complete information can be collected in different ways, either by acquiring many longitudinal **OCT** images (**B-scans**) at different en-face positions or by many en-face **OCT** images (**C-scans**) at different depth positions.

t-test (*Synonym*: student's **t-test**): Test for determining whether an observed sample mean differs significantly from a hypothetical normal population mean.

tubular structure: Structure consisting of tubes.

tumor: An abnormal or diseased swelling in any part of the body, especially a more or less circumscribed overgrowth of new **tissue** that is autonomous, differs more or less in structure from the part in which it grows, and serves no useful purpose. See, also **neoplasm**.

tumorigenicity: Capable of causing **tumors**.

tunable laser: **Laser** in which one can vary the **wavelength** over some limited spectral range. See, for example, **swept-laser source**.

turbidity: Cloudiness or haziness of material (biological fluid or **tissue**) caused by individual particles (suspended **scatterers**) that are generally invisible to the naked eye, producing a milky appearance.

turbidity suppression by optical phase conjugation (TSOPC): In **tissues**, optical **wave** propagation is dominated by elastic (static) **light scattering**, which randomizes the optical wavefront and limits optical measurements to superficial depths because of strong **backscattering** due to **multiple scattering**; thus, direct **optical imaging** through **tissues** is strongly limited. Nevertheless, the elastic **scattering** of an optical **wave** is a deterministic and time-reversible process. It was demonstrated that holographic recording of the transmission of a single-mode **laser** through **tissue**, followed by an **optical phase conjugation (OPC)** playback, can allow an optical **wave** to retrace the **scattering** path. This process, termed **turbidity suppression by optical phase conjugation (TSOPC)**, allows one to perform images through ≤ 7-mm-thick excised chicken-**tissue** sections ($\mu_s l \sim 10\text{--}13$, where μ_s is the **scattering coefficient** and l is the **tissue** sample thickness). The applicability for *in vivo* investigations depends on the relative time scales between the optical realization of **TSOPC** and **tissue** variation that can perturb the time-reversal process, because **scatterer** motion during and after the recording time reduces the portion of the optical **wave** that is efficiently time reversed. Unlike **scattering**, **tissue absorption** is an irreversible process and can be categorized as a loss mechanism that eliminates parts of the input **light** field from phase conjugation considerations.

turbulent flow: Flow regime characterized by chaotic, stochastic property changes. This includes low momentum **diffusion**, high momentum convection, and rapid variation of **pressure** and velocity in space and time. Flow that is not turbulent is called **laminar flow**. The dimensionless **Reynolds number (Re)** characterizes whether flow conditions lead to laminar or **turbulent flow**, e.g., for pipe flow, **Re** above about 2300 will be turbulent.

two-frequency Zeeman laser: **Laser** with the active medium placed in the axial magnetic field. The **laser** produces two **laser** lines with a small **frequency** separation (about 250 kHz) and mutually orthogonal linear **polarizations**. Due to a high degree of mutual coherence (a constant **phase shift** between two optical fields), it can be used for direct measurements of the **amplitude scattering matrix** (**S-matrix** or **Jones matrix**) of anisotropic **tissues**.

541

two-photon fluorescence microscopy (TPF microscopy): **Microscopy** that employs both **ballistic photons** and scattered **photons** at the **wavelength** of the two-photon **fluorescence** of **radiation** coming to a wide-**aperture photodetector** exactly from the focal area of the excitation beam. A powerful tool for **non-invasive**, free of **exogenous labeling**, 3D imaging of **collagen** and other **tissue** components, as well as for precise microvascular imaging using fluorescent **labeling** techniques. **TPF microscopy** is a **laser**-scanning imaging technique based on a nonlinear optical process in which a molecule can be excited by simultaneous **absorption** of two **photons** in the same quantum event. It offers two large advantages with respect to conventional **fluorescence** techniques: (1) the **fluorescence** signal depends nonlinearly on the density of **photons**, providing an **absorption** volume spatially confined to the **focal point**; and (2) for both **tissue autofluorescence** and commonly used **fluorescence** probes, two-photon **absorption** occurs in the near-**IR wavelength** range, allowing deeper penetration into highly **scattering media** with respect to the equivalent single-photon techniques. The localization of the excitation is maintained even in strong **scattering tissues** because the scattered **photon** density is too low to generate a significant signal. For these reasons, nonlinear **microscopy** allows **micron**-scale resolution in deep **tissue**. **TPF microscopy** has already been successfully used as a powerful technique for many imaging applications in life science, including fluorescent-**protein** investigation and **spectroscopy**, and for studying biological mechanisms inside **cells** and **tissues**. It has also been applied to *in vivo* imaging using common microscopes or combined with **optical fibers** to realize movable or endoscopic microscopes. **TPF microscopy** is particularly useful in human **tissue** imaging and **optical biopsy**. Human **tissues** intrinsically contain many different fluorescent molecules that allow them to be imaged without any exogenously added probe. **Tissue** intrinsic **fluorophores**, as **NADH**, keratins, flavins, **melanin**, **elastin**, and cholecalciferol (vitamin D_3) can be excited by two- or three-**photon absorption** using the **Ti:Sapphire laser wavelength** (typically between 700 and 1000 nm), which consists of the so-called optical **therapeutic/diagnostic window** of **tissues**. The major practical advantage is a versatility of fluorescent probes available; however, **photobleaching** and inefficient **labeling** may be limitations. See also nonlinear **optical imaging** and **endoscopic nonlinear optical imaging**.

two-wavelength fiber optical coherence tomography (OCT): Multi-**wavelength** images are very helpful to detect an abnormality within the optically sampled **tissue**. The sensitivity and recognition range of such systems may be very high because **scattering** and **absorption** properties of normal **tissue** and **pathological** inclusions depend on the probing **wavelength** in different ways. It is very important to acquire **OCT** images at different **wavelengths** simultaneously using the same **interferometer** and focusing system. The typical **two-wavelength fiber OCT** system contains two **SLDs** with central **wavelengths** of 830 and 1300 nm, spectral **bandwidths** of 25 nm and 50 nm (corresponding axial **coherence lengths** of 13 μm and 19 μm), and **power** of 1.5 mW and 0.5 mW, respectively. The **light** from both **SLDs** is coupled to a fiber optic **Michelson interferometer**. The most challenging problem to compensate for simultaneously, the **wave dispersion** for two different **wavelengths** in **interferometer** arms, is solved by inserting into one of the arms of the **interferometer** an additional piece of **fiber** whose **dispersion** properties are quite different from those of the principal **fiber**. The attained in-depth **spatial resolution** for the **wavelengths** 830 nm and 1300 nm is 15 μm and 34 μm, respectively.

tympanic membrane: **Membrane** separating the tympanium or middle **ear** from the passage of the external **ear**.

type I collagen: Most abundant **collagen** of the human body. It is present in **scar tissue**, the end product when **tissue** heals by repair. It is found in **tendons**, the endomysium of **myofibrils**, and the organic part of **bone**.

tyrosine: Crystalline amino acid resulting from the hydrolysis of **proteins**.

ulcer: Sore that is open either to the surface of the body or to a natural cavity, and accompanied by the disintegration of **tissue**, the formation of pus, etc.

ultrahigh-resolution OCT: The typical axial resolution of **OCT** imaging systems with such universally adopted broadband **light** sources as **SLDs** or **mode-locked lasers** varies from 10–15 μm (**SLD**) to 4–5 μm (short-pulse **laser** sources such as organic-dye and **Ti:sapphire lasers**). To provide significantly higher axial resolution (e.g., on the subcellular level), the broadband **light** sources covering a few hundred **nanometers** in the **visible** and **NIR** range are required. Such **ultrahigh-resolution OCT** instruments for *in vivo* imaging provide longitudinal resolution on the order of 1 μm. A Kerr-lens **mode-locked** (KLM) **femtosecond Ti:sapphire laser** is typically used as an illuminating source. It emits sub-two-cycle pulses corresponding to **bandwidths** of up to 350 nm with a center **wavelength** at 800 nm. Such high performance is achieved with specially designed double-chirped mirrors with a high-reflectivity **bandwidth** and controlled **dispersion** response in combination with low-**dispersion calcium fluoride prisms** for intracavity **dispersion compensation**. A pair of fused-silica **prisms** and razor blades are used to spectrally disperse the **laser beam** and spectrally shape the **laser** output. The optical scheme of the low-coherence **interferometer** should be optimized for the ultrabroad **bandwidth** of the illuminating source. Usually, specially designed **lenses** with a 10-mm **focal length** and a **numerical aperture** of 0.30 in combination with **single-mode fibers** and special broadband **fiber couplers** are used. **Polarization** controllers are also used to exclude the broadening of the shape of the **interference** envelope due to **polarization** mismatch. **Dispersion** is matched by use of a variable-thickness fused-silica and **BK7 prism** in order to reach a uniform group-delay **dispersion**. The optimized **OCT** system can support optical spectra of up to 260 nm (**FWHM**) and a 1.5-μm longitudinal resolution in free space, corresponding to 1-μm resolution in **tissue**. The *in vivo* subcellular-level resolution (1 μm × 3 μm, longitudinal × transverse) tomograms of an **African frog** (*Xenopus laevis*) tadpole were obtained to demonstrate the potential of the **ultrahigh-resolution OCT** instrument. Obtained images clearly depict the multiple mesanchymal cells of various sizes and nuclear-to-cytoplasmatic ratios, olfactory tract and intracellular morphology, as well as **mitosis** of several **cells**. For a super-resolution **OCT**, broadband **light** sources based on **photonic crystal fibers (PCFs)** at **femtosecond laser** excitation are very promising (see **supercontinuum**).

ultrashort laser pulse: Pulses usually produced by **mode-locked** lasers (**picosecond** and subpicosecond range) or their modifications, such as synchronously optically pumped or colliding-pulse mode-locked (CPM) dye lasers (**femtosecond** range), or the **titanium–sapphire laser** with passive **mode-locking** via a Kerr-lens mode-locking (KLM) **laser** (10–100 fs).

ultrasonic transducer: Device that converts **energy** into **ultrasound**. It refers to a **piezoelectric transducer** that converts electrical **energy** into sound. Alternative methods for creating and detecting **ultrasound** include magnetostriction and capacitive actuation. It is used in many applications including medical **ultrasonography** and nondestructive testing.

ultrasonography: An **ultrasound**-based, medical diagnostic imaging technique used to visualize **subcutaneous** body structures including **tendons**, **muscles**, joints, **vessels**, and internal organs for possible pathology or **lesions**. Obstetric **ultrasonography** is commonly used during pregnancy. It is also often used in clinical studies using optical instrumentation as a subsidiary technique.

ultrasound (US): Mechanical vibrations with frequencies in the range of 2×10^4 to 10^7 Hz.

ultrasound gel: Viscous **gel** for medical **ultrasound** transmission used for diagnostic and therapeutic **ultrasound** applications. It acoustically corrects US **energy** transmission for the frequencies used.

ultraviolet (UV):   See **light wavelength range**.

ultraviolet A (UVA):   See **light wavelength range**.

ultraviolet B (UVB):   See **light wavelength range**.

ultraviolet (UV) filter: Optical filter that blocks **UV radiation** but lets **visible light** through. They are widely used in physiological optics and other biomedical applications.

ultraviolet (UV) skin filter: **Sunscreen** cream or lotion based on chemical formulations and/or reflecting **nanoparticles** that filter broadband **UV radiation** and help shield the **skin** from the **UVA** and **UVB** rays that produce **skin** damage.

uniaxial crystal: **Anisotropic crystal** that exhibits two refractive indices, an "ordinary" index (n_o) for **light** polarized in the x- or y-directions, and an "extraordinary" index (n_e) for **polarization** in the z-direction. A **uniaxial crystal** is "positive" if $n_e > n_o$ and "negative" if $n_e < n_o$. **Light** polarized at some angle to the axes will experience a different phase velocity for different **polarization** components and cannot be described by a single **index of refraction**. This is often depicted as an index ellipsoid.

unsaturated fatty acid: **Fatty acid** in which there are one or more double bonds in the **fatty acid** chain. A **fat** molecule is monounsaturated if it contains one double bond and polyunsaturated if it contains more than one double bond. Where double bonds are formed, hydrogen atoms are eliminated. Thus, a saturated **fat** is "saturated" with hydrogen atoms. The greater the degree of unsaturation in a **fatty acid** (i.e., the more double bonds in the **fatty acid**), the more vulnerable it is to **lipid** peroxidation (rancidity). Antioxidants can protect unsaturated **fat** from **lipid** peroxidation. Unsaturated **fats** also have a more enlarged shape than saturated **fats**.

urea (*Synonym*: carbamide): An organic compound of carbon, nitrogen, **oxygen**, and hydrogen with the formula CON_2H_4 or $(NH_2)_2CO$.

urinary bladder: Sac for storing **urine**. It is a diverticulum of the hindgut. **Urine** is conducted to the **bladder** by a ureter. The exit to the **bladder** is closed by a sphincter **muscle**.

urine: Yellowish, slightly acid, watery fluid. Waste matter excreted by the **kidneys**.

urocanic acid: 4-imidazoleacrylic acid, found in the **skin epidermis**. It has a high **absorption** in the **UV** with a peak at 260 nm.

uroporphyrin: Any of several **porphyrins** produced by oxidation of uroporphyrinogen. One or more are excreted in excess in the **urine** in several of the porphyries.

uterine: Related to the **uterus**, e.g., the **uterine** walls.

uterus: An organ in which the **embryo** develops and is nourished. It has walls of unstriated **muscle** that increase greatly in thickness during pregnancy and whose contractions expel the **embryo** at birth. The **uterus** is lined with endometrium, which undergoes modification during pregnancy and is also modified under control of sex **hormones** during the estrus cycle. The **uterus** is connected through the **cervix** to the vagina. The plural is uteri.

vacuole: (1) A cavity within a **cell**, often containing a watery liquid or secretion; (2) a minute cavity or **vesicle** in organic **tissue**.

vacuolization: Irreversible **tissue** damage by vapor bubble formation during heating, $T \geq 100\ °C$. It is the basis for photo-induced mechanical **tissue** destruction.

valve: Structure that allows fluids to flow through it in one direction only. This is done by closing the **vessel**, or canal, to stop backward flow [see **lymphatic vessels (lymphatics)**].

van de Hulst approximation: Simple and accurate approximation introduced by van de Hulst to describe **optical reflectance** from a semi-infinite turbid medium at diffuse illumination, $R_d = (1 - s)(1 - 0.139s)/(1 + 1.17s)$, where the similarity parameter s is defined as $s^2 = (1 - \Lambda')$ and Λ' is the **transport albedo**. This expression has an error of less than 0.003 for any **albedo** Λ and **scattering anisotropy factor** g. This functional form is convenient because it has the correct limiting behavior for small and large transport (reduced) **albedos** $R \to 0$ as $\Lambda' \to 0$ and $R \to 1$ as $\Lambda' \to 1$.

van Gieson stain: Mixture of **picric acid** and acid **fuchsine**. It is the simplest method of differential staining of **collagen** and other **connective tissue**.

vaporization: Irreversible **tissue** damage at heating accompanied by **tissue dehydration** and vapor bubble formation (**vacuolization**), $T \geq 100$ °C. It is the basis for photo-induced mechanical **tissue** destruction.

variable optical attenuator (VOA): An optical attenuator is needed to reduce optical power when an optical signal with an excessive **power** level greater than an allowed **power** level is directed to a **tissue** and/or to an optical signal receiver. **VOAs** are used to permit dynamic control of optical power levels throughout a network and diminish differences of optical **power** between **wavelength** channels in **wavelength-division multiplexing (WDM)** optical networks, and maintain the **SNRs** of the channels. **VOAs** are commonly used to provide **gain** equalization in optical **amplifiers** or to monitor and distribute optical **power** of a cross-connected network dynamically in a dense **WDM** system. They are generally formed of a blocking structure disposed in a free-space region between an input **waveguide** and an output **waveguide**.

variance: Square of the **standard deviation**.

vascular: Related to **vessels**.

vascularization: Consisting of or containing that which conducts **blood** and **lymph**.

vascular-targeted photodynamic therapy (VT-PDT): PDT procedure that causes extensive **vascular** damage due to the photosensitizers that stay exclusively within the **vascular** network, such as **TOOKAD®**.

vasculature: Arrangement of **blood vessels** in the body, or in an organ or body part. The **vascular** network of an organ.

vasoconstriction: Constriction of the **blood** or **lymphatic vessels**, as by the action of a **nerve**.

vasodilation: Where **blood vessels** in the body become wider following the relaxation of the smooth **muscle** in the **vessel** wall. This will reduce **blood pressure** since there is more room for **blood**. **Vasodilation** also occurs in superficial **blood vessels** of warm-blooded animals when their ambient environment is hot. This process diverts the flow of heated **blood** to the **skin** of the animal, where heat can be more easily released into the atmosphere. The opposite physiological process is **vasoconstriction**.

vector radiation-transfer equation (VRTE): Radiation-transfer equation **(RTE)** accounting for **polarization** properties of **light** and its interaction with a **scattering** medium.

vector radiation-transfer theory (VRTT): Radiation-transfer theory **(RTT)** accounting for **polarization** properties of **light** and its interaction with a **scattering** medium.

vehicles: Nonliving means of transportation. Pertaining to transportation of drugs by various solutes.

vein: **Blood vessel** that conducts **blood** from the **tissues** and organs back to the **heart**. The **vein** is lined with **endothelium** (smooth flat **cells**) and surrounded by muscular and **fibrous tissue**. The walls are thin and the diameter large compared to an **artery**. The **vein** contains **valves** that allow **blood** to flow only toward the **heart**.

vein femoralis: Femoral **vein** pertaining to the thigh or femur.

ventricle: Chamber in the **brain** or **heart**. In a **heart**, it is a chamber that collects **blood** from an **atrium** (another **heart** chamber that is smaller than a **ventricle**) and pumps it out of the **heart**.

venule: Small **vein** that collects **blood** from **capillaries**. It joins other venules to form a **vein**. A **venule** has more **connective tissue** than a **capillary muscle**. The permeability of the **venule** wall to **blood** is similar to that of a **capillary** wall.

verografin: **Water**-soluble colorless liquid usually used at concentrations of 60 or 76% as an intravenous **x-ray** contrasting agent. **Verografin** is a very good agent for **optical clearing** of **fibrous tissue** owing to its high **osmolarity** and high **index of refraction**. It is an analog of **trazograph**.

vertical-cavity surface-emitting laser (VCSEL): A type of **diode laser** that emits a **light beam** at right angles to the chip.

vesicle: Relatively small and enclosed compartment, separated from the **cytosol** by at least one **lipid bilayer**. If there is only one **lipid bilayer**, they are called unilamellar vesicles, otherwise they are called multilamellar. Vesicles store, transport, or digest cellular products and waste.

vessel: Tube or **duct**, such as an **artery**, **vein**, or the like, containing or conveying **blood** or some other body fluid.

vibrational spectrum: See **vibrational transition**.

vibrational modes: In general, a molecule composed of n atoms has $3n$ degrees of freedom for motion, six of which are translational and rotational of the molecule itself, and the rest $(3n - 6)$ [or $(3n - 5)$ for linear molecules] are vibrational. Molecular **vibrational modes** are usually described as stretching, bending, scissoring, rocking, wagging, and twisting, all of which describe a type of motion. **Infrared spectroscopy** is possible because these chemical bonds have specific frequencies at which they vibrate corresponding to **energy** levels. Simple diatomic (linear) molecules have only one bond, which may stretch. More complex molecules may have many bonds, and vibrations can be conjugated, leading to infrared absorption at characteristic frequencies that may be related to chemical groups. The atoms in an H_2O molecule, which is a nonlinear triatomic molecule, can vibrate in three different ways: symmetrical stretching (**symmetric vibrational mode**), asymmetrical stretching, and bending. The atoms in a CH_2 group, commonly found in organic compounds, can vibrate in six different ways: symmetrical and asymmetrical stretching, bending, rocking, wagging, and twisting. Infrared spectra do not normally display separate absorption signals for each of the $(3n-6)$ fundamental **vibrational modes** of a molecule. The exact frequency at which a given vibration occurs is determined by the strengths of the bonds involved and the mass of the component atoms. The number of observed **absorption bands** may be increased by additive and subtractive interactions, leading to combination tones and overtones of the fundamental vibrations. The number of observed **absorption bands** may be decreased by molecular symmetry and spectroscopic selection rules. One selection rule that defines the intensity of infrared bands is that a change in **dipole moment** should occur for a vibration to absorb effectively infrared **energy**, and therefore **absorption bands** associated with C=O bond stretching are usually very strong. Stretching frequencies are higher than corresponding bending frequencies because it is easier to bend a bond than to stretch or compress it.

vibrational transition: Denotes an energetic transition of a molecule with the change of vibrational quantum number (energetic state or level). At **vibrational transitions**, only absorbing or emitting **infrared light** (**vibrational spectrum**) is possible.

vibrometer: An instrument for measuring amplitudes and frequencies of the mechanical vibrations of an object.

vibronic spectrum: See **vibronic transition**.

vibronic transition: Denotes the simultaneous change of vibrational and electronic quantum number (energetic state, or level) in a molecule. According to the separability of electronic and nuclear motion in the Born–Oppenheimer approximation, the **vibrational transition** and **electronic transition** may be described separately. The selection rule for **vibrational transitions** is described by the **Franck–Condon principle**. Most processes that lead to the **absorption** and emission of a relatively broad band of **visible light** (vibronic spectra), and, therefore, the colorful world around us, are due to **vibronic transitions**.

videokeratoscope: Keratoscope fitted with a video camera. A keratoscope is an instrument marked with lines or circles by means of which the corneal reflex can be observed.

virus: Infectious agent too small to be seen directly with a **light microscope**. They are not made of **cells** and can only replicate inside the **cells** of another organism (the viruses' host). **Viruses** infect all types of organisms. There are millions of different types of **viruses**, with about 5,000 already described in detail. The study of **viruses** is known as virology, a subspecialty of microbiology. **Viruses** consist of two or three parts, all **viruses** have **genes** made from either **DNA** or **RNA**, all have a **protein** coat that protects these **genes**, and some have an envelope of **fat** that surrounds them when they are outside a **cell**. **Viruses** vary from simple helical and icosahedral shapes to more complex structures. Most **viruses** are about one hundred times smaller than an average bacterium. Viral infections in animals provoke an **immune response** that usually eliminates the infecting **virus**.

viscosity of the medium: Viscosity arises from the friction between one layer of a fluid in motion relative to another layer of the fluid. It is caused by the cohesive forces between molecules. The viscosity of **glycerol** is high, but the viscosity of **water** or **ethanol** is low.

visible: See **visible wavelength range** and **light wavelength range**.

visible wavelength range: Wavelengths of **light** that are seen by a naked human eye. The **wavelengths** range from 400 to 780 nm (see **light wavelength range**).

visual acuity: Acuteness or clarity of vision, especially form vision, which is dependent on the sharpness of the retinal focus within the eye, the sensitivity of the nervous elements, and the interpretative faculty of the **brain**.

Visudyne®: Verteporfin for injection is a **PDT photosensitizer**, that contains **benzoporphyrin derivative** monoacid ring A (**BPD-MA**). It requires **laser light** of a specific **wavelength** of 693 nm for activation. **Visudyne®** is typically used in **photodynamic therapy (PDT)** to eliminate the abnormal **blood vessels** in the eye associated with conditions such as the wet form of macular degeneration. Verteporfin accumulates in these abnormal **blood vessels**, and the **laser** activates the drug in a targeted area of the eye, resulting in local damage to the **endothelium** and blockage of the **vessels**.

vital activity: Also called vital function, any function of the body, **tissue**, **cell**, etc., that is essential for life.

vitality: Peculiarity distinguishing the living from the nonliving; the capacity to live and develop.

vitamin A: See **retinol**.

vitamin B$_2$: See **riboflavin**.

vitreopathy: Pathology of vitreous body.

vitreous humor: Transparent gelatinous substance filling the **eyeball** behind the **crystalline lens**; it is also called vitreous body.

vocal chord: Either of the two pairs of folds of **mucous membrane** projecting into the cavity of the **larynx**.

volar: Pertaining to both the palm and feet sole.

volatile solvents: Liquids that vaporize at room temperature. These organic solvents can be inhaled for psychoactive effects and are present in many domestic and industrial products such as glue, aerosol, paints, industrial solvents, lacquer thinners, gasoline, and cleaning fluids. Some substances are directly toxic to the **liver**, **kidney**, or **heart**, and some produce peripheral neuropathy (**nerve** damage usually affecting the feet and legs) or progressive **brain** degeneration.

volume fraction: Dealing with mixtures in which there is a large disparity between the sizes and **refractive indices** of the various kinds of molecules or particles. This fraction provides an appropriate way to express the relative amounts of various components. In any ideal mixture, the total volume is the sum of the individual volumes prior to mixing. In nonideal cases, the additivity of volume is no longer guaranteed. Volumes can contract or expand upon mixing, and molar volume becomes a function of both concentration and temperature. This is why **mole** fractions are a safer unit to use.

waist of a laser beam: Narrowest part of a **Gaussian light beam**.

water (H_2O): A unique polar solvent, and its properties have a vast impact on the behavior of biological molecules. A wide range of time scales (10^{-18}–10^3 s) of **water** dynamics are important to understanding its biological function. The range of time scales includes such features as the elastic collisions of **water** at ultra-fast times ($\sim 10^{-15}$ s) to the macroscopic hydrodynamic processes observed in **blood flow** at much lower times on the order of seconds. In biomedical research and applications, purified **water** with physically removed impurities is used. **Distilled water** and **deionized water** have been the most common forms of purified **water**, but **water** can also be purified by other processes including reverse osmosis, carbon filtration, microporous filtration, ultrafiltration, **UV light** oxidation, or electrodialysis. A combination of the above processes allows one to produce **water** of such high purity that its trace contaminants are measured in parts per billion (ppb) or parts per trillion (ppt).

water absorption band: Bands of **water** are related to molecular vibrations involving various combinations of the **water** molecule's three fundamental vibrational modes of the covalent bonds: v_1—symmetric stretch, v_2—bending, and v_3—asymmetric stretch. In the **visible** and **IR**, **water** vapor absorbs mostly at 600 nm, 720 nm, 820 nm, 940 nm, 1100 nm, 1380 nm, 1870 nm, 2700 nm, 3200 nm, and 6300 nm. In liquid **water**, as a result of molecular interactions, the **absorption bands** due to fundamental vibrational-rotational transitions are much more broadened in comparison with those in **water** vapor; rotations tend to be hindered by hydrogen bonds, leading to librations, or rocking motions. Stretching vibrations are shifted to a lower **frequency** while the bending **frequency** increases due to hydrogen bonding. The relation between **absorption** intensities of these modes are $a(v_1):a(v_2):a(v_3)$ = 0.07:1.47:1.00 for **water** vapor and 0.87:0.33:1.00 for liquid **water**. For pure liquid **water**, the strongest **absorption bands** in the **visible-IR** range are between 2300 and 8000 nm. The band formed by combined fundamental mode v_1 and mode v_3 transitions peaks at 2900–3000 nm and is the strongest in the **IR**; another strong band is peaked at 4650 nm, which is a combination band of molecular bending (v_2) and librations (L_2). Less intensive, but sometimes more important for **biophotonics**, are the **absorption bands** near 970 nm that are attributed to a ($2v_1 + v_3$) combination; 1200 nm, to a ($v_1 + v_2 + v_3$) combination; 1450 nm, to a ($v_1 + v_3$) combination; and 1950 nm, to a ($v_2 + v_3$) combination. For pure liquid **water**, the strongest peaks near $1400, 1950, 2500$ nm; $2950, 4700$, and 6100 nm; and three minor ones at $750, 970$ and 1200 nm that are characteristic in the **visible** and **IR** range. For the short **wavelengths** in UV, the strongest band is very broad, with the central **wavelength** at 65 nm and the **absorption coefficient** of 10^6 cm^{-1}, while two other less intensive peaks are at 115 and 180 nm. In **tissues**, **water** bands are also slightly corrected due to interactions with the surrounding organic molecules and in many **tissues** seen as **absorption** at the following **wavelengths** <300, ~980, ~1180, ~1450, ~1950, ~2500, and ~2910–3050 nm.

water dispersion function: **Wavelength** dependence of **water index of refraction**. In the **visible** and **NIR**, it is described as $n_w(\lambda) = 1.31848 + [6.662/(\lambda - 129.2)] \cong 1.3199 + (6878/\lambda^2) - (1.132 \cdot 10^9/\lambda^4) + (1.11 \cdot 10^{14}/\lambda^6)$, where λ is in **nanometers** (see **dispersion**).

water-binding mode: Denotes biological molecule interaction with **water** molecules and corresponding changes in molecular-**water** complex spectra.

watt: Unit of **power**; 1 **watt** is equal to 1 **joule** per second.

wave: Disturbance that propagates through space and time, usually with transference of **energy**. A mechanical **wave** is a **wave** that propagates or travels through a medium due to the restoring forces it produces upon **deformation**. **Electromagnatic waves** can travel through free space (vacuum). Waves travel and transfer **energy** from one point to another, often with no permanent displacement of the particles of the medium (that is, with little or no associated mass transport). They consist instead of oscillations or vibrations around almost fixed locations.

waveguide: Structure that guides waves, such as **electromagnetic waves** or **sound waves**. There are different types of **waveguides** that differ in their geometry and can confine **energy** in one dimension such as in slab **waveguides**, two dimensions as in **fiber** or channel **waveguides**, and three dimensions as in **photonic crystal fibers**.

waveguide dispersion: Propagation constant β of a guided mode of a **fiber** is determined both by the parameters of the **fiber**, such as its **refractive index** profile and core diameter $2a$, and by the material properties. Therefore, the **frequency** (**wavelength**) dependence of β of a particular mode has mixed contributions from material **dispersion** and **waveguide dispersion**. The effective **refractive index** n_β, the effective **group refractive index** $n_{g\beta}$, and the effective **group-velocity dispersion** D_β for the mode are $n_\beta = c\beta/\omega, n_{g\beta} = c(d\beta/d\omega) = n_\beta - \lambda(dn_\beta/d\lambda)$, and $D_\beta = c\omega(d^2\beta/d\omega^2) = \lambda^2(d^2 n_\beta/d\lambda^2)$. The exact **frequency** (**wavelength**) dependence of these parameters depends on the **fiber waveguide parameter** V, the normalized index difference $\Delta \cong (n_1 - n_2)/n_1$ (see **fiber numerical aperture**), and, in the case of the **graded-index fiber** with a power-law profile, the parameter α. For the fundamental mode of a step-index germania–silica (13.5 mol % GeO_2) **fiber** with an index step of $n_1 - n_2 = 0.006$ and a core diameter of $2a = 6$ μm, the point of zero **dispersion** is shifted from that of the germania–silica material at 1.383 μm to 1.5 μm because of the **waveguide** contribution.

wavelength: Distance between two adjacent peaks in a **wave**. **Light wavelengths** are typically measured in **nanometers** (nm) or **micrometers** (μm): 1 nm is 10^{-9} meter (m) and 1 μm is 10^{-6} m.

wavelength-division multiplexing (WDM) (*Synonym*: multiwavelength multiplexing): Technology that multiplexes multiple optical carrier signals on a single **optical fiber** by using slightly different **wavelengths** of **laser light** to carry different signals. This allows for a multiplication in capacity in addition to enabling bidirectional communications over one strand of **fiber**.

wavelet transformation: Refers to the representation of a signal in terms of scaled and translated copies (known as "daughter wavelets") of a finite length or fast-decaying oscillating waveform (known as the "mother wavelet"). In formal terms, this representation is a wavelet series that is a representation of a square-integrable (real or complex-valued) function by a certain orthonormal series generated by a wavelet.

wavenumber: See **propagation constant of electromagnetic wave (EMW)**. $\tilde{v} = 1/\lambda$; this unit, measured in cm^{-1}, is used in **Raman spectroscopy** and **infrared spectroscopy**.

weakly scattering random-phase screen (RPS): RPS whose **variance** in induced-phase fluctuations in the scattered field is much less than unity.

white blood cell (WBC): See **leukocyte**.

white fiber: See **white fibrous tissue**.

white fibrous tissue: **Connective tissue** that consists of a matrix of very fine, white wavy **fibers** arranged parallel to each other, in bundles and unbranching, with **fibroblasts** embedded in the bundle. The **tissue** is tough and inelastic, and is found pure in **tendons**. The **white fibers** are composed of **collagen**.

white matter: **Nervous tissue** found in the **central nervous system**. It consists of tracts of medullated **nerve fibers** in the **brain** and **spinal cord**. It also contains **blood vessels** and **neuroglia**. It is mainly external to **gray matter**, but it is internal to **gray matter** in the cerebral hemispheres and in the **cerebellum**. The medullated **fibers** give the **tissue** its shiny white appearance.

white noise: Random signal (or process) with a flat **power** spectral density. The signal's **power** spectral density has equal **power** in any band, at any center **frequency** having a given **bandwidth**. **White noise** is considered analogous to white **light**, which contains all frequencies.

whole blood: **Blood** containing all its natural components: **blood cells** and **plasma**.

Wien's displacement law: It states that the **wavelength** distribution of radiated heat **energy** from a **blackbody** at any temperature has essentially the same shape as the distribution at any other temperature, except that each **wavelength** is displaced, or moved over, on the graph. There is an inverse relationship between the **wavelength** of the peak of the emission of a **blackbody** λ_{max} and its **absolute temperature** T, $\lambda_{max} = b/T$, where b is a constant of proportionality called Wien displacement constant, equal to 2.8977685 (51) $\times$ 10^{-3} m $\cdot$ K or b = 2, 897, 768.5 (51) nm $\cdot$ K; the two digits between the parentheses denote the uncertainty (the **standard deviation** at 68.27% confidence level).

Wigner phase space distribution function: Complex function that defines the coherence property of an optical field for a given position depending on the **wave** vector.

Wistar rat: Strain of albino rats developed at the Wistar Institute in 1906 for use in biological and medical research. It is the first rat strain developed to serve as a model organism and currently one of the most popular rat strains used for laboratory research. It is characterized by its wide **head**, long **ears**, and having a tail length that is always less than its body length. The **Sprague Dawley rat** and **Long–Evans rat** strains were developed from **Wistar rats**.

Wollaston prism (WP): An optical device, invented by William Hyde Wollaston, that manipulates **polarized light**. It separates randomly **polarized** or unpolarized **light** into two orthogonal, linearly polarized outgoing beams. The **prism** consists of two orthogonal calcite **prisms** cemented together at their base (typically with Canada balsam) to form two right triangle **prisms** with perpendicular **optical axes**. Outgoing **light beams** diverge from the **prism**, giving two polarized rays with the angle of divergence determined by the prisms' wedge angle and the

wavelength of the **light**. Commercial **prisms** are available with divergence angles from 15 deg to about 45 deg.

working distance: In **microscopy**, it is the distance between the front **lens** of the **objective** and the coverslip (or uncovered object) when the **lens** is focused on the specimen.

wound: Type of physical **trauma** wherein the **skin** is torn, cut, or punctured (an open **wound**), or where blunt force **trauma** causes a contusion (a closed **wound**). In pathology, it specifically refers to a sharp **injury** that damages the **dermis** of the **skin**.

Wright–Giemsa stain: Buffered **Wright stain** for which specific instructions depend on the used solutions. It uses such dyes as **eosin** Y, **azure** B, and **methylene blue**.

Wright stain: Histologic stain that facilitates the differentiation of **blood cell** types. It is used primarily to stain peripheral **blood smears** and **bone marrow aspirates** that are examined under a **light** microscope. In cytogenetics, it is used to stain **chromosomes** to facilitate diagnosis of syndromes and diseases. This is a modification of the **Romanowsky stain**. A Wright stain easily distinguishes between **blood cells**, thus it became widely used for performing differential **white blood cell** counts, which are routinely ordered when infections are expected.

wrinkle: Ridge or crease of a surface. It usually refers to the **skin** of an organism. In **skin**, a **wrinkle** or fold may be permanent. Skin **wrinkles** typically appear as a result of aging processes such as **glycation** or, temporarily as the result of prolonged (more than a few minutes) immersion in **water**. Wrinkling in **skin** is caused by habitual facial expressions, aging, sun damage, smoking, poor **hydration**, and various other factors.

wrist: In human anatomy, the **wrist** is the flexible and narrower connection between the **forearm** and the **hand**. The **wrist** is essentially a double row of small short **bones**, called carpals, intertwined to form a malleable hinge.

xenon arc lamp: Discharge arc lamp filled with xenon. It gives out very bright **UV** and **visible light** in the range from 200 nm to >1.0 μm.

xenon flash lamp: Pulsed **xenon arc lamp**.

xerostomia: See **dry mouth**.

x ray (*Synonym*: Röntgen rays): Form of **electromagnetic radiation** with a **wavelength** in the range of 10 to 0.01 nm. Primarily used for diagnostic radiography and crystallography, it is a form of **ionizing radiation**, and as such can be dangerous.

x-ray computed tomography (CT): Medical imaging method employing **tomography** created by computer processing. Digital geometry processing is used to generate a 3D image of the inside of an object from a large series of 2D **x-ray** images taken around a single axis of rotation. **CT** produces a volume of data that can be manipulated, through a process known as "windowing," in order to demonstrate various bodily structures based on their ability to block the **x-ray** beam.

x-ray contrast: **Exogenous** substance used to alter the **contrast** in **x-ray** imaging by affecting the **attenuation** of **x rays**. Introduction of gases (air, CO_2) into hollow viscera, cavities, **vessels**, or surrounding structures will reduce the **attenuation** of **x rays**. Such substances are called negative **contrast media**; examples include use of air in double-**contrast** examinations of the **gastrointestinal tract**, air encephalography, and CO_2 digital subtraction angiography. The majority of **x-ray contrast media** are positive or radiopaque, i.e., they increase the **attenuation** of **x rays**. The increased **attenuation** is accomplished by two different atoms: barium, which is used in the form of insoluble barium sulphate for examinations of the **gastrointestinal tract**, and iodine, which is the main component of all other **x-ray contrast media**. Iodinated **contrast media** may be divided into **water**-soluble, **water**-insoluble, and oily **contrast media**. All

561

water-soluble iodinated **contrast media** developed are derivatives of tri-iodinated benzoic acid, such as oral cholegraphic **contrast** and uro/angiographic **media**. The uro/angiographic **media** are all salts of derivatives of tri-iodinated benzoic acid with the cations mainly either sodium or meglumine, or a mixture of both. Sodium salts are generally more toxic to the **vascular endothelium** and to the **blood–brain** barrier and neural **tissue** than meglumine. A mixture of sodium and meglumine has lower cardiotoxicity than either salt alone. Some manufacturers have partially replaced sodium with calcium and magnesium to reduce toxicity.

x-ray diffraction: Finds the geometry or shape of a molecule using **x rays**. This method is based on the elastic **scattering** of **x rays** from structures that have long-range order. Single-crystal **x-ray diffraction** is a technique used to solve the complete structure of **crystalline** materials, ranging from simple inorganic solids to complex **macromolecules**, such as **proteins**. Powder **diffraction** is a technique used to characterize the crystallographic structure, crystallite size (grain size), and preferred orientation in polycrystalline or powdered solid samples.

yeast: Eukaryotic micro-organisms classified in the kingdom Fungi, with about 1,500 species currently described. They are unicellular, although some species with **yeast** forms may become multicellular through the formation of a string of connected budding **cells** known as pseudohyphae as seen in most molds. Their size can vary greatly depending on the species, typically measuring 3–4 μm in diameter, although some **yeasts** can reach over 40 μm. **Yeast** is also extremely important as a model organism in modern **cell** biology research, and is one of the most thoroughly researched eukaryotic microorganisms. Other species of **yeast**, such as *Candida albicans*, are opportunistic pathogens and can cause infections in humans.

yellow elastic tissue: **Connective tissue** that consists of a matrix of coarse yellow elastic **fibers** that branch regularly and anastomose, with **fibroblasts** in the matrix. **Elastin** is the principal constituent of this **tissue**. The **tissue** rarely occurs pure and usually contains **white fibers** as well. Yellow elastic **fibers** are numerous in the **lungs** and in the walls of **arteries**, where elastic supporting **tissues** are required. **Yellow elastic tissue** occurs in **ligaments** where an extensible **tissue** is required.

yellow fiber: See **yellow elastic tissue**.

ytterbium:yttrium aluminium garnet (Yb:YAG) laser: Solid-state **laser** whose lasing medium is the crystal **Yb:YAG** emitting in the **NIR** at 1030 nm. Ytterbium lasing ions have a smallest **photon energy** difference between the pumping **diode laser** with the **wavelength** of 808 nm and the generated **wavelength** of 1030 nm, thus less pumping **energy** is converted to heat (approximately twice less than that for **Nd:YAG laser** with 1064 nm). It often works as a disc **laser**.

Yucatan micropig: Strain of hairless small animals widely used in experimental studies.

zigzag photon (*Synonym*: snake photon): Low-angle scattered **photon** with a zigzag (or snake) trajectory.

zinc oxide (ZnO): **Semiconductor** material. Its electronic **energy** structure is represented by two bands, namely, conduction band and valence band with an **energy** gap (**bandgap**) between them. Being excited by a **photon**, an electron from the valence band goes to the conduction band, generating a positive-charged hole in the valence band. Only **photons** with energies larger than the **bandgap** can be absorbed. The formed charged carriers can recombine either radiatively (by emitting a **photon**) or nonradiatively (releasing **energy** as heat). Electrons and holes can recombine on a particle surface, reducing or oxidizing surrounding molecules, thus producing **radicals**. **ZnO** is a wide **bandgap semiconductor** of 3.37 eV at room temperature. The interband transition is direct. It is used in **sunscreens** in the form of insoluble nano-sized particles, the protective efficiency of which depends on their size being an optimal diameter of 20–30 nm. Because particles scatter **UV** and not **visible light**, the **sunscreen** appears to be transparent. **ZnO** is commonly used in the form of particles of 30–200-nm in diameter with the surface covered by inert coating materials, such as SiO_2 or Al_2O_3, to improve their **dispersion** in **sunscreen** formulations and prevent radical generation at **light-tissue** interaction mediated by **nanoparticles** via the **photocatalytic effect**.

zinc selenide (ZnSe) crystal: Crystal for **ATR (attenuated total reflectance) spectroscopy** that is insoluble with a **refractive index** of 2.4, long-**wavelength** cut-off **frequency** of 525 cm^{-1}, depth of penetration at 1000 cm^{-1} of 1.66 μm, and **pH** range of samples under study of 5–9.

z-scan: See **A-scan**.

Zucker rat: Genetic model for research on **obesity** and hypertension. It is named after Lois M. Zucker and Theodore F. Zucker, pioneer researchers in the study of the **genetics** of **obesity**. There are two types of rats, lean and fatty. The fatty rat type is capable of weighing more than twice the average weight, up to 1 kg. They have high levels of **lipids** and **cholesterol** in the **blood**, are resistant to **insulin** without being hyperglycemic, and **gain** weight from an increase in both the size and number of **fat cells**.

Laser Specifications:

Laser	Wavelength λ, nm	Wavenumber $\frac{1}{\lambda} \cdot 10^3$, cm^{-1}	Photon energy, $h\nu$	
			10^{-19}, J	eV
Excimer (ArF)	193	51.8	10.29	6.42
Excimer (XeCl)	308	32.5	6.45	4.03
Excimer (XeF)	350	28.6	5.67	3.54
N$_2$ (nitrogen)	337.1	29.7	5.89	3.68
He–Cd (helium cadmium)	325.0	30.8	6.11	3.82
	441.6	22.6	4.50	2.81
Ar (argon) ion	351.1	28.5	5.66	3.53
	363.8	27.5	5.46	3.41
	488.0	20.5	4.07	2.54
	514.5	19.4	3.86	2.41
He–Ne (helium neon)	543.3	18.4	3.65	2.28
	632.8	15.8	3.14	1.96
	1152.3	8.7	1.72	1.08
	3391.2	2.9	0.59	0.37
Rhodamine dye	600	16.7	3.31	2.07
Kr (krypton) ion	647.1	15.5	3.07	1.92
Ruby	694.3	14.4	2.86	1.79
Alexandrite	755	13.2	2.63	1.65
Ti:sapphire	800	12.5	2.48	1.55
GaAs (diode)	830	12.0	2.39	1.49
Nd:YAP (perovskite)	1054	9.4	1.88	1.17
Nd:YAG (neodymium)	1064	9.4	1.87	1.17
Ho:YAG (holmium)	2088	4.8	0.95	0.59
Er:YAG (erbium)	2940	3.4	0.68	0.42
CO (carbon monoxide)	5500	1.8	0.36	0.22
CO$_2$ (carbon dioxide)	9600	1.0	0.21	0.13
	10600	0.9	0.19	0.12
CH$_3$I	$1.25 \cdot 10^6$	$8 \cdot 10^{-3}$	$1.6 \cdot 10^{-3}$	$9.9 \cdot 10^{-4}$

Bibliography:

P. Agache and P. Humbert, Eds., *Measuring the Skin*, Springer, Berlin (2004).

G. Ahluwalia, Ed., *Light Based Systems for Cosmetic Application*, William Andrew, Norwich, CT (2009).

R. R. Anderson and J. A. Parrish, "Optical properties of human skin," in *The Science of Photomedicine*, J. D. Regan and J. A. Parrish, Eds., pp. 147–194, Plenum Press, New York (1982).

D. L. Andrews, *Encyclopedia of Applied Spectroscopy*, Wiley-VCH Verlag GmbH & Co. KGaA, Weinheim (2009).

ANSI, *American National Standard for the Safe Use of Lasers*, ANSI Z136.1-2007, Laser Institute of America, Orlando, FL (2007).

E. Baron, *Light-Based Therapies for Skin of Color*, Springer, New York (2009).

H.-P. Berlien and G. J. Müller, Eds., *Applied Laser Medicine*, Springer, Berlin (2003).

D. A. Boas, C. Pitris, and N. Ramanujam, Eds., *Handbook of Biomedical Optics*, CRC Press, Taylor & Francis Group, London (2011).

C. F. Bohren and D. R. Huffman, *Absorption and Scattering of Light by Small Particles*, John Wiley & Sons, New York (1983).

M. Born and E. Wolf, *Principles of Optics, 7th Edition*, Cambridge University Press, Cambridge, UK (1999).

S. Bown and G. Buonaccorsi, Eds., "Special issue on VI biennial meeting of the International Photodynamic Association," *Lasers Med. Sci.* **12**, 180–284 (1997).

S. E. Braslavsky and K. Heihoff, "Photothermal methods," in *Handbook of Organic Photochemistry*, J.C. Scaiano, Ed, CRC Press, Boca Raton, FL (1989).

J. M. Chalmers and P. R. Grifiths, Eds., *Handbook of Vibrational Spectroscopy*, John Wiley & Sons, Chichester (2002).

B. Chance, Ed., *Photon Migration in Tissue*, Plenum, New York (1989).

B. Chance, M. Cope, E. Gratton, N. Ramanujam, and B. Tromberg, "Phase measurement of light absorption and scatter in human tissue," *Rev. Sci. Instrum.* **69**(10), 3457–3481 (1998).

A. Chmyrov, "Photo-induced dark states in fluorescence spectroscopy—investigations and applications," Ph.D Thesis, Royal Institute of Technology, Stockholm, Sweden (2010).

R. Cicchi, L. Sacconi, and F. S. Pavone, "Morpho-functional nonlinear laser imaging of tissues," in *Intern. Conf. Laser Applications in Life Sciences* (LALS-2010), Book of Abstracts, p. 92, University of Oulu Press, Finland (2010).

J. C. Dainty, Ed., *Laser Speckle and Related Phenomena, 2nd Edition*, Springer-Verlag, New York (1984).

B. B. Das, F. Liu, and R. R. Alfano, "Time-resolved fluorescence and photon migration studies in biomedical and random media," *Rep. Prog. Phys.* **60**, 227–292 (1997).

A. Diaspro, Ed., *Confocal and Two-Photon Microscopy: Foundations, Applications, and Advances*, Wiley-Liss, New York (2002).

W. Drexler and J. G. Fujimoto, Eds., *Optical Coherence Tomography: Technology and Applications*, Springer, Berlin (2008).

R. G. Driggers, Ed., *Encyclopedia of Optical Engineering*, Marcel-Dekker, New York (2003).

F. A. Duck, *Physical Properties of Tissue: Comprehensive Reference Book*, Academic Press, London (1990).

B. M. Eley and J. D. Manson, *Periodontics, 5th Edition*, Elsevier, Philadelphia (2004).

K. Flaig and M. Wilkens, Eds., *Photonics21: Second Strategic Research Agenda in Photonics. Light the Way Ahead* (Executive Summary, 2nd Edition), The European Technology Platform Photonics21, Stuttgart, Germany (January, 2010); www.Photonics21.org.

K. Frank and M. Kessler, Eds, *Quantitative Spectroscopy in Tissue*, pmi Verlag, Frankfurt am Main (1992).

A. Godman and E. M. F. Payne, *Longman Dictionary of Scientific Usage* (reprint edition), Longman Group, Harlow, UK (1979).

H. Gross, H. Zugge, M. Peschka, and F. Blechinger, *Aberration Theory and Correction of Optical Systems: Handbook of Optical Systems*, Vol. 3, H. Gross (ed.), Wiley-VCH Verlag GmbH & Co. KGaA, Weinheim, Germany (2007).

M. Hamblin and P. Mroz, Eds., *Advances in Photodynamic Therapy: Basic, Translational and Clinical*, Artec, Boston (2008).

J. A. Harrington, *Infrared Fibers and Their Applications*, SPIE Press, Bellingham, WA (2004) [doi:10.1117/3.540899].

B. W. Henderson and T. J. Dougherty, Eds., *Photodynamic Therapy: Basic Principles and Clinical Applications*, Marcel Dekker, Inc, New York (1992).

P. Herman, *Physics of the Human Body*, Springer, Berlin (2007).

A. Ishimaru, *Wave Propagation and Scattering in Random Media*, Academic Press, New York (1978).

K. Jimbow, W.C. Quevedo, T. B. Fitzpatrick, and G. Szabo, "Biology of melaninocytes," in *Dermatology in General Medicine*, T. B. Fitzpatrick, A. Z. Eisen, K. Wolff, I. M. Freedberg, and K. F. Austen, Eds., pp. 261–288, McGraw-Hill, New York (1993).

T. I. Karu, *Photobiology of Low-Power Laser Therapy*, Harwood Academic, New York (1989).

A. Katzir, *Lasers and Optical Fibers in Medicine*, Academic Press, San Diego (1993).

A. Kishen and A. Asundi, Eds., *Photonics in Dentistry: Series of Biomaterials and Bioengineering*, Imperial College Press, London (2006).

J. R. Lakowicz, *Principles of Fluorescence Spectroscopy, 3rd Edition*, Springer, New York (2006).

V. S. Letokhov, "Laser biology and medicine," *Nature* **316** (6026) 325–328 (1985).

K. Licha, *Contrast Agents for Optical Imaging: Topics in Current Chemistry Series*, vol. 222, Springer, Berlin (2002).

J.-M. Liu, *Photonic Devices*, Cambridge University Press, Cambridge, UK (2005).

A. Mahadevan–Jansen and R. Richards-Kortum, "Raman spectroscopy for detection of cancers and precancers," *J. Biomed. Opt.* **1**(1), 31–70 (1996).

B. R. Masters, *Confocal Microscopy and Multiphoton Excitation Microscopy: The Genesis of Live Cell Imaging*, SPIE Press, Bellingham, WA (2006) [doi:10.1117/3.660403].

B. R. Masters and P. T. C. So, Eds., *Handbook of Biomedical Nonlinear Optical Microscopy*, Oxford University Press, New York (2008).

M. I. Mishchenko, J.W. Hovenier, and L. D. Travis, Eds., *Light Scattering by Nonspherical Particles*, Academic Press, San Diego (2000).

M. I. Mishchenko, L.D. Travis, and A. A. Lacis, *Multiple Scattering of Light by Particles: Radiative Transfer and Coherent Backscattering*, Cambridge University Press, New York (2006).

M. I. Mishchenko, L. D. Travis, and A. A. Lacis, *Scattering, Absorption, and Emission of Light by Small Particles*, Cambridge University Press, Cambridge, UK (2002).

L. Moss-Salentijn and M. Hendricks-Klyvert, *Dental and Oral Tissues, An Introduction, 3rd Edition*, Lea & Febiger, Philadelphia (1990).

G. Müller and A. Roggan, Eds., *Laser-Induced Interstitial Thermotherapy and Contact Laser Probe Surgery*, SPIE Press, Bellingham, WA (1995).

G. Müller et al., Eds., *Medical Optical Tomography: Functional Imaging and Monitoring*, SPIE Press, Bellingham, WA (1993).

M. H. Niemz, *Laser-Tissue Interactions: Fundamentals and Applications, 3rd Edition*, Springer-Verlag, Berlin (2007).

R. Paschotta, *Encyclopedia of Laser Physics and Technology*, vols. 1 and 2, Wiley-VCH, Berlin (2008); www.rp-photonics.com.

L. Pavesi, Ph. M. Fauchet, Eds., *Biophotonics (Biological and Medical Physics, Biomedical Engineering)*, Springer-Verlag, Berlin (2010).

F. S. Pavone, Ed., *Laser Imaging and Manipulation in Cell Biology*, Wiley-VCH Verlag GmbH & Co. KGaA, Weinheim, Germany (2010).

M. Pederson, A. Bardow, S. Beier Jensen, and B. Nauntofte, "Saliva and gastrointestinal functions of taste, mastication, swallowing and digestion," *Oral Diseases* **8**, 117–129 (2002).

K.-E. Peiponen, R. Myllylä, and A. V. Priezzhev, *Optical Measurement Techniques, Innovations for Industry and the Life Sciences*, Springer-Verlag, Berlin (2009).

J. Popp and M. Strehle, Eds., *Biophotonics: Visions for Better Health Care*, Wiley-VCH Verlag GmbH & Co. KGaA (2006).

J. Popp, V. V. Tuchin, A. Chiou, and S. H. Heinemann, Eds., *Handbook of Biophotonics: Basics and Techniques*, vol.1, Wiley-VCH Verlag GmbH & Co. KGaA, Weinheim (2011).

J. Popp, V. V. Tuchin, A. Chiou, and S. H. Heinemann, Eds., *Handbook of Biophotonics: Photonics for Health Care*, vol. 2, Wiley-VCH Verlag GmbH & Co. KGaA, Weinheim (2011).

P. Prasad, *Introduction to Biophotonics*, Wiley-Interscience, Hoboken, NJ (2003).

V. Priezzhev, V. V. Tuchin, and L. P. Shubochkin, *Laser Diagnostics in Biology and Medicine*, Nauka, Moscow (1989).

M. Prokhorov, Ed., *Physical Encyclopedia*, vol. 1, Soviet Encyclopedia, Moscow (1988).

M. Prokhorov, Ed., *Physical Encyclopedia*, vol. 2, Soviet Encyclopedia, Moscow (1990).

M. Prokhorov, Ed., *Physical Encyclopedia*, vol. 3, Big Russian Encyclopedia, Moscow (1992).

M. Prokhorov, Ed., *Physical Encyclopedia*, vol. 4, Big Russian Encyclopedia, Moscow (1994).

M. Prokhorov, Ed., *Physical Encyclopedic Dictionary*, Soviet Encyclopedia, Moscow (1983).

G.J. Puppels, "Confocal Raman Microspectroscopy," in *Fluorescent and Luminescent Probes for Biological Activity*, W. Mason, Ed., pp. 377–406, Academic Press, London (1999).

S. M. Rytov, Y. A. Kravtsov, and V. I. Tatarskii, "Wave Propagation through Random Media," vol. 4 of *Principles of Statistical Radiophysics*, Springer-Verlag, Berlin (1989).

S. S. Saliterman, *Fundamentals of BioMEMS and Medical Microdevices*, Wiley Interscience, SPIE Press, Bellingham, WA (2006) [doi:10.1117/3.631781].

G. C. Salzmann, S. B. Singham, R. G. Johnston, and C. F. Bohren, "Light scattering and cytometry," *Flow Cytometry and Sorting, 2nd Edition*, M.R. Melamed, T. Lindmo, and M.L. Mendelsohn, Eds., pp. 81–107, Wiley-Liss, New York (1990).

E. F. Schubert, *Light-Emitting Diodes*, Cambridge University Press, Cambridge, UK (2003).

J. W. Shim, *Measurement of Cell/Tissue-Biomaterial Interface Strength: The Laser Spallation Technique for Measurement of Tensile Strength of Cell/Tissue-Biomaterial Interface and its Applications*, VDM Verlag, Berlin (2009).

J. A. Ship, S. R. Pillemer, and B. J. Baum, "Xerostomia and the geriatric patient," *J. Am. Geriatr. Soc.* **50**, 535–543 (2002).

D. H. Sliney and S. L. Trokel, *Medical Lasers and Their Safe Use*, Academic Press, New York (1993).

R. Splinter and B. A. Hooper, *An Introduction to Biomedical Optics*, Taylor & Francis, New York (2007).

Stedman's Medical Dictionary, Williams & Wilkins, Baltimore, MD (1995).

S. Tanev, B. C. Wilson, V. V. Tuchin, and D. Matthews, Eds., "Special issue on biophotonics," *Adv. Opt. Technol.* (2008) [doi:10.1155/2008/134215].

A. T. Tu, *Raman Spectroscopy in Biology*, John Wiley & Sons, New York (1982).

V. V. Tuchin, *Lasers and Fiber Optics in Biomedical Science, 2nd Edition*, Fizmatlit, Moscow (2010).

V. V. Tuchin, "Lasers and fiber optics in biomedicine," *Laser Physics* **3**(4–5), 767–820, 925–950 (1993).

V. V. Tuchin, *Optical Clearing of Tissues and Blood*, SPIE Press, Bellingham, WA (2006) [doi:10.1117/ 3.637760].

V. V. Tuchin "Optical spectroscopy of biological materials," Chapter 16 in *Encyclopedia of Applied Spectroscopy*, D. L. Andrews, Ed., Wiley-VCH Verlag GmbH & Co. KGaA, Weinheim, Germany (2009).

V. V. Tuchin, *Tissue Optics: Light Scattering Methods and Instruments for Medical Diagnosis, 2nd Edition*, SPIE Press, Bellingham, WA (2007) [doi:10.1117/3.684093].

V. V. Tuchin, Ed., *Advanced Optical Cytometry: Methods and Disease Diagnoses*, Wiley-VCH Verlag GmbH & Co. KGaA, Weinheim, Germany (2010).

V. V. Tuchin, Ed., *Coherent-Domain Optical Methods: Biomedical Diagnostics, Environmental and Material Science*, vols. 1 and 2, Kluwer, Boston (2004).

V. V. Tuchin, Ed., *Handbook of Optical Biomedical Diagnostics*, SPIE Press, Bellingham, WA (2002) [doi:10.1117/3.433220].

V. V. Tuchin, Ed., *Handbook of Optical Sensing of Glucose in Biological Fluids and Tissues*, CRC Press, Taylor & Francis Group, London (2009).

V. V. Tuchin, Ed., *Handbook of Photonics for Biomedical Science*, CRC Press, Taylor & Francis Group, London (2011).

V. V. Tuchin, Ed., *Selected Papers on Tissue Optics: Applications in Medical Diagnostics and Therapy*, SPIE Press, Bellingham, WA (1994).

V. V. Tuchin, R. Drezek, S. Nie, and V. P. Zharov, Eds., "Special section on nanophotonics for diagnostics, protection, and treatment of cancer and inflammatory diseases," *J. Biomed. Opt.* **14**(2), 020901 (2009).

V. V. Tuchin, A. Tarnok, and V. P. Zharov, Eds., "Special issue on toward *in vivo* flow cytometry," *J. Biophoton.* **2**(8–9), 457–458 (2009).

V. V. Tuchin, L. V. Wang, and D. A. Zimnyakov, *Optical Polarization in Biomedical Applications*, Springer-Verlag, Berlin (2006).

V. V. Tuchin, A. N. Yaroslavsky, S. L. Jacques, and R. Anderson, Eds., "Special issue on biophotonics for dermatology: science and applications," *J. Biophoton.* **3**(1–2), 9–10, 15–88 (2010).

H. C. Van de Hulst, *Light Scattering by Small Particles*, Dover, New York (1981).

H. C. Van de Hulst, *Multiple Light Scattering*, Academic Press, New York (1980).

R. Vij and K. Mahesh, Eds., *Lasers in Medicine*, Kluwer, Boston (2002).

T. Vo-Dinh, Ed., *Biomedical Photonics Handbook*, CRC Press, Boca Raton, FL (2003).

T. A. Waigh, *Applied Biophysics: Molecular Approach for Physical Scientists*, John Wiley & Sons, Chichester, UK (2007).

L. Wang, Ed, *Photoacoustic Imaging and Spectroscopy*, CRC Press, Taylor & Francis Group, London (2009).

L. V. Wang and H.-I Wu, *Biomedical Optics: Principles and Imaging*, Wiley-Interscience, Hoboken, NJ (2007).

Webster's New Universal Unabridged Dictionary, Macmillan, New York (1994).

J. Welch and M. J. C. van Gemert, Eds., *Optical-Thermal Response of Laser Irradiated Tissue*, Plenum Press, New York (1995).

J. Welch and van M. C. J. Gemert, Eds., *Tissue Optics*, Academic Press, New York (1992).

B. Wilson, V. V. Tuchin, and S. Tanev, *Advances in Biophotonics*, NATO Science Series I. Life and Behavioural Sciences, 369, IOS Press, Amsterdam (2005).

B. Woźniak and J. Dera, *Light Absorption in Sea Water*. Atmospheric and Oceanographic Sciences Library, vol. 33, Springer, Berlin (2007).

X.-C. Zhang and J. Xu, *Introduction to THz Wave Photonics*, Springer, New York (2010).

V. P. Zharov and V. S. Letokhov, *Laser Opto-Acoustic Spectroscopy*, Springer Verlag, New York (1989).

http://agrc.ucsf.edu/supplements/pulmonary/12_oxy-hemoglobin_curve.html.

http://biology.about.com/library/organs/heart/blmicrocirc.htm.

http://www.biophotonics.com/.

http://www.biophotonicsworld.org.

http://www.burnsurvivor.com/scar_types.html.

http://cbst.ucdavis.edu/news.

http://colorusage.arc.nasa.gov/luminance_cont.php.

http://www.disabled-world.com/artman/publish/glossary.shtml.

http://www.dmso.org.

http://en.wikipedia.org.

http://encyclopedia.thefreedictionary.com/.

http://www.faculty.londondeanery.ac.uk/.

http://freespace.virgin.net/ahcare.qua/index4.html.

http://gaul.sourceforge.net/intro.html.

http://www.infraredcamerasinc.com/thermal-imaging-terms.html.

http://www.medterms.com.

http://www.nsf.gov/news/.

http://omlc.ogi.edu/classroom/.

http://www.online-medical-dictionary.org/link.asp.

http://www.scipress.org/journals/forma/pdf/1503/15030227.pdf.

http://www.standa.lt/products/catalog/optical_tables.

http://www.stedmans.com/.

http://www.thorlabs.com/tutorials/tables.cfm.

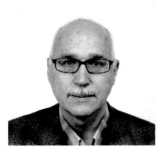

Valery V. Tuchin was born February 4, 1944. He received his degrees MS in Radiophysics and Electronics (1966), Candidate of Sciences in Optics (PhD, 1973), and Doctor of Science in Quantum Radiophysics (1982) from Saratov State University, Saratov, Russia. He is a Professor and holds the Optics and Biomedical Physics Chair, and he is a director of Research-Educational Institute of Optics and Biophotonics at Saratov State University. Prof. Tuchin also heads the Laboratory of Laser Diagnostics of Technical and Living Systems of Precision Mechanics and Control Institute, Russian Academy of Sciences. He was dean of the Faculty of Physics of Saratov University from 1982 to 1989.

His research interests include biomedical optics, biophotonics and laser medicine, nonlinear dynamics of laser and biophysical systems, physics of optical and laser measurements. He has authored more than 300 peer-reviewed papers and books, including his latest, *Handbook of Optical Biomedical Diagnostics* (SPIE Press, Vol. PM107, 2002; Translation to Russian, Fizmatlit, Moscow, 2007), *Coherent-Domain Optical Methods for Biomedical Diagnostics, Environmental and Material Science* (Kluwer Academic Publishers, Boston, USA, vol. 1 & 2, 2004), *Optical Clearing of Tissues and Blood* (SPIE Press, Vol. PM 154, 2005), and *Optical Polarization in Biomedical Applications*, Springer, 2006 (Lihong Wang, and Dmitry Zimnyakov – co-authors). He is a holder of more than 25 patents.

Prof. Tuchin currently teaches courses on optics, tissue optics, laser and fiber optics in biomedicine, optical measurements in biomedicine, laser dynamics, biophysics and medical physics for undergraduate and postgraduate students. Since 1992, Prof. Tuchin has been the instructor of SPIE and OSA short courses on biomedical optics for an international audience of engineers, students and medical doctors; and he is an editorial board member of *J. of Biomedical Optics* (SPIE), *Lasers in the Life Sciences*, *J. of X-Ray Science and Technology*, *J. of Biophotonics, J. on Biomedical Photonics* (China), and the Russian journals *Izvestiya VUZ, Applied Nonlinear Dynamics, Quantum Electronics* and *Laser Medicine*. He is a member of the Russian Academy of Natural Sciences and the International Academy of Informatization, a member of the board of SPIE/RUS and a fellow of SPIE. He has been awarded the title and scholarship "Soros Professor" (1997–1999), and the Russian Federation Scholarship for the outstanding scientists (1994–2003); and Honored Science Worker of the Russian Federation (since 2000). Since 2005 Prof. Tuchin is a vice-president of Russian Photobiology Society. In 2007 he has been awarded by SPIE Educator Award.